Autoimmune Bullous Diseases

Naveed Sami
Editor

Autoimmune Bullous Diseases

Approach and Management

Springer

Editor
Naveed Sami, MD, FAAD
Department of Dermatology
University of Alabama at Birmingham
Birmingham, AL
USA

ISBN 978-3-319-26726-5 ISBN 978-3-319-26728-9 (eBook)
DOI 10.1007/978-3-319-26728-9

Library of Congress Control Number: 2016931996

Springer Cham Heidelberg New York Dordrecht London

Printed on acid-free paper

Springer International Publishing AG Switzerland is part of Springer Science+Business Media (www.springer.com)

This book is wholeheartedly dedicated to the following:
To my devoted parents, for their boundless wisdom and prayers in continually encouraging me to make a contribution and difference in the lives of those who seek remedy for their illnesses, and comfort from ailments.
To my lovely wife, Abira, and precious daughters, Eshal and Inaya, who have been graciously supportive in allowing me to dedicate the time and energy in completing this endeavor.
To my memorable teachers for their guidance and indispensable mentorship.
To all of the patients and their families who have entrusted me with their lives and care. They have taught me not only about the management of complex diseases, but so much more including the essence of the art of medicine, and the virtue of patience. It is the unfeigned desire to make a difference in patients' lives that has fueled my motivation to continue the unending search for better solutions.

Preface

The objective of this book is to provide a coherent synopsis on the treatment and management of autoimmune blistering diseases, with one chapter focusing on each of these rare conditions. Many of these disorders can have irreversible consequences, and in some cases the potential to be fatal. Each chapter has endeavored to summarize the present-day literature on currently available therapies, and how they may fit into various feasible treatment algorithms. The contributing authors are individuals who have devoted their careers to understanding these diseases and have invested countless hours in their research laboratories and clinical settings. The ideas presented by this text do not intend to serve as the de facto treatment approach. Instead, it is our aspiration that the information and algorithms presented may help serve clinicians by providing some direction and assistance in the management of their patients. There is a large amount of overlap in the conventional treatments of these complex ailments. To help better stratify therapeutic strategies to specific diseases, the authors have provided expert opinions based on their vast sum of experiences. This serves to add an angle in balancing evidence based science with the "art of medicine" in patient care. This includes practical matters in disease management, and an algorithm based on various factors such as severity indices, side effect profiles, and the authors' personal preferences based on anecdotal observations.

While the overall focus of this text has been on the more common autoimmune blistering diseases afflicting adults, there are four chapters which separately address other important topics, including: the more rare blistering diseases, systemic corticosteroids, supportive and topical care, and blistering diseases in children. The sections on systemic corticosteroids and supportive care add two components of management which can often be overlooked, as clinicians search for the appropriate long-term treatment for their patient. It is my hope and desire that this book may serve as a guide in assisting my colleagues to develop their approach to treatment. However, as many of us have come to realize, the overall strategy will need to be individualized to each patient, and may evolve based on numerous factors in the patients' long-term care.

Lastly, with sincere gratitude, I would like to thank Springer for recognizing the importance of dedicating a book to the treatment of this rare group of diseases. This has been an amazing experience!

Birmingham, AL Naveed Sami, MD, FAAD

Acknowledgments

I would like to acknowledge all my esteemed senior colleagues (basic scientists and clinicians alike) who have invested their efforts and dedicated their careers in helping us reach our current understanding of the pathogenesis and treatment of these diseases.

Finally, I would like to express my genuine and deep appreciation to all of the authors who have contributed their time and effort in completing a momentous accomplishment. I am truly humbled by this team of authors who have a steadfast dedication to their careers as researchers, teachers, and clinicians.

Contents

Contributors

Christine S. Ahn, MD Department of Dermatology, Wake Forest University School of Medicine, Winston Salem, NC, USA

Lawrence S. Chan, MD Department of Dermatology, University of Illinois College of Medicine, Chicago, IL, USA

Mei Chen, PhD Department of Dermatology, University of Southern California, Los Angeles, CA, USA

Julia A. Curtis, MD Department of Dermatology, University of Utah School of Medicine, Salt Lake City, UT, USA

Salma Faghri de la Feld, MD, FDDA Department of Dermatology, Emory University School of Medicine, Atlanta, GA, USA

Brittney K. DeClerck, MD Department of Pathology and Dermatology, Keck School of Medicine of the University of Southern California, Los Angeles, CA, USA

Swetha Dhanireddy, MD, BS Department of Ophthalmology, Massachusetts Eye Research and Surgery Institution, Cambridge, MA, USA

Janet A. Fairley, MD Department of Dermatology, The University of Iowa, Iowa City, IA, USA

C. Stephen Foster, MD, FACS, FACR Department of Ophthalmology, Ocular Immunology and Uveitis Foundation/Massachusetts Eye Research and Surgery Institution, Cambridge, MA, USA

Kara Heelan, MBBCH, BAO, MRCPI Department of Dermatology, University College London Hospital (UCLH), London, UK

William W. Huang, MD, MPH Department of Dermatology, Wake Forest University School of Medicine, Winston Salem, NC, USA

Michael Kasperkiewicz, MD Department of Dermatology, University of Lübeck, Lübeck, Germany

Neil J. Korman, MD, PhD Department of Dermatology, University Hospitals Case Medical Center, Cleveland, OH, USA

Young Kwak, MD, CSM Department of Dermatology, University of Alabama at Birmingham, Birmingham, AL, USA

Olivia Y. Lai, BS Department of Dermatology, USC Keck School of Medicine, Los Angeles, CA, USA

Phillip Laws, MBChB Department of Dermatology, Chapel Allerton Hospital, University of Leeds, Leeds, West Yorkshire, UK

Armin Maghsoudlou, MD Department of Uveitis, Massachusetts Eye Research and Surgery Institution (MERSI), Cambridge, MA, USA

Elizabeth M. Moore, BA Department of Dermatology, University of Pennsylvania, Philadelphia, PA, USA

P. Régine Mydlarski, MD, FRCPC, DABD Division of Dermatology, Department of Medicine, University of Calgary, Calgary, AB, Canada

Richmond Road Diagnostic and Treatment Centres, Calgary, AB, Canada

Megan H. Noe, MD, MPH Department of Dermatology, The University of Iowa, Iowa City, IA, USA

Timothy Patton, DO Department of Dermatology, University of Pittsburgh, Pittsburgh, PA, USA

Janine M. Preble, MS Department of Ophthalmology, Ocular Immunology and Uveitis Foundation/Massachusetts Eye Research and Surgery Institution, Cambridge, MA, USA

Malinga D. Ratwatte, BA (Cantab) School of Clinical Medicine, University of Cambridge, Cambridge, Cambridgeshire, UK

Naveed Sami, MD, FAAD Department of Dermatology, University of Alabama at Birmingham, Birmingham, AL, USA

Neil H. Shear, MD, FRCPC Division of Dermatology, Department of Medicine (Clinical Pharmacology), Sunnybrook Health Sciences Centre/University of Toronto, Toronto, ON, Canada

Ilya Shoimer, MD Division of Dermatology, University of Calgary, Calgary, AB, Canada

Amy Theos, MD Department of Dermatology, University of Alabama at Birmingham, Birmingham, AL, USA

Henry B. Townsend, MD Rheumatology Associates PC, Birmingham, AL, USA

Anthony M. Turkiewicz, MD Clinical Research Unit, Rheumatology Associates, Birmingham, AL, USA

Scott Walsh, MD, PhD Division of Dermatology, Department of Medicine, Sunnybrook Health Sciences Centre/University of Toronto, Toronto, ON, Canada

Victoria P. Werth, MD Department of Dermatology, Corporal Michael J. Crescenz Veterans Affairs Medical Center, University of Pennsylvania, Philadelphia, PA, USA

Department of Dermatology, Perelman Center for Advanced Medicine, Philadelphia, PA, USA

Xena A. Whittier, MD Rheumatology, University of Alabama at Birmingham, Birmingham, AL, USA

Russell X. Wong, MD Division of Dermatology, University of Calgary, Calgary, AB, Canada

David T. Woodley, MD Department of Dermatology, Keck School of Medicine, University of Southern California, Los Angeles, CA, USA

John J. Zone, MD Department of Dermatology, University of Utah School of Medicine, Salt Lake City, UT, USA

Chapter 1
Pemphigus Vulgaris

Ilya Shoimer, Russell X. Wong, and P. Régine Mydlarski

Abstract Pemphigus vulgaris (PV) is an autoimmune mucocutaneous blistering disorder for which early recognition and treatment are necessary to achieve a favourable prognosis. A multidisciplinary, patient-centred approach is required to optimize therapeutic outcomes. Systemic corticosteroids remain first-line treatment for PV patients, yet their optimal dosing regimen remains unknown. Further, various steroid-sparing adjuvants play an important role in the treatment of PV. As clinical trials in the field are limited by small sample sizes and a lack of standardized outcome measures, a therapeutic algorithm is presented to guide the management of PV patients.

Keywords Pemphigus vulgaris • Systemic steroids • Dapsone • Azathioprine • Mycophenolate mofetil • Cyclophosphamide • Methotrexate • Rituximab • Tumor Necrosis Factor-α Inhibitors • Intravenous Immunoglobulin

Introduction

Pemphigus refers to a group of autoimmune bullous disorders that are characterized by blistering of the skin, mucous membranes or both. The two main types of pemphigus are pemphigus vulgaris (PV) and pemphigus foliaceus (PF), each with its own clinical subtypes. Less common variants include paraneoplastic autoimmune multiorgan syndrome (or paraneoplastic pemphigus), IgA pemphigus, and pemphigus herpetiformis. This chapter will focus on PV, a prototypical organ-specific autoimmune disorder.

I. Shoimer, MD • R.X. Wong, MD
Division of Dermatology, University of Calgary, Calgary, AB, Canada

P.R. Mydlarski, MD, FRCPC, DABD (✉)
Division of Dermatology, Department of Medicine,
University of Calgary, Calgary, AB, Canada

Richmond Road Diagnostic and Treatment Centres,
1820 Richmond Road SW, Calgary, AB T2T 5C7, Canada
e-mail: regine.mydlarski@ucalgary.ca

N. Sami (ed.), *Autoimmune Bullous Diseases: Approach and Management*,
DOI 10.1007/978-3-319-26728-9_1

The estimated incidence of PV is between one and five cases per million population per year [1]. The prevalence of PV is higher in individuals of Ashkenazi Jewish, Mediterranean, Indian, Malaysian, Chinese and Japanese descent [1, 2]. PV has no gender predilection and has an average age of onset of between 40 and 60 years [2]. Though rare, childhood cases have been reported [1, 2].

Mucosal disease precedes cutaneous involvement in the majority of cases. The oral mucosa is most frequently involved, with lesions affecting the hard and soft palate, tongue, floor of the mouth and labial mucosa. Occasionally, PV patients may present with a desquamative gingivitis. Conjunctival, nasal, pharyngeal, laryngeal, esophageal, genital and anal involvement are less common. Patients may complain of cutaneous (i.e., pain, pruritus), mucosal (i.e., dysphagia, dysuria, anogenital or ocular concerns) and/or systemic (i.e., weight loss) symptoms.

Skin disease is characterized by multiple, painful erosions, vesicles, or flaccid bullae (Fig. 1.1). The Nikolsky sign may be elicited by applying a shearing force on intact skin and inducing blister formation. The Asboe-Hansen sign, also known as the Nikolsky II or indirect Nikolsky sign, is demonstrated by applying lateral pressure on the edge of a blister and extending the blister into clinically unaffected skin. The most commonly affected areas include the scalp, face, trunk and intertriginous regions. Rarely, nail involvement has been reported.

Pemphigus vegetans, a rare subtype of PV, is typified by a localized vegetative or papillomatous response. There are two types of pemphigus vegetans: the Hallopeau type and the Neumann type [3]. In pemphigus vegetans of Hallopeau, pustular lesions predominantly involve the folds and heal into localized verrucous, hyperkeratotic plaques. Pemphigus vegetans of Neumann is more extensive, characterized by periorificial papillomas and results in the formation of excess granulation tissue.

In 1964, Beutner and Jordan demonstrated the presence of anti-epidermal antibodies in the serum of pemphigus patients [4]. Anhalt et al. confirmed that passive transfer of PV immunoglobulin G (IgG) induced a pemphigus phenotype in neonatal mice [5]. Circulating IgG autoantibodies against the cadherins, desmogleins 1 (Dsg1) and 3 (Dsg3), were subsequently characterized [6]. By 1997, Koch et al. established that the disruption of desmoglein 3 in mice resulted in the loss of kera-

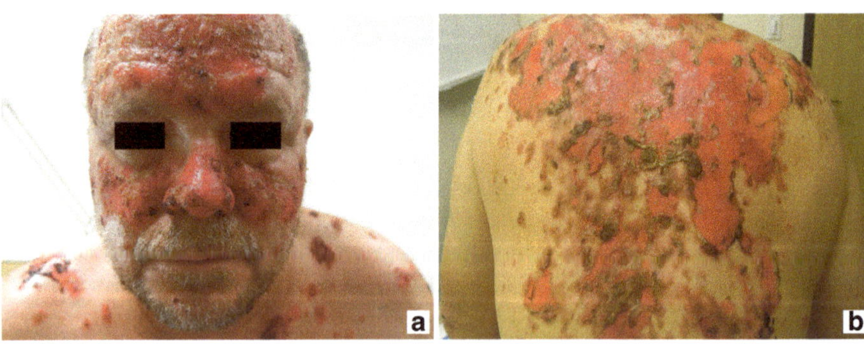

Fig. 1.1 Clinical features of pemphigus vulgaris. Flaccid blisters, erosions and crusting on the face (**a**) and back (**b**) of a 55-year-old man

tinocyte cell-cell adhesion and a PV phenotype [7]. The collective data support the pathogenicity of these antibodies in pemphigus patients.

PV is a complex polygenic disorder involving multiple genetic loci, many of which remain unknown. Association studies link HLA class II genes to PV, as over 95 % of patients carry either the DRB1*0402 or DQB1*0503 alleles [2]. Though rare, familial cases of the disease have been reported [8].

Up to 25 % of patients with pemphigus have another underlying immunologic disease [9]. Pemphigus is associated with autoimmune thyroid disease, type I diabetes, rheumatoid arthritis and systemic lupus erythematosus [10]. Further, the association between pemphigus and myasthenia gravis is well established [11]. These findings suggest that common genetic factors from clinically distinct disorders may underlie the susceptibility to autoimmune disease.

Genetic predisposition alone is not sufficient to cause the development of PV. Environmental factors seem to be required to initiate and perpetuate the disease process. However, an inducing agent cannot be identified in most patients. Occasionally, drugs, physical agents, contact allergens, viral infections, vaccinations, and diet have been implicated in the disease [11]. For instance, drug-induced pemphigus may occur with thiols (i.e., penicillamine, captopril), phenols (i.e., aspirin, rifampin) and non-thiol, non-phenol drugs (i.e., non-steroidal anti-inflammatories, nifedipine) [11].

If left untreated, PV has a mortality rate ranging from 60 to 90 % [12]. Overwhelming sepsis, fluid and electrolyte imbalances, impaired thermoregulation, as well as cardiac and renal failure are possible life-threatening complications of the disease. Systemic corticosteroids and adjuvant therapies have reduced the mortality rate of PV patients to approximately 10 %; yet, treatment-related complications are now the leading cause of morbidity and mortality. By understanding the molecular mechanisms that underlie pemphigus, researchers are developing novel targeted therapies for the management of PV.

Diagnosis

During the initial clinical encounter, the physician should look for signs and symptoms to support a diagnosis of pemphigus. A thorough evaluation for potential risk factors, triggers and comorbidities must be elicited. Validated scoring systems, such as the Autoimmune Bullous Skin Intensity and Severity Score (ABSIS) and the Pemphigus Disease Area Index (PDAI), may be used to measure the extent and distribution of lesions.

To confirm the diagnosis of PV, biopsies must be performed for both routine pathology and direct immunofluorescence (DIF). A 4.0 mm punch excision from an early, small vesicle or the periphery of a larger blister should be obtained for histopathologic analysis. Routine histology reveals loss of cellular cohesion (acantholysis) in the suprabasilar layer of the epithelium (Fig. 1.2a). A classical "tombstone" appearance of basal keratinocytes is commonly described (Fig. 1.2b). Direct immu-

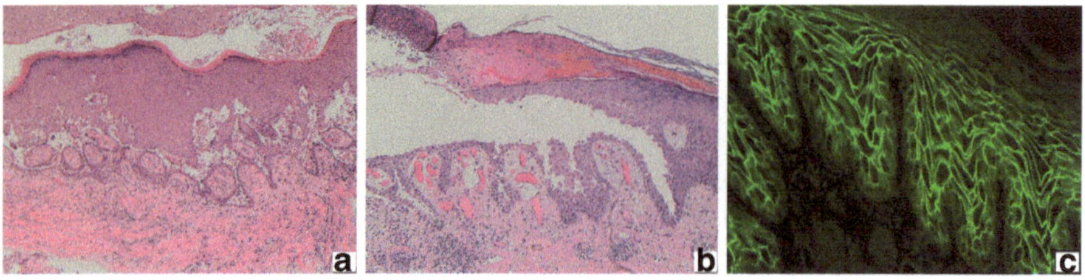

Fig. 1.2 Immunohistology of pemphigus vulgaris. Suprabasilar clefting, blister formation (**a**) and acantholysis (**b**) in a "tombstone" pattern (H&E, 100× magnification). Circulating intercellular IgG autoantibodies revealing a "chicken-wire," "honey-comb," or "fishnet" pattern on indirect immunofluorescence (**c**)

nofluorescence of perilesional skin demonstrates intercellular deposition of IgG and/or C3. Since antibodies correlate with disease activity in most patients, indirect immunofluorescence (IIF) assays are frequently used to semi-quantitatively measure circulating antibody levels. Using monkey or guinea pig esophagus as a substrate for IIF, an intercellular staining pattern may be visualized. The findings resemble a 'chicken-wire', 'honeycomb' or 'fishnet' appearance (Fig. 1.2c). Enzyme-linked immunosorbent assays (ELISA) are a more sensitive method for measuring antibodies to desmoglein 1 and desmoglein 3. Lastly, immunoblot and immunoprecipitation may be used to identify specific autoantibody profiles.

Management

A multidisciplinary approach is required to optimize patient care and outcomes. An experienced dermatologist must work closely with the patient's general practitioner. Other specialists may play a supportive role for PV patients, including oral pathologists, otolaryngologists, ophthalmologists, gynecologists, urologists, internists and psychiatrists, among others [13].

Allied health care professionals often work with patients to minimize their comorbidities. Educated wound care specialists are particularly helpful in providing non-adhesive dressing recommendations. Proper dental care and good oral hygiene are required. A dietician may provide nutritional support for patients with severe oral disease and resultant malnutrition, as well as those with steroid-related complications (i.e., diabetes, hypertension, obesity). If needed, analgesics should be ordered to ensure adequate pain control. Infections should be promptly recognized and treated aggressively.

If a potential triggering agent is identified on history, every effort must be made to eliminate the precipitating factor. As drug-induced pemphigus is a well-described phenomenon, a close review of the patient's medication history is required. Other reported exogenous triggers include: (1) infections, such as herpes simplex virus; (2) physical agents, such as ultraviolet or ionizing radiation; (3) contact allergens, such as 1,3-dichloropropene; and (4) dietary factors, such as members of the *Allium* species (i.e., garlic, leeks, onions, chives) [2].

An extensive work-up is required prior to initiating corticosteroid and/or immunosuppressive therapies [13]. Recommended investigations include:

- Complete blood count and differential;
- Serum electrolytes, creatinine, urea;
- Liver panel;
- Fasting glucose, cholesterol and triglycerides;
- Hepatitis B, Hepatitis C and HIV serologies;
- Serum β–HCG on all woman of childbearing age;
- Screening Mantoux test (or quantiFERON® test) for tuberculosis;
- Chest X-ray;
- Baseline bone density;
- Baseline ocular examination.

If indicated, additional bloodwork may be requested to determine a patient's candidacy for select therapies. For instance, thiopurine methyltransferase (TPMT) or glucose-6-phosphate dehydrogenase (G6PD) should be ordered prior to initiating treatment with azathioprine or dapsone, respectively. Further screening bloodwork and/or radiologic investigations should be considered on a case-by-case basis. Vaccinations (i.e., seasonal influenza, H1N1, tetanus, hepatitis B) should be brought up-to-date. However, live vaccinations are contraindicated in patients on immunosuppressive therapies.

The main objectives of therapy are to heal existing lesions, prevent the formation of new blisters and improve the patient's quality of life. The goal of management is to induce and maintain remission with the lowest possible doses of medication, so as to minimize the risk of serious and potentially life-threatening drug-related adverse events. Though the optimal therapeutic strategy for PV patients has yet to be established, systemic corticosteroids remain the cornerstone of treatment.

Therapeutic Interventions

Systemic corticosteroids and immunosuppressive therapies are the mainstay of treatment in PV patients. Given the rarity of this disease, studies are limited by small sample size, varied methodologies and a lack of standardized outcomes. As a result, there is a paucity of high-quality, randomized controlled trials (RCTs). Herein, we present a thorough review on the safety and efficacy of the therapeutic interventions for PV (Table 1.1).

Topical Therapies

Baths containing antiseptics (i.e., chlorhexidine) are often recommended to reduce the risks of secondary infections in patients with extensive skin involvement [11]. Potent topical corticosteroids (i.e., clobetasol proprionate 0.05 %) and calcineurin inhibitors (i.e., tacrolimus 0.1 % ointment and pimecrolimus 1 % cream) are

Table 1.1 Therapeutic options for the treatment of pemphigus vulgaris

Drug class	Medication	Route	Dose
Systemic corticosteroids	Dexamethasone	Oral or IV pulse	50–200 mg/d for 3–5 d
	Methylprednisolone	IV pulse	500–1000 mg/d for 3–5 d
	Prednisone	Oral	0.5–2 mg/kg/d
Immunosuppressive & anti-inflammatory therapies	Azathioprine[a]	Oral	0.5–2.5 mg/kg/d
	Cyclophosphamide	Oral	2–3 mg/kg/d
		IV pulse	0.5–1 g/m^2 monthly
		Immunoablative high-dose IV	50 mg/kg/d for 4 d
	Cyclosporine	Oral	2–5 mg/kg/d
	Dapsone	Oral	25–200 mg/d
	Gold	IM	25–50 mg/biweekly
		Oral	6–9 mg/d
	Methotrexate	Oral or SC	10–25 mg/week
	Mycophenolate mofetil	Oral	2–3 g/d
	Pentoxifylline	Oral	1500 mg/d
	Sulfasalazine	Oral	1200 mg/d
Biologics	Etanercept	SC	50 mg weekly
	Infliximab	IV	5 mg/kg/cycle
	IVIG[b]	IV	1–2 g/kg/cycle
	Rituximab	IV	375 mg/m^2 weekly for 4 weeks or 1000 mg on days 1 and 15

Adapted from Prajapati et al. [81], with permission from Skin Therapy Letter
IV intravenous, *IM* intramuscular, *SC* subcutaneous, *mg* milligrams, *kg* kilograms, *d* days
[a]Azathioprine should be dosed in accordance with thiopurine methyltransferase (TPMT) levels
[b]*IVIG* Intravenous Immunoglobulin

beneficial in the treatment of localized skin and/or mucous membrane lesions [13–15]. For vegetative plaques, intralesional corticosteroids (i.e., triamcinolone acetonide 2.5–10 mg/ml) may provide symptomatic relief [13]. Oral topical formulations (i.e., triamcinolone acetonide 0.1 % paste) and inhaled corticosteroids (i.e., mometasone furoate monohydrate nasal spray) can also be used to enhance the delivery of corticosteroids to mucosal surfaces. The use of dental trays improves the efficacy of topical therapies for lesions affecting the gumlines and hard palate. Topical epidermal growth factor (EGF) has also been shown to hasten the healing of PV lesions [16].

Nicotine, a cholinergic agonist, has been proven to induce T cell anergy and improve antibody-mediated acantholysis in pemphigus [17, 18]. Further, remission may be achieved sooner in smokers than in non-smokers [19]. Given the many harmful effects caused by smoking, cigarette smoking is not recommended to PV patients. However, 4 % pilocarpine gel, a cholinomimetic, has been shown to improve the lesional rates of re-epithelialization in PV patients [20].

Systemic Glucocorticoids

Systemic steroids remain the first-line treatment for PV patients. Though the dose of prednisone has been the subject of debate, Ratnam's RCT suggests that low-dose (i.e., 45–60 mg/day) is as effective as high-dose (i.e., 120–180 mg/day) prednisone [21]. This study, which included 22 participants, did not demonstrate a difference in any of the reported outcomes, including disease control, relapse and death. An RCT of 20 patients further demonstrated that adjuvant pulsed oral dexamethasone treatments provided no additional benefit to conventional first-line therapies [22]. Moreover, significant adverse events occurred more commonly in the pulsed steroid group.

Most expert opinions suggest the initial use of prednisone 1 mg/kg/day, though ranges in dose from 0.5 to 1.5 mg/kg/day have been proposed [13, 23, 24]. If control is not obtained within 2 weeks, a higher dose of prednisone (2 mg/kg/day) may be considered [13]. The approach to steroid dosage must be dynamic and adjusted according to disease severity, underlying patient co-morbidities and response to treatment.

Patients treated with systemic corticosteroids should receive calcium and vitamin D supplementation. To prevent steroid-induced osteoporosis, bisphosphonates (i.e., alendronate, risendronate) should be considered in at-risk patients [25]. The prophylactic use of H2-blockers or proton pump inhibitors for steroid-induced peptic ulcers remains controversial, and treatment should be individualized to the patient [26]. Annual ophthalmologic examinations are recommended to screen for steroid-related ocular complications (i.e., cataracts, glaucoma). Systemic antibacterial, antifungal and antiviral therapies are recommended when clinically indicated [13].

Adjuvant Immunomodulatory Therapies

Azathioprine

Azathioprine, a purine analog which inhibits DNA/RNA synthesis, has long been known to have immunosuppressive and anti-inflammatory effects. In RCTs of pemphigus patients, azathioprine has been compared to corticosteroids alone, mycophenolate mofetil (MMF), cyclophosphamide and tacrolimus [24–31]. Chams-Davatchi et al. conducted a landmark, multi-arm RCT (n = 120) which compared prednisolone alone to three adjuvant therapies: MMF, azathioprine and pulsed cyclophosphamide [27]. Azathioprine demonstrated a steroid-sparing effect when compared to prednisolone alone [27, 28]. Though MMF appeared more effective than azathioprine at achieving disease control, azathioprine showed superior steroid-sparing properties [27, 30]. When compared to cyclophosphamide, azathioprine again demonstrated superior steroid-sparing effects; however, its effect on disease control was inconclusive [27, 29]. In the only trial comparing azathioprine to tacrolimus, there was no significant benefit in any outcome measures [31]. In a meta-analysis of PV therapies, azathioprine was considered to be a steroid-sparing treatment option that had no effect on remission, relapse rate or death [32].

The functional enzyme assay for TPMT should guide physicians when dosing azathioprine. Genetic polymorphisms have been associated with high, intermediate, low and very low levels of TPMT activity. The awareness of these phenotypes allows the physician to: (1) minimize the risk of myelosuppression, and (2) optimally dose azathioprine according to the patient's TPMT level [33, 34]. Azathioprine should be dosed in accordance with the following recommendations:

- Very low TPMT levels (i.e., <5.0 U): azathioprine contraindicated;
- Low TPMT levels (i.e., between 5.0 and 13.7 U): up to 0.5 mg/kg/day;
- Intermediate TPMT levels (i.e., between 13.7 and 19.0 U): up to 1.5 mg/kg/day;
- High TPMT levels (i.e., >19.0 U): up to 2.5 mg/kg/day.

If TPMT functional assays are not routinely available, patients should be started on low-dose (i.e., 50 mg/day) azathioprine. The dose should be slowly increased and blood counts must be closely monitored throughout.

Cyclophosphamide

A derivative of nitrogen mustard, cyclophosphamide is an alkylating agent that acts by cross-linking DNA. Cyclophosphamide preferentially targets B over T lymphocytes, and has potent immunosuppressive properties. Studies have compared cyclophosphamide to corticosteroids alone, azathioprine, MMF and cyclosporine [27, 29, 35, 36]. As a steroid-sparing treatment, cyclophosphamide appears to be more effective than MMF, but less effective than azathioprine [27]. There were no significant benefits for patients receiving pulse dexamethasone-cyclophosphamide as compared to oral methylprednisolone-azathioprine therapy [29]. In a randomized trial to assess the efficacy of adjuvant pulse intravenous cyclophosphamide therapy, there were trends towards fewer relapses and reduced times to remission in the cyclophosphamide-treated group [36]. However, in the meta-analysis by Atzmony et al., cyclophosphamide was found to have no effect on remission rate, relapse rate or time-to-disease control [32]. Though one PV patient died of sepsis during cyclophosphamide therapy, the overall rates of withdrawal due to adverse events were similar among the various treatment groups [32, 36].

The long-term use of cyclophosphamide is associated with significant adverse effects, including infertility, carcinogenicity and hemorrhagic cystitis. Given the lack of evidence and the potential for drug-related toxicities, cyclophosphamide should be reserved for cases that have failed conventional therapies. When treatment with cyclophosphamide is indicated, it may be administered intravenously (i.e., 0.5–1.0 g/m^2) or orally (i.e., 2 mg/kg/day) [13]. Few case reports suggest a potential role for immunoablative high-dose cyclophosphamide without stem cell rescue [37].

Cyclosporine

Cyclosporine, a calcineurin inhibitor, is a potent immunosuppressant widely used in transplantation to prevent organ rejection. The efficacy of cyclosporine in the treatment of PV has been evaluated in two small RCTs [35, 38]. As compared to steroids (i.e., prednisone, methylprednisolone) or cyclophosphamide, cyclosporine offers no significant benefit in terms of cumulative corticosteroid dose, disease control, remission, or relapse rates. Adverse events were similar in all treatment groups. Given the lack of evidence, cyclosporine is not routinely recommended in the treatment of PV.

Dapsone

Dapsone, an antibiotic commonly used in the treatment of leprosy, has potent anti-inflammatory and immunomodulatory properties. The efficacy of dapsone has been studied in one small RCT of 19 pemphigus patients who were unable to taper their dose of prednisone below 15 mg/day [39]. While a trend towards efficacy of dapsone was demonstrated, the study was underpowered and the data were inconclusive. There was no significant effect of dapsone on the rate of remission. No patients withdrew from the study because of adverse events. In patients with a normal G6PD level, dapsone is typically dosed between 100 and 150 mg daily.

Intravenous Immunoglobulin

Derived from purified human plasma, intravenous immunoglobulin (IVIG) contains supraphysiologic levels of IgG as well as traces of other immunoglobulins. It exerts a variety of immunomodulatory effects and has been used in the treatment of immunodeficiencies, autoimmune disorders and infections. Though multiple case series suggest a role for IVIG in the treatment of PV, there is only one RCT which evaluates its efficacy in pemphigus patients [40]. A total of 61 PV or PF patients, resistant to treatment with prednisolone, were randomized to receive a single course of adjuvant IVIG (400, 200 or 0 mg/kg/day) for 5 consecutive days. In the three groups, a dose-response relationship was observed. The duration of response, as measured by time to escape from protocol, was significantly improved in the 400 mg group as compared to placebo. There was a significant reduction in the pemphigus activity scores and the ELISA levels in the 400 mg group. No significant differences in safety end points were noted.

Due to the risk of fluid overload, congestive heart failure and renal failure are relative contraindications to the use of IVIG. Patients with IgA deficiency and those with hypercoagulable states are at increased risk for anaphylaxis and thromboembolic events, respectively. Further, treatment with IVIG may predispose patients with rheumatoid arthritis and cryoglobulinemia to renal disease. Screening bloodwork prior to initiating treatment with IVIG includes: a complete blood count, liver and renal panels, IgA level, rheumatoid factor, cryoglobulins, as well as hepatitis B, hepatitis C and HIV serologies. The typical dosing regimen for IVIG is 2 g/kg/month, with the infusions divided over 2–5 days [41, 42].

Methotrexate

Methotrexate, a folic acid antagonist, has anti-inflammatory and immunosuppressive effects. Though methotrexate has been used as a treatment for PV since the 1960s, there are no RCTs evaluating its efficacy. Case series support the use of methotrexate as a steroid-sparing option for PV [43–45]. In the most recent retrospective chart review of 23 PV patients, Tran et al. demonstrated a steroid-sparing effect for methotrexate [46]. Sixteen patients (70 %) were able to taper and ultimately discontinue prednisone within a median time of 18 months. An additional 23 % of patients demonstrated a partial steroid-sparing effect. Methotrexate was only discontinued in two patients (9 %) due to adverse events.

Methotrexate is typically dosed between 10 and 25 mg/week, and may be administered orally or subcutaneously. The use of folic acid supplementation to reduce gastrointestinal adverse effects and pancytopenia remains controversial.

Mycophenolate Mofetil

Mycophenolate mofetil (MMF) is a non-competitive inhibitor of inosine monophosphate dehydrogenase, an important enzyme in the *de novo* purine synthesis pathway. As this pathway is the major route of purine synthesis for T- and B-lymphocytes, MMF has potent immunosuppressive properties. Studies have compared MMF to corticosteroids alone, azathioprine and cyclophosphamide [27, 30, 47, 48]. As compared to corticosteroids alone, MMF demonstrated a faster and more durable response [47]. Though Ioannides et al. found no significant difference in relapse rate, another study suggested that the time to relapse was delayed in patients treated with MMF [47, 48]. Further, MMF-treated PV patients demonstrated a complete response more rapidly than azathioprine-treated patients [30]. In terms of steroid-sparing effects, MMF showed inferiority to both azathioprine and cyclophosphamide [27, 30]. There were no significant differences noted between the study groups on remission, death or withdrawals due to adverse events.

The typical dosing regimen for MMF is between 2 and 3 g/day. Though the efficacy of enteric coated-mycophenolate sodium in PV patients has yet to be established, it may prove useful in patients presenting with MMF-induced gastrointestinal symptoms.

Plasmapheresis, Immunoadsorption and Extracorporeal Photopheresis

Plasmapheresis has been used to treat a variety of autoimmune disorders that require the rapid removal of disease-causing autoantibodies from the circulation. Guillaume et al. studied the role of plasmapheresis in a multicenter randomized trial of 40 pemphigus patients [49]. As compared to prednisolone alone, the plasmapheresis/prednisolone group showed no significant improvement in disease control, cumulative steroid dose or serum antibody titers. While there was no significant difference in mortality rates, 4 of 22 patients in the intervention group died of thromboembolism or infection.

Immunoadsorption (IA) has been used to successfully treat PV patients who have failed conventional therapies [50–55]. Recent studies have suggested that IA is most effective when used in combination with immunosuppressive agents, including corticosteroids, azathioprine, MMF and rituximab [50, 54, 55]. Case reports also document the use of extracorporeal photopheresis for the treatment of severe, recalcitrant PV [56–59].

Rituximab

Rituximab may be considered the most promising new therapy for the treatment of pemphigus. It is a chimeric IgG1 monoclonal antibody against CD20, a marker expressed on the surface of pre-B and mature B lymphocytes. Several studies have established the efficacy of rituximab using the lymphoma dosing schedule of 375 mg/m^2 weekly for 4 consecutive weeks [60–62]. In a phase II clinical trial of 45 PV patients, participants received four doses of intravenous rituximab 375 mg/m^2 weekly and concomitant prednisolone [63]. Clinical improvement was noted after an average of 6.4 weeks, with marked improvement being noted by a mean of 10.1 months. Approximately 47 % of patients had a sustained clinical response after one treatment cycle, with subsequent infusions increasing the rates of remission. Furthermore, there was a significant decrease in cumulative steroid dose. However, 22.5 % of patients experienced complications including infections (i.e., sepsis, lung and skin infections), thrombosis (i.e., cavernous sinus thrombosis, deep vein thrombosis) and Stevens-Johnson syndrome. Ahmed et al. suggested using a combination of rituximab and high-dose monthly IVIG to minimize the risks of infection [64].

In 2006, a weight-independent dosing regimen was approved for the treatment of rheumatoid arthritis [65]. Several retrospective studies subsequently demonstrated high remission rates in patients treated with rituximab using two 1000 mg infusions within a 2-week interval [66–69]. In a large retrospective study of 47 PV patients, remission rates of 76 % were obtained after one treatment cycle of biweekly 1 g infusions [67]. With repeated cycles of rituximab, remission rates increased to 91 % [67]. The rheumatoid arthritis dosing schedule for rituximab had relatively few adverse events. A modified fixed-dose rituximab protocol was also studied in a retrospective cohort study of 92 pemphigus patients [66]. Participants received 1000 mg intravenously on days 1 and 15, followed by either 500 mg intravenously or repeated full dosing if clinically warranted at 6-month intervals. At final follow-up, 61 % of patients were in complete remission off therapy, whereas 28 % were in complete remission on adjuvant treatments. There were no significant infectious complications.

Kanwar et al. carried out an RCT (n=22) comparing high-dose (1000 mg biweekly) and low-dose (500 mg biweekly) rituximab treatments in PV [70]. Complete remission was achieved in 95 % of participants. There were no significant differences in rates of remission, relapse, cumulative steroid dose or study drop-out due to adverse events. However, the low-dose intervention group had significantly higher Dsg1 and Dsg3 antibody levels post-treatment. They also received a higher cumulative dose of azathioprine.

Some authors have suggested that rituximab become a first-line treatment option for pemphigus [71, 72]. Given the risks of infection, such as progressive multifocal leukoencephalopathy, and the lack of high-quality RCTs, rituximab should be reserved for severe or recalcitrant PV cases. Rituximab may be optimally dosed at 1000 mg on days 1 and 15. Subcutaneous veltuzumab, a humanized anti-CD20 antibody that recently gained FDA orphan drug status for pemphigus, may also play a role in the treatment of refractory PV [73]. Other anti-CD20 therapies, such as ofatumumab, obinutuzumab and ocrelizumab, hold therapeutic potential.

Tumour Necrosis Factor-α Inhibitors

Studies have shown that serum tumour necrosis factor-α (TNF-α) levels correlate with disease activity, and that TNF-α may play a role in the process of acantholysis [74, 75]. Several trials have examined the role of TNF-α inhibition in the treatment of PV.

Etanercept

Etanercept, a recombinant fusion protein of TNF-α receptor 2 and the constant portion of human IgG1, acts as a competitive inhibitor for TNF-α [76], The efficacy of etanercept was evaluated in one small RCT (n = 8) of PV patients [76]. Patients were randomized to etanercept (50 mg) or saline subcutaneously once weekly for 16 weeks. The study was underpowered and the data were inconclusive. No serious adverse events were noted.

Infliximab

Infliximab, a chimeric monoclonal antibody against TNF-α, was compared to prednisone alone in a multi-centered randomized trial [77]. Twenty patients with PV were randomized to receive infliximab (5 mg/kg at 0, 2, 6 and 14 weeks) and prednisone, or prednisone alone. Though a reduction in anti-Dsg1 and Dsg3 antibodies was noted, infliximab was shown to be ineffective in the treatment of PV patients.

Sulfazalazine/Pentoxifylline

The low-cost anti-tumour necrosis factor-alpha (TNF-α) therapies, sulfasalazine and pentoxifylline, were studied as adjuvant treatments for PV [78]. All 64 patients participating in the RCT received a combination of steroids and cyclophosphamide. Patients were then randomized to receive additional sulfasalazine and pentoxifylline, or placebo. Patients receiving adjuvant therapy had a significant clinical improvement and reduction in serum TNF-α levels. The dosing regimen used in the study was pentoxifylline 500 mg t.i.d. and sulfasalazine 400 mg t.i.d.

Therapeutic Algorithm

Although strong evidence in the form of RCTs is lacking, the authors propose the following therapeutic algorithm to guide the management of PV patients (Fig. 1.3). Systemic corticosteroids remain the cornerstone of treatment. Once the diagnosis of PV has been confirmed, patients should receive prednisone 1 mg/kg/day. For individuals with mild disease, prednisone alone may be sufficient to achieve disease control. However, many experts advocate the early use of steroid-sparing therapies to minimize the risk of side effects associated with the prolonged use of corticosteroids [79, 80]. Azathioprine and MMF are considered first-line steroid-sparing treatment options. While MMF-treated patients seem to demonstrate a complete response more rapidly, azathioprine may have superior steroid-sparing properties. As there have been no studies that clearly demonstrate superiority of one treatment regimen over the other, the low cost of azathioprine is frequently taken into consideration. Thiopurine methyl transferase levels should guide the physician when dosing azathioprine. Alternatively, MMF can be administered at a starting dose of 2 g/day. In select patients, methotrexate or dapsone may be an alternative to azathioprine or MMF. Once disease control is obtained, the dose of prednisone can be tapered in accordance with previous recommendations [39]. As steroid-sparing adjuvants frequently take months to demonstrate full therapeutic efficacy, a slow prednisone taper is recommended to prevent a rebound flare of the disease (Table 1.2). For patients with severe or recalcitrant pemphigus, IVIG (2 g/kg/month) or rituximab (1000 mg biweekly) may be warranted. Should conventional therapies fail, consideration may be given to cyclophosphamide, plasmapheresis, immunoadsorption or extracorporeal photopheresis.

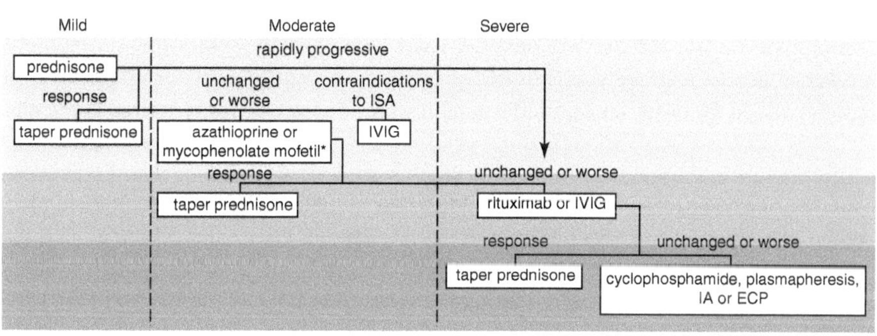

Fig. 1.3 Therapeutic algorithm for the treatment of pemphigus vulgaris. *ECP* extracorporeal photopheresis, *IA* immunoadsorption, *ISA* immunosuppressive agents, *IVIG* intravenous immunoglobulin. * In select patients, methotrexate or dapsone may be an alternative to azathioprine or MMF

Table 1.2 Glucocorticoid taper schedule

Prednisone dosage, mg/d × 7 days (total taper over 15 weeks)[a]		
40	17.5	5
35	15	4
30	12.5	3
25	10	2
20	7.5	1
Prednisone, mg every other day × 8 days (total taper over 34 weeks)[b]		
40-35	40-4	12.5-1
40-30	40-3	12.5-0
40-25	35-3	10-0
40-20	30-3	7.5-0
40-17.5	30-2	6-0
40-12.5	25-2	5-0
40-10	20-2	4-0
40-7.5	17.5-2	3-0
40-6	17.5-1	2-0
40-5	15-1	1-0

Adapted from Table 1, Ref. [39]. With permission from the American Medical Association

[a]Presents a daily prednisone tapering schedule below 40 mg/d. Thus, if the starting dosage is 40 mg/d, the patient will taper to 35 mg/d on week 2, 30 mg/d on week 3 and so on. Assuming disease stability, the prednisone will be discontinued by the end of week 15

[b]Presents an every other day prednisone tapering schedule below 40 mg/d. Thus, "40-35" means 40 mg one day, 35 mg the next day, 40 mg the next day, and so forth for a total of 8 days. The dose of prednisone would then be reduced to 40/30 for 8 days, 40/25 for 8 days and so on until discontinued over 34 weeks

Conclusion and Future Directions

Pemphigus is a life-threatening disorder for which early recognition and treatment are necessary to achieve a favourable prognosis. A multidisciplinary approach is recommended in order to optimize patient care. Systemic corticosteroids are the mainstay of treatment, though their optimal dosing regimen remains unknown. Clinical trials in the field are limited by small sample sizes and the lack of standardized outcome measures. Yet, multiple treatment modalities exist, thus requiring the choice of treatment to be individualized to the patient. Given the efficacy of rituximab, other anti-CD20 treatments, such as veltuzumab, ofatumumab, obinutuzumab and ocrelizumab, hold therapeutic promise. The earlier introduction of biologics into the therapeutic algorithm has the potential improve overall outcomes, reduce drug-related complications and be cost-effective. With the development of validated scoring systems, consensus definitions and defined outcome parameters, smaller clinical studies will be combined into powerful meta-analyses. By understanding the mechanisms of disease, researchers will continue to develop novel targeted therapies for the treatment of PV. The foundations have been laid to enhance the quality of RCTs in hope of providing PV patients with an evidence-based therapeutic approach.

References

1. Joly P, Litrowski N. Pemphigus group (vulgaris, vegetans, foliaceus, herpetiformis, brasiliensis). Clin Dermatol. 2011;29:432–6.
2. Ruocco V, Ruocco E, Lo Schiavo A, Brunetti G, Guerrera LP, Wolf R. Pemphigus: etiology, pathogenesis, and inducing or triggering factors: facts and controversies. Clin Dermatol. 2013;31:374–81.
3. Zaraa I, Sellami A, Bouguerra C, et al. Pemphigus vegetans: a clinical, histological, immunopathological and prognostic study. J Eur Acad Dermatol Venereol. 2011;25:1160–7.
4. Beutner EH, Jordon RE. Demonstration of skin antibodies in sera of pemphigus vulgaris patients by indirect immunofluorescent staining. Proc Soc Exp Biol Med. 1964;117:505–10.
5. Anhalt GJ, Labib RS, Voorhees JJ, Beals TF, Diaz LA. Induction of pemphigus in neonatal mice by passive transfer of IgG from patients with the disease. N Engl J Med. 1982;306:1189–96.
6. Amagai M, Klaus-Kovtun V, Stanley JR. Autoantibodies against a novel epithelial cadherin in pemphigus vulgaris, a disease of cell adhesion. Cell. 1991;67:869–77.
7. Koch PJ, Mahoney MG, Ishikawa H, et al. Targeted disruption of the pemphigus vulgaris antigen (desmoglein 3) gene in mice causes loss of keratinocyte cell adhesion with a phenotype similar to pemphigus vulgaris. J Cell Biol. 1997;137:1091–102.
8. Yamamoto T, Ikeda K, Sasaoka S, et al. Human leukocyte antigen genotypes and antibody profiles associated with familial pemphigus in Japanese. J Dermatol. 2011;38:711–6.
9. Mohan MP, Ramesh TC. Multiple autoimmune syndrome. Indian J Dermatol Venereol Leprol. 2003;69:298–9.
10. Parameswaran A, Attwood K, Sato R, Seiffert-Sinha K, Sinha AA. Identification of a new disease cluster of pemphigus vulgaris with autoimmune thyroid disease, rheumatoid arthritis, and type I diabetes. Br J Dermatol. 2015;172(3):729–38.
11. Ruocco E, Wolf R, Ruocco V, Brunetti G, Romano F, Lo Schiavo A. Pemphigus: associations and management guidelines: facts and controversies. Clin Dermatol. 2013;31:382–90.
12. Bystryn JC, Rudolph JL. Pemphigus. Lancet. 2005;366:61–73.
13. Hertl M, Jedlickova H, Karpati S, et al. Pemphigus. S2 guideline for diagnosis and treatment – guided by the European Dermatology Forum (EDF) in cooperation with the European Academy of Dermatology and Venereology (EADV). J Eur Acad Dermatol Venereol. 2015;29(3):405–14.
14. Iraji F, Asilian A, Siadat AH. Pimecrolimus 1% cream in the treatment of cutaneous lesions of pemphigus vulgaris: a double-blind, placebo-controlled clinical trial. J Drugs Dermatol. 2010;9:684–6.
15. Cohen SN, Lim RP, Paul CJ, Abdullah A. Equal efficacy of topical tacrolimus and clobetasone butyrate in pemphigus foliaceus. Int J Dermatol. 2006;45:1379.
16. Tabrizi MN, Chams-Davatchi C, Esmaeeli N, et al. Accelerating effects of epidermal growth factor on skin lesions of pemphigus vulgaris: a double-blind, randomized, controlled trial. J Eur Acad Dermatol Venereol. 2007;21:79–84.
17. Geng Y, Savage SM, Razani-Boroujerdi S, Sopori ML. Effects of nicotine on the immune response. II. Chronic nicotine treatment induces T cell anergy. J Immunol. 1996;156:2384–90.

18. Nguyen VT, Arredondo J, Chernyavsky AI, Pittelkow MR, Kitajima Y, Grando SA. Pemphigus vulgaris acantholysis ameliorated by cholinergic agonists. Arch Dermatol. 2004;140: 327–34.
19. Valikhani M, Kavusi S, Chams-Davatchi C, et al. Impact of smoking on pemphigus. Int J Dermatol. 2008;47:567–70.
20. Iraji F, Yoosefi A. Healing effect of Pilocarpine gel 4% on skin lesions of pemphigus vulgaris. Int J Dermatol. 2006;45:743–6.
21. Ratnam KV, Phay KL, Tan CK. Pemphigus therapy with oral prednisolone regimens. A 5-year study. Int J Dermatol. 1990;29:363–7.
22. Mentink LF, Mackenzie MW, Toth GG, et al. Randomized controlled trial of adjuvant oral dexamethasone pulse therapy in pemphigus vulgaris: PEMPULS trial. Arch Dermatol. 2006;142:570–6.
23. Martin LK, Werth VP, Villaneuva EV, Murrell DF. A systematic review of randomized controlled trials for pemphigus vulgaris and pemphigus foliaceus. J Am Acad Dermatol. 2011;64:903–8.
24. Frew JW, Martin LK, Murrell DF. Evidence-based treatments in pemphigus vulgaris and pemphigus foliaceus. Dermatol Clin. 2011;29:599–606.
25. Grossman JM, Gordon R, Ranganath VK, et al. American College of Rheumatology 2010 recommendations for the prevention and treatment of glucocorticoid-induced osteoporosis. Arthritis Care Res (Hoboken). 2010;62:1515–26.
26. Guslandi M. Steroid ulcers: any news? World J Gastrointest Pharmacol Ther. 2013;4:39–40.
27. Chams-Davatchi C, Esmaili N, Daneshpazhooh M, et al. Randomized controlled open-label trial of four treatment regimens for pemphigus vulgaris. J Am Acad Dermatol. 2007;57:622–8.
28. Chams-Davatchi C, Mortazavizadeh A, Daneshpazhooh M, et al. Randomized double blind trial of prednisolone and azathioprine, vs. prednisolone and placebo, in the treatment of pemphigus vulgaris. J Eur Acad Dermatol Venereol. 2013;27:1285–92.
29. Rose E, Wever S, Zillikens D, Linse R, Haustein U, Bröcker E. Intravenous dexamethasone-cyclophosphamide pulse therapy in comparison with oral methylprednisolone-azathioprine therapy in patients with pemphigus: results of a multicenter prospectively randomized study. J Dtsch Dermatol Ges J Dtsc Dermatol Ges. 2005;3:200–6.
30. Beissert S, Werfel T, Frieling U, et al. A comparison of oral methylprednisolone plus azathioprine or mycophenolate mofetil for the treatment of pemphigus. Arch Dermatol. 2006;142:1447–54.
31. Dastgheib L, Sadati MS, Baghernejhad M. Assessment of the adjuvant effect of tacrolimus in the management of pemphigus vulgaris: A randomized controlled trial. J Dermatolog Treat. 2015;26(1):90–3.
32. Atzmony L, Hodak E, Gdalevich M, Rosenbaum O, Mimouni D. Treatment of pemphigus vulgaris and pemphigus foliaceus: a systematic review and meta-analysis. Am J Clin Dermatol. 2014;15:503–15.
33. Meggitt S, Anstey A, Mohd Mustapa M, Reynolds N, Wakelin S. British Association of Dermatologists' guidelines for the safe and effective prescribing of azathioprine 2011. Br J Dermatol. 2011;165:711–34.
34. Badalamenti S, Kerdel F. Azathioprine. Comprehensive dermatologic drug therapy. Wolverton SE, editor. Philadelphia: WB Saunders Co; 2001. p. 165–79.
35. Chrysomallis F, Ioannides D, Teknetzis A, Panagiotidou D, Minas A. Treatment of oral pemphigus vulgaris. Int J Dermatol. 1994;33:803–7.
36. Sharma V, Khandpur S. Evaluation of cyclophosphamide pulse therapy as an adjuvant to oral corticosteroid in the management of pemphigus vulgaris. Clin Exp Dermatol. 2013;38:659–64.
37. Hayag MV, Cohen JA, Kerdel FA. Immunoablative high-dose cyclophosphamide without stem cell rescue in a patient with pemphigus vulgaris. J Am Acad Dermatol. 2000;43:1065–9.
38. Ioannides D, Chrysomallis F, Bystryn J. Ineffectiveness of cyclosporine as an adjuvant to corticosteroids in the treatment of pemphigus. Arch Dermatol. 2000;136:868–72.
39. Werth VP, Fivenson D, Pandya AG, et al. Multicenter randomized, double-blind, placebo-controlled, clinical trial of dapsone as a glucocorticoid-sparing agent in maintenance-phase pemphigus vulgaris. Arch Dermatol. 2008;144(1):25–32.

40. Amagai M, Ikeda S, Shimizu H, et al. A randomized double-blind trial of intravenous immunoglobulin for pemphigus. J Am Acad Dermatol. 2009;60:595–603.
41. Mydlarski P, Mittmann N, Shear N. Intravenous immunoglobulin: use in dermatology. Skin Therapy Lett. 2004;9:1–6.
42. Mydlarski PR, Ho V, Shear NH. Canadian consensus statement on the use of intravenous immunoglobulin therapy in dermatology. J Cutan Med Surg. 2006;10:205–21.
43. Baum S, Greenberger S, Samuelov L, et al. Methotrexate is an effective and safe adjuvant therapy for pemphigus vulgaris. Eur J Dermatol. 2012;22:83–7.
44. Gürcan H, Ahmed AR. Analysis of current data on the use of methotrexate in the treatment of pemphigus and pemphigoid. Br J Dermatol. 2009;161:723–31.
45. Smith TJ, Bystryn J. Methotrexate as an adjuvant treatment for pemphigus vulgaris. Arch Dermatol. 1999;135:1275–6.
46. Tran K, Wolverton J, Soter N. Methotrexate in the treatment of pemphigus vulgaris: experience in 23 patients. Br J Dermatol. 2013;169:916–21.
47. Beissert S, Mimouni D, Kanwar AJ, Solomons N, Kalia V, Anhalt GJ. Treating pemphigus vulgaris with prednisone and mycophenolate mofetil: a multicenter, randomized, placebo-controlled trial. J Invest Dermatol. 2010;130:2041–8.
48. Ioannides D, Apalla Z, Lazaridou E, Rigopoulos D. Evaluation of mycophenolate mofetil as a steroid-sparing agent in pemphigus: a randomized, prospective study. J Eur Acad Dermatol Venereol. 2012;26:855–60.
49. Guillaume J, Roujeau J, Morel P, et al. Controlled study of plasma exchange in pemphigus. Arch Dermatol. 1988;124:1659–63.
50. Kolesnik M, Becker E, Reinhold D, et al. Treatment of severe autoimmune blistering skin diseases with combination of protein A immunoadsorption and rituximab: a protocol without initial high dose or pulse steroid medication. J Eur Acad Dermatol Venereol. 2014;28:771–80.
51. Mlynek A, Meurer M. Immunoadsorption in the treatment of pemphigus. Atheroscler Suppl. 2009;10:107–9.
52. Pfutze M, Eming R, Kneisel A, Kuhlmann U, Hoyer J, Hertl M. Clinical and immunological follow-up of pemphigus patients on adjuvant treatment with immunoadsorption or rituximab. Dermatology. 2009;218:237–45.
53. Günther C, Laske J, Frind A, Julius U, Pfeiffer C. Successful therapy of pemphigus vulgaris with immunoadsorption using the TheraSorb™ adsorber. J Dtsch Dermatol Ges J Dtsch Dermatol Ges. 2008;6:661–3.
54. Kasperkiewicz M, Shimanovich I, Meier M, et al. Treatment of severe pemphigus with a combination of immunoadsorption, rituximab, pulsed dexamethasone and azathioprine/mycophenolate mofetil: a pilot study of 23 patients. Br J Dermatol. 2012;166:154–60.
55. Behzad M, Möbs C, Kneisel A, et al. Combined treatment with immunoadsorption and rituximab leads to fast and prolonged clinical remission in difficult-to-treat pemphigus vulgaris. Br J Dermatol. 2012;166:844–52.
56. Kaiser J, Kaatz M, Elsner P, Ziemer M. Complete remission of drug-resistant Pemphigus vegetans treated by extracorporeal photopheresis. J Eur Acad Dermatol Venereol. 2007;21:843–4.
57. Wollina U, Lange D, Looks A. Short-time extracorporeal photochemotherapy in the treatment of drug-resistant autoimmune bullous diseases. Dermatology. 1999;198:140–4.
58. Gollnick HP, Owsianowski M, Taube KM, Orfanos CE. Unresponsive severe generalized pemphigus vulgaris successfully controlled by extracorporeal photopheresis. J Am Acad Dermatol. 1993;28:122–4.
59. Rook AH, Jegasothy BV, Heald P, et al. Extracorporeal photochemotherapy for drug-resistant pemphigus vulgaris. Ann Intern Med. 1990;112:303–5.
60. Kim J, Kim Y, Kim M, Kim S. Clinical efficacy of different doses of rituximab in the treatment of pemphigus: a retrospective study of 27 patients. Br J Dermatol. 2011;165:646–51.
61. Schmidt E, Goebeler M, Zillikens D. Rituximab in severe pemphigus. Ann N Y Acad Sci. 2009;1173:683–91.
62. Joly P, Mouquet H, Roujeau J, et al. A single cycle of rituximab for the treatment of severe pemphigus. N Engl J Med. 2007;357:545–52.

63. Kamran B, Maryam D, Somayeh K, Mostafa M, Mahsa H, Cheyda C. Adjuvant rituximab in the treatment of pemphigus vulgaris: a phase II clinical trial. Int J Dermatol. 2013;52:862–7.
64. Ahmed AR, Spigelman Z, Cavacini LA, Posner MR. Treatment of pemphigus vulgaris with rituximab and intravenous immune globulin. N Engl J Med. 2006;355:1772–9.
65. Cohen SB, Emery P, Greenwald MW, et al. Rituximab for rheumatoid arthritis refractory to anti–tumor necrosis factor therapy: results of a multicenter, randomized, double-blind, placebo-controlled, phase III trial evaluating primary efficacy and safety at twenty-four weeks. Arthritis Rheum. 2006;54:2793–806.
66. Heelan K, Al-Mohammedi F, Smith MJ, et al. Durable remission of pemphigus with a fixed-dose rituximab protocol. JAMA Dermatol. 2014;150:703–8.
67. Leshem YA, Hodak E, David M, Anhalt GJ, Mimouni D. Successful treatment of pemphigus with biweekly 1-g infusions of rituximab: a retrospective study of 47 patients. J Am Acad Dermatol. 2013;68:404–11.
68. Lunardon L, Tsai KJ, Propert KJ, et al. Adjuvant rituximab therapy of pemphigus: a single-center experience with 31 patients. Arch Dermatol. 2012;148:1031–6.
69. Cianchini G, Lupi F, Masini C, Corona R, Puddu P, De Pità O. Therapy with rituximab for autoimmune pemphigus: results from a single-center observational study on 42 cases with long-term follow-up. J Am Acad Dermatol. 2012;67:617–22.
70. Kanwar AJ, Vinay K, Sawatkar G, et al. Clinical and immunological outcomes of high-and low-dose rituximab treatments in patients with pemphigus: a randomized, comparative, observer-blinded study. Br J Dermatol. 2014;170:1341–9.
71. Ingen-Housz-Oro S, Valeyrie-Allanore L, Cosnes A, et al. First-line treatment of pemphigus vulgaris with a combination of rituximab and high-potency topical corticosteroids. JAMA Dermatol. 2015;151(2):200–3.
72. Cho Y, Lee F, Chu C, Wang L. First-line combination therapy with rituximab and corticosteroids is effective and safe for pemphigus. Acta Derm Venereol. 2014;94:472–3.
73. Ellebrecht CT, Choi EJ, Allman DM, et al. Subcutaneous veltuzumab, a humanized anti-CD20 antibody, in the treatment of refractory pemphigus vulgaris. JAMA Dermatol. 2014;150:1331–5.
74. Ragab N, Abdallah M, El-Gohary E, Elewa R. Stress and serum TNF-alpha levels may predict disease outcome in patients with pemphigus: a preliminary study. Cutis. 2011;87:189–94.
75. Feliciani C, Toto P, Wang B, Sauder DN, Amerio P, Tulli A. Urokinase plasminogen activator mRNA is induced by IL-1alpha and TNF-alpha in in vitro acantholysis. Exp Dermatol. 2003;12:466–71.
76. Fiorentino DF, Garcia MS, Rehmus W, Kimball AB. A pilot study of etanercept treatment for pemphigus vulgaris. Arch Dermatol. 2011;147:117–8.
77. Hall R, Fairley J, Woodley D, et al. A multi-centered randomized trial of the treatment of pemphigus vulgaris patients with infliximab and prednisone compared to prednisone alone. Br J Dermatol. 2015;172(3):760–8.
78. El-Darouti M, Marzouk S, Abdel Hay R, et al. The use of sulfasalazine and pentoxifylline (low-cost antitumour necrosis factor drugs) as adjuvant therapy for the treatment of pemphigus vulgaris: a comparative study. Br J Dermatol. 2009;161:313–9.
79. Strowd LC, Taylor SL, Jorizzo JL, Namazi MR. Therapeutic ladder for pemphigus vulgaris: emphasis on achieving complete remission. J Am Acad Dermatol. 2011;64:490–4.
80. Daniel BS, Murrell DF. Management of pemphigus. F1000Prime Rep. 2014;6:32.
81. Prajapati V, et al. Advances in pemphigus therapy. Skin Therapy Lett. 2008;13:4–7.

Chapter 2
Pemphigus Foliaceus

Kara Heelan, Scott Walsh, and Neil H. Shear

Abstract Pemphigus foliaceus is a rare autoimmune disease that results in blistering of the skin. It is caused by autoantibodies directed against cell-surface antigens on keratinocytes, which when targeted lose their cellular adhesion properties and separate from one another to form blisters within the epidermis. The disease has two predominant types: endemic and sporadic. In pemphigus foliaceus the blisters are high in the epidermis, just below the stratum corneum, and are associated with antibodies against desmoglein-1. The disease is diagnosed based on its clinical manifestations (flaccid blisters and erosions on skin), histology (epidermal acantholysis), and immunological abnormalities (circulating and tissue-fixed antibodies against keratinocyte surface antigens). This chapter summarizes the epidemiology, clinical features and diagnostic techniques. An in-depth review of treatment modalities reported in the literature is presented and includes topical agents, anti-inflammatory agents, immunosuppressant and biologic therapy. We also present a treatment approach based on the authors' experience of treating this rare disease.

Keywords Pemphigus foliaceus • Dapsone • Methotrexate • Azathioprine • Mycophenolate mofetil • Intravenous immunoglobulin • Cyclophosphamide • Plasmapheresis • Rituximab • Plaquenil • Colchicine • Tetracyclines • Treatment algorithm for pemphigus foliaceus

K. Heelan, MB BCH, BAO, MRCPI (✉)
Department of Dermatology, University College London Hospital (UCLH), 250 Euston Road, London NW1 2PG, UK
e-mail: karaheelan@yahoo.com

S. Walsh, MD, PhD
Division of Dermatology, Department of Medicine, Sunnybrook Health Sciences Centre/University of Toronto, Toronto, ON, Canada
e-mail: scott.walsh@sunnybrook.ca

N.H. Shear, MD, FRCPC
Division of Dermatology, Department of Medicine (Clinical Pharmacology), Sunnybrook Health Sciences Centre/University of Toronto, Toronto, ON, Canada
e-mail: Neil.Shear@sunnybrook.ca

N. Sami (ed.), *Autoimmune Bullous Diseases: Approach and Management*,
DOI 10.1007/978-3-319-26728-9_2

Abbreviations

AIBD	Autoimmune bullous disorders
CR	Complete remission off therapy
CROT	Complete remission on therapy
DCP	Dexamethasone and cyclophosphamide pulse therapy
DIF	Direct immunofluorescence
dsg	Desmoglein
ELISA	Enzyme-linked immunosorbent assay
G-6PD	Glucose-6-phosphate dehydrogenase
IIF	Indirect immunofluorescence
IVIg	Intravenous immunoglobulin
LE	Lupus erythematosus
MMF	Mycophenolate mofetil
MTX	Methotrexate
PE	Pemphigus erythematosus
PF	Pemphigus foliaceus
PH	Pemphigus herpetiformis
PR	Partial remission off therapy
PROT	Partial remission on minimal therapy
PV	Pemphigus vulgaris
RTX	Rituximab
TPMT	Thiopurine methyl transferase

Introduction

Pemphigus foliaceus (PF) is a rare acquired autoimmune blistering disease caused by IgG autoantibodies directed against desmoglein (dsg)-1, an intercellular adhesion glycoprotein. Dsg-1 is found predominantly in the granular cell layer of the epidermis. The binding of these IgG autoantibodies can cause eosinophilic spongiosis, acantholysis and the formation of subcorneal blisters within the epidermis [1].

Clinical Presentation

There are two predominant types of PF: sporadic and endemic. Rarer forms within the sporadic grouping include pemphigus erythematosus (PE, Senear-Usher syndrome), pemphigus herpetiformis (PH) and drug-induced PF. Clinical presentations of both sporadic and endemic PF include fragile erythematous plaques and superficial bullae that easily rupture leading to shallow erosions, and tend to favour a seborrheic distribution. Multiple pruritic, eroded and crusted plaques (Fig. 2.1a) typically present on the upper torso (Fig. 2.1b, c), axillae (Fig. 2.2) face (Fig. 2.3)

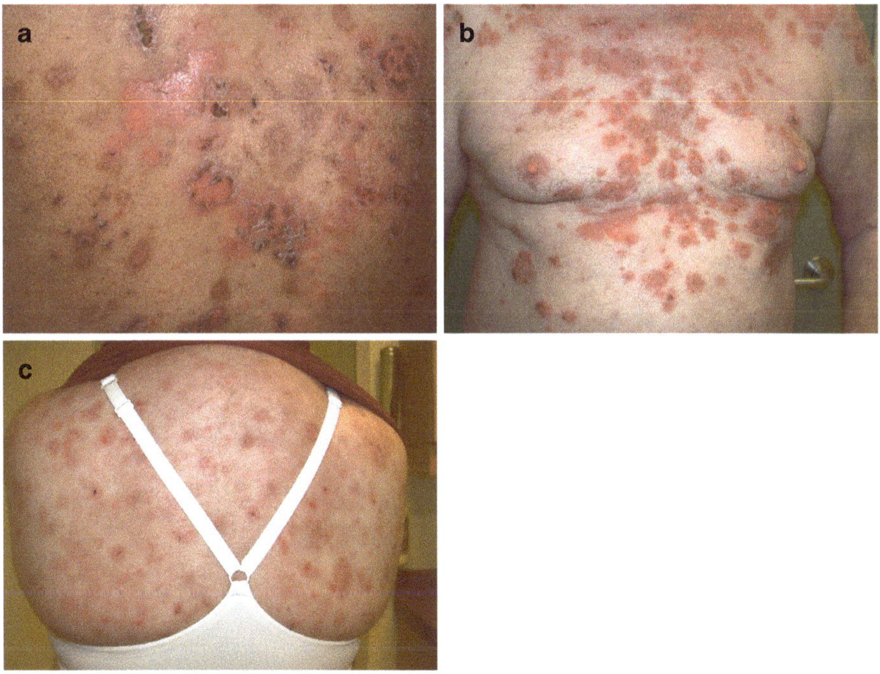

Fig. 2.1 (**a**) Typical pruritic, eroded and crusted plaques. (**b**) Typical pruritic, crusted plaques on the chest in a seborrheic distribution. (**c**) Erosions and erythematous plaques on the back of a woman with pemphigus foliaceus

and scalp (Fig. 2.4). Lesions can appear to become confluent (Fig. 2.5a) or can appear circinate and geometric with pronounced peripheral scale (Fig. 2.5b). Untreated lesions do not heal, and over weeks to months increase in number. In more severe cases, the lesions can coalesce and resemble an exfoliative erythroderma, involving the entire skin surface. In contrast with pemphigus vulgaris (PV), oral involvement is absent. PE is characterized by an erythematosus scaly-to-crusted rash often in a butterfly distribution that resembles lupus erythematosus (LE) and is localized to the face (Fig. 2.6a, b). PH is characterized by erythematous, edematous well-demarcated plaques (Fig. 2.7a) sometimes with grouped vesicles or pustules (Fig. 2.7b), but generally with heavy eosinophilic spongiosis and minimal acantholysis [2].

Demographics

In Europe and the USA the sporadic form is most common with an incidence of about a fifth to a tenth that of PV. The susceptibility genes associated are HLA DRB1*0102 and 0404 [3]. The average age of onset is between 40 and 60 years, has an equal gender distribution and can affect all races and ethnicities [1].

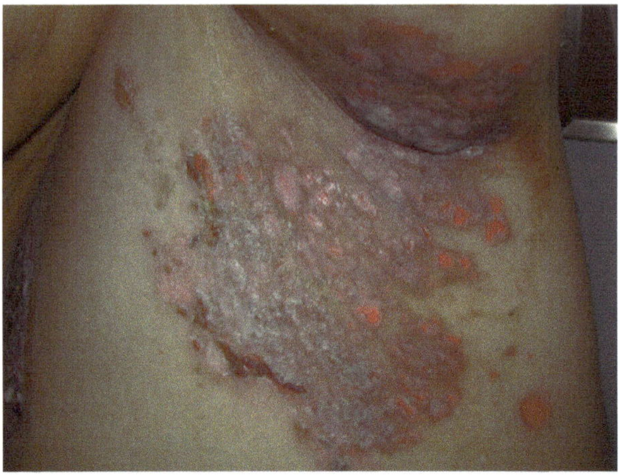

Fig. 2.2 Well-demarcated eroded plaques in the axilla of a patient with pemphigus foliaceus

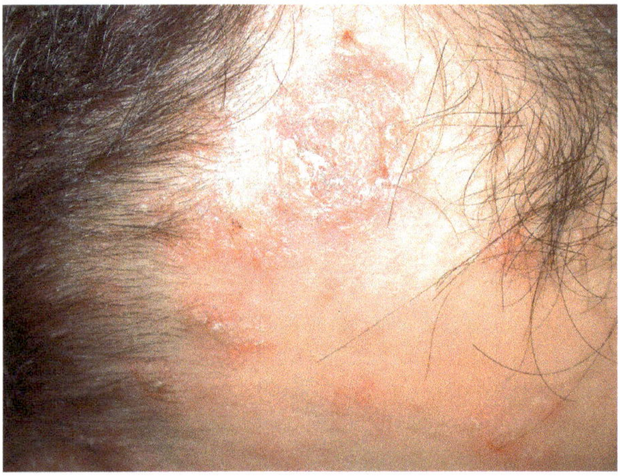

Fig. 2.3 Hyperkeratotic, slightly eroded plaques on the forehead, temple and hairline of a patient with pemphigus foliaceus

The endemic form (also known as fogo selvagem and Brazilian PF) is most often diagnosed in certain parts of Brazil, Tunisia and Colombia, typically arising at the interface between developing and non-developed areas. Younger individuals in their teens and twenties and multiple members of the same family can be affected. Epidemiological studies suggest an environmental cause which is as yet unidentified, although an insect vector is highly suspected [4]. It seems that as an area becomes more urbanized the disease disappears [5]. The associated susceptibility genes are HLA DRB1*0102, 0404, 1402, and 1406 [6]. Clinically and histologically, both forms of the disease are similar. Globally the incidence and prevalence of PF is very low, however due to the endemic variant and depending on the geographic area being studied, figures may vary significantly.

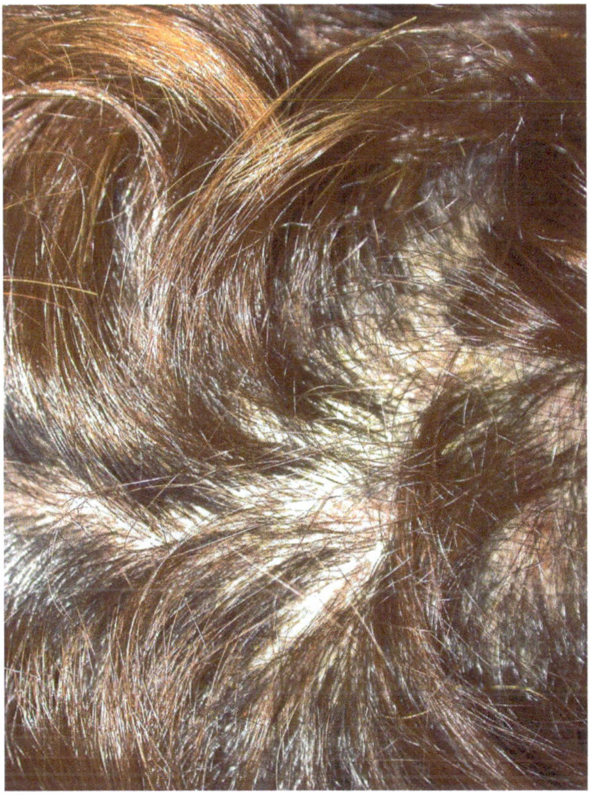

Fig. 2.4 Scalp involvement with pemphigus foliaceus

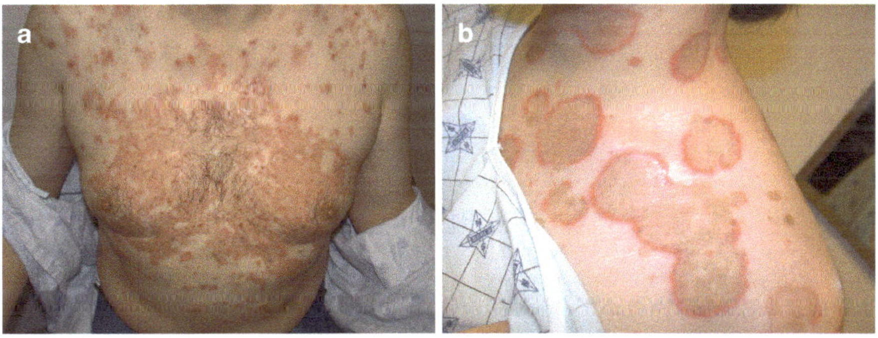

Fig. 2.5 (**a**) Confluence of erythematous plaques with small erosions in a patient with pemphigus foliaceus. (**b**) Annular, circinate and geographic plaques with peripheral erosions in this morphological variant of pemphigus foliaceus

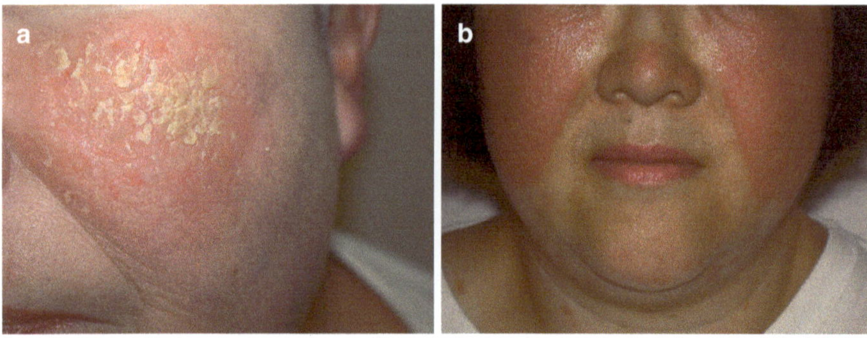

Fig. 2.6 (**a**) Hyperkeratotic plaque with subtle surface erosions in a patient with pemphigus erythematosus. (**b**) Bilateral erythematous plaques with light non-confluent scale over the malar cheeks in a patient with pemphigus herpetiformis

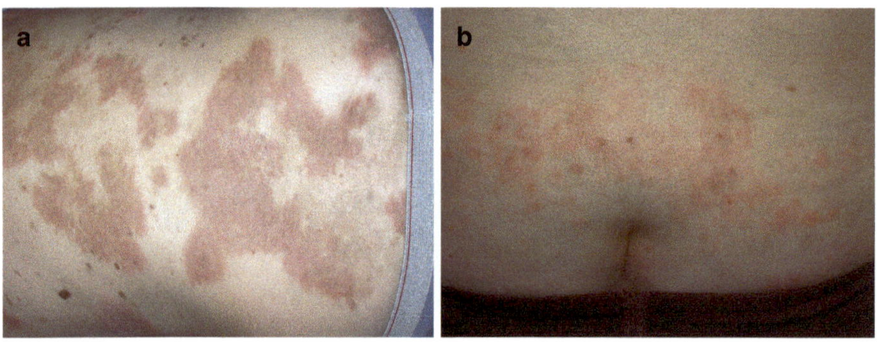

Fig. 2.7 (**a**) Indurated confluent plaques with an urticarial quality over the back in a patient with pemphigus herpetiformis variant. (**b**) Urticarial plaques over the gluteal cleft with small vesicles in a patient with pemphigus herpetiformis variant

Diagnosis

Diagnosis is based on a combination of clinical features, histopathological findings and the presence of autoantibodies on direct immunofluorescence (DIF) and indirect immunofluorescence (IIF). ELISA studies can also be sought. None of these tests are exclusively diagnostic and the diagnosis of PF is based on a combination of the above along with a strong clinical suspicion. Histology and DIF require skin biopsies. The biopsy for DIF should be perilesional, normal-appearing skin adjacent to a representative lesion. IIF and ELISA require serum samples.

Histopathology

A superficial bulla with the split high in the granular layer or directly beneath the stratum corneum is typical of an established PF lesion [1]. The bullae contains fibrin, neutrophils, and scattered acantholytic keratinocytes [7]. Early findings include the formation of vacuoles in the intercellular spaces in the upper layers of the epidermis [8]. These can expand, leading to cleft formation. Eosinophilic spongiosis can be seen as a precursor lesion, or as the prominent lesion in the PH variant [9]. Neutrophilic spongiosis is a rare occurrence in PF [10, 11]; and is usually related to the deposition of IgA. Neutrophilic pustules are also an uncommon finding [12]. Later findings include subcorneal blisters in the upper epidermis, which may contain neutrophils and fibrin. The epidermis may be hyperplastic, with overlying focal parakeratosis and some orthokeratosis [13]. Dyskeratotic cells with hyperchromatic nuclei reminiscent of the 'grains' found in Darier's disease can sometimes be found in the granular layer [14]. The superficial dermis is edematous with a mixed inflammatory cell infiltrate (eosinophils and neutrophils predominantly) [13]. Follicular plugging may be present and is important to note for if little else is evident but a clinical suspicion of PF exists [1].

Direct Immunofluorescence (DIF)

The DIF staining shows an intercellular pattern positive for IgG and C3 in both affected and normal skin [15]. This gives a "chicken wire" appearance to the epidermis. The intensity is generally greater in the upper epidermis and sometimes is localized to this level [16]. PE may stain both the intercellular spaces and the basement membrane zone if there is true overlap with systemic lupus erythematosus [17]. Most commonly, PE simply demonstrates the findings of PF (IgG and C3 intercellularly) and appears confined to a clinical distribution seen in acute LE.

IIF Indirect Immunofluorescence (IIF)

IIF uses patient serum to identify antibodies directed against an antigen on a specific substrate. IIF demonstrates circulating antibodies in nearly 90 % of cases of non-endemic PF depending on the substrate utilized [18]. Human skin has a greater density of dsg-1 and therefore has been found to be more sensitive than monkey or guinea-pig esophagus for PF diagnosis [19, 20]. The use of both however increases sensitivity to close to 100 % [21]. Similar to DIF, IIF will show intercellular staining with most fluorescence in the upper epidermis [22]. IIF titers can be used to assess disease activity [23]. Higher titres generally depict more severe disease and vice versa.

Enzyme-Linked Immunosorbent Assay (ELISA)

ELISA uses purified recombinant human dsg-1 to detect PF IgG autoantibodies in patient serum [24]. ELISA also provides a method of measuring the amount of circulating antibodies and hence, can be useful in monitoring a response to treatment

[25]. Unfortunately, ELISA and IIF both, are not restricted to the detection of only pathogenic antibody, and will detect any circulating antibodies present to dsg-1.

Systemic Treatment

Dapsone

Dapsone is a sulfone derived antibacterial agent initially used for the treatment of leprosy [26]. It is predominantly used in dermatological conditions with an abnormal accumulation of myeloid cells as it inhibits neutrophil and eosinophil activation and recruitment [27]. It is also used in some autoimmune bullous disorders (AIBD), however its mechanism of action in antibody-mediated diseases e.g. PF remains unclear. As one of the earliest changes observed in PF can be eosinophilic spongiosis, dapsone may be advantageous in the therapeutic armentarium. Adverse effects particularly in patients who are glucose-6-phosphate dehydrogenase (G-6PD) deficient (relative or functional) include methaemoglobinemia and anemia. More rare and serious side-effects can include agranulocytosis and dapsone hypersensitivity syndrome [26]. Gurcan and Ahmed [28] performed a retrospective review of 18 PF patients treated with dapsone. This included a case series of 9 patients reported by Basset et al. [29] and a remaining 9 individual case reports. Overall, 14 of 18 patients responded to dapsone alone (dose-range 100–300 mg/day) or in combination with prednisolone (dose-range 25–75 mg/day). Four patients did not respond. A total of 6-patients developed adverse effects, in 2 this necessitated discontinuation of treatment [28]. Several cases of pediatric sporadic PF including 3 in the Gurcan and Ahmed [28] review responsive to dapsone have been reported [30, 31]. Similarly, the variant PH with heavy eosinophilic spongiosis appears to be very dapsone-responsive [32].

Methotrexate

Methotrexate (MTX) is a folate antagonist initially used in the treatment of malignant disease and later used as an immunosuppressive agent [33]. MTX was one of the first immunosuppressive agents to be used in AIBD. High doses, up to 150 mg weekly, were used leading to severe side-effects [34]. Subsequently MTX use fell out of favour but has been re-emerging more recently. Gurcan and Ahmed [35] analyzed the data to date regarding MTX and PF. In three studies [36–38], a combination of systemic corticosteroids and MTX were used. Twenty patients were treated in total, with a dose range between 12.5 and 37.5 mg weekly. Fifteen patients showed clinical improvement when treated with 20–37.5 mg weekly for 1–27 weeks. At the time of reporting all patients were still on MTX. Four deaths were recorded in this group (3 bronchopneumonia, 1 cerebral thrombosis). Five patients did not improve on MTX. The dosages at the conclusion of MTX were not provided so a corticosteroid-sparing effect could not be determined.

Azathioprine

Azathioprine is a purine analog and prodrug of 6-mercaptopurine. It is metabolized to 6-thioguanine and can block purine synthesis, thus inhibiting rapidly-dividing cells in both de novo and salvage pathways, causing immunosuppression. Testing for normal thiopurine methyl transferase (TPMT) levels can minimize potential bone marrow toxicity with this drug. There are no studies examining the effect of azathioprine in PF alone. Any existing literature is for both PV and PF. Beissert et al. [39] examined 38 pemphigus patients (7 PF). They found no significant difference between azathioprine or mycophenolate mofetil (MMF) both in combination with corticosteroids. However, they subsequently scrutinized this in relation to remission of disease and corticosteroid sparing effects. The patients who were treated with azathioprine received a mean steroid dose of 8.916 ± 29.844 mg. The mean duration of follow-up was 438-days. The duration to disease control in 50 % of patients was less in the azathioprine treated patients as compared to the MMF group (30 vs. 75 days). After 200-days of treatment the remission rate was 75 % in the azathioprine group.

Rose et al. [40] compared dexamethasone/cyclophosphamide pulse therapy with oral methylprednisolone/azathioprine therapy in 22 patients (6 PF). Two patients with PF were examined in the methylprednisolone/azathioprine group. A trend was found in favour of methylprednisolone/azathioprine for remissions and for dexamethasone/cyclophosphamide for side-effect profile. Overall no significant differences were found regarding safety and efficacy.

van Dijk and van Velde [41] reported a case series of ten patients with either pemphigus or pemphigoid treated with azathioprine. Two patients with PF were graded as having a very good response to treatment without severe side-effects. Roenigk and Deodhar [42] also reported a case series of pemphigus patients (1 PF) treated with azathioprine. The PF patient had an excellent response with no side-effects reported.

Mycophenolate Mofetil

MMF is the 2-morpholinoethyl ester of mycophenolic acid. By inhibiting inosine monophosphate dehydrogenase in the de novo purine synthesis pathway, it has the ability to inhibit T and B-cell proliferation, induce T-cell apoptosis and inhibit B-cell antibody production [43–46]. In a study to investigate the safety and efficacy of oral methylprednisolone combined with azathioprine or MMF for the treatment of pemphigus, Beissert et al. [39] assigned 21 pemphigus patients to the MMF group (17 PV, 4 PF). The dose regimen was MMF 2 g/day plus methylprednisolone 2 mg/kg/day, the mean duration of follow-up was 438-days. Complete healing of the lesions and disease remission was noted in 20 (95 %) of 21 MMF patients. One patient (5 %) was noncompliant, discontinued treatment prematurely and did not achieve remission. Complete remission was seen after a mean of 91 ± 113 days. The mean disease-free interval from the time when complete remission was achieved until recurrence of lesions was 123 ± 103 days. Overall it was found that both immunosuppressants (MMF and azathioprine) had a similar efficacy and safety.

Powell et al. [47] described their experience of the addition of MMF to prednisolone in the management of 17 severe refractory pemphigus patients (12 PV, 4 PF, 1 paraneoplastic pemphigus). The regimen used was MMF 750 mg–3.5 g/day plus prednisolone 15–60 mg/day. At the time of reporting only one of the PF cases had clinically inactive disease. Two cases have experienced improved disease control and one case has clinically active disease responding recently to the addition of monthly-pulsed intravenous immunoglobulin 2 mg/kg/month to a combination of prednisolone 20 mg/day and MMF 3 g/day. The average doses of prednisolone prior to commencing MMF therapy and currently for this group are 35 mg and 8 mg daily, respectively.

Mimouni et al. [48] examined 42 patients with pemphigus (31 PV, 11 PF) who had relapses during prednisolone taper or were unable to tolerate side effects from previously used drugs. With MMF, complete remission was achieved in 22 PV and 5 PF patients and partial remission in 1 PV and 4 PF patients. Two treatment failures were recorded in the PF group. The median treatment/follow-up period was 22-months (range: 4–49 months) and the median time to remission was 9-months (range: 1–13 months). There was no statistical difference in the number of complete/partial remission or adverse effects between PV and PF patients.

Several other isolated cases of PF treated successfully with MMF are reported in the literature. Nousari et al. [49] reported a case of a 55-year-old male with only partial response to prednisolone and hepatoxicity to azathioprine. MMF was commenced at a dose of 1 g/twice daily, progressive improvement within 5-weeks of therapy was noted which allowed a gradual taper of prednisolone. At 6-months he was in complete remission receiving prednisolone 10 mg/day and MMF 1 g twice daily with no reported side-effects. Katz et al. [50] reported a 37-year-old female with PF initially treated with doses of prednisolone up to 60 mg/day and azathioprine 250 mg/day resulting only in partial remission. She was switched to MMF 1 g twice daily and prednisolone was continued at 40 mg/day. The patient improved over a 6-week period but flared when prednisolone was tapered below 20 mg/day. MMF was increased to 1.5 g twice daily and prednisolone was successfully tapered to 7.5 mg/day. At 9-months the patient remained clear with no flares.

Bongiorno et al. [51] investigated the efficacy of enteric-coated mycophenolate sodium (EC-MPS) 1440 mg daily and prednisolone 75 mg daily, in ten patients with active, refractory PV or PF over 18-months. A single PF patient was included, at 18-months had clinically quiescent disease. By 6-months the EC-MPS dose had been reduced to 720 mg/day and prednisolone 15 mg/day, this regimen continued at 18-months.

Intravenous Immunoglobulin

Intravenous immunoglobulin (IVIg) is made from IgG fractionated from pooled plasma via whole blood donors or by plasmapheresis and is usually administered in a monthly dose [52]. IVIg blocks fetal Fc receptors resulting in catabolism of circulating antibodies. As IVIg does not contain pemphigus antibodies, the patient ends up preferentially breaking down the pathogenic pemphigus antibodies as normal antibodies are being replaced. To prevent rebound auto-antibody production when fetal Fc receptors again become exposed, IVIg is often used with a systemic immunosuppressive agent capable of suppressing antibody production. Generally the use of IVIg is restricted to patients who: fail conventional therapy; have side-effects or contraindications to conventional therapy; and/or have rapidly progressive disease; have a very high indirect antibody titer [53]. The majority of the reported cases of IVIg use in pemphigus utilize the 2 g/kg/cycle dose [54]. Amagai et al. [55] in a randomized, double-blinded, placebo-controlled trial investigated the therapeutic effect of a single cycle of IVIg compared to conventional therapy with systemic corticosteroids in 61 patients with either PV or PF. If pemphigus lesions improved, patients were allowed to stay on protocol; patients not responding to therapy were removed from the study. Those randomized to receive IVIg, stayed in the study significantly longer, showed clinical improvement and suppression of autoantibody levels, compared to those randomized to conventional therapy. The follow up period was 90-days. The authors concluded that a single cycle of IVIg is rapidly effective in the treatment of pemphigus. However, most clinicians utilize multiple courses of IVIg to maintain disease control. In their consensus statement on IVIg use, Ahmed and Dahl [56] proposed its use at a dose of 2 g/kg divided over 3–5 days every 4-weeks until disease control is obtained. They recommend the interval between infusions is then slowly increased to 6, 8, 10, 12, 14, and 16-weeks and then stopped. If the disease flares, the frequency of infusions is increased until control is obtained and then the tapering regimen is again resumed. Jolles [57] reported that AIBD seem to have a better response to IVIg when used concomitantly with other treatments. IVIg in combination with systemic corticosteroids and/or immunosuppressive agents exhibited 91 % response rate compared to 56 % response rate when used as monotherapy, likely due to increased synthesis or rebound of pathogenic antibody. The addition of cytotoxic agents e.g. cyclophosphamide appears to make IVIg even more effective, as this agent is one of the strongest suppressors of antibody production from B-cells [52].

Cyclophosphamide

Cyclophosphamide is a nitrogen mustard with potent effects upon B-cells and strong suppression of antibody production. Pasricha et al. [58] first described the use of high-dose dexamethasone and cyclophosphamide pulse therapy (DCP) for pemphigus patients. The treatment regimen was divided into four-phases. Phase I consisted of monthly 100 mg intravenous (I.V.) dexamethasone on 3-consecutive days and 500 mg of intravenous cyclophosphamide on one of the days plus daily oral cyclophosphamide (50 mg). This was repeated until clinical remission was achieved (phase I) and then a further 6-months of DCP treatment was given (phase II). If remission was maintained DCP treatments were stopped and oral cyclophosphamide was continued for a further year (phase III); all treatment was withdrawn thereafter if patients remained in remission. Pasricha et al.'s [58–64] data suggested that this regimen was highly effective in inducing remission with minimal toxicity.

Between 1982 and 1998, 500 patients (PV 444, PF 33, PE 18, and pemphigus vegetans 5), with an almost equal sex ratio (251 males, 249 females) were enrolled for DCP regimen. The patient ages varied; 44 patients <20 years, 246 patients between 20 and 40 years, 190 patients between 40 and 60 years and 20 >60 years. Of these, 97 patients could not complete treatment, 19 patients died due to a variety of causes, most of which were unrelated to the disease or its treatment, or causes that were preventable with better patient management. The remaining 384 patients recovered from the disease and at the time of reporting were living without any disease and without any maintenance treatment [64]. Pasricha et al. conclude that pemphigus can be controlled in almost every patient and if a patient strictly follows the DCP regimen, a cure can be achieved.

In a multicenter, prospectively randomized study, Rose et al. [40] compared efficacy and side-effects of DCP with a methylprednisolone-azathioprine (M/A) therapy in 22 pemphigus patients, 6 of whom had PF. Eleven received DCP. This consisted of 100 mg I.V. dexamethasone per day on 3 consecutive days with cyclophosphamide (500 mg) day 1. Initially pulses were repeated every 2–4 weeks and then at increasing intervals. In between pulses, oral cyclophosphamide (50 mg) was given daily for 6-months. The results showed that within 24-months after treatment initiation, 5 of the 11 patients of the DCP group had a remission (complete remissions after discontinuation of therapy in 3 patients) and 6 of the 11 patients had a progression. There were more relapses in M/A therapy after remission than in DCP therapy. Side-effects were more common in the M/A group. These differences were not significant. The authors concluded that due to the high number of progressions in patients treated with DCP, the encouraging results of earlier reports about DCP could not be confirmed. However DCP was better tolerated and, in the case of primary efficacy, was associated with fewer recurrences than M/A therapy.

Saha et al. [65] presented a retrospective review of 21 patients (2 PF) treated with pulsed cyclophosphamide and high-dose methylprednisolone over a 10-year period. These patients had all been refractory to steroid and adjuvant either azathioprine or MMF. Of the treated patients the responses were: 7 excellent, 2 good, 5 moderate, 6 minimal and 1 had no clinical response. Four patients achieved complete clinical remission and the number of pulses for these patients varied between 11 and 22. All patients were able to reduce their prednisolone dose from a pre-pulsing median dose of 40–10 mg at the last pulse with a median dose reduction of 66 % ($p<0.001$). The most common adverse effect was transient lymphopenia (12 patients), nonlife-threatening sepsis (7 patients) and pre-mature ovarian failure (2 patients). The authors concluded that pulsed cyclophosphamide can be an effective treatment for refractory pemphigus but its adverse effects should be considered prior to therapy and closely monitored in patients on treatment. Longer-term risks from cyclophosphamide should also be taken into account including risk for bladder cancer and acute myelogenous leukemia that would not have been found in the short time frame of these studies.

Plasmapheresis

Guillaume et al. [66] reported the results of a multicenter randomized study examining the efficacy of plasmapheresis in 40 pemphigus patients (7 PF). Eighteen patients were treated with prednisolone alone and 22 with prednisolone and plasmapheresis. There was no difference in outcome between the treated group and control patients regarding disease control, cumulative corticosteroid dose or serum antibody titers. Four deaths were documented in the treatment group. It was concluded that plasmapheresis in association with low steroid doses are not effective in the treatment of pemphigus and may even promote sepsis.

Rituximab

Rituximab (RTX) is a chimeric murine/human monoclonal antibody that recognizes the B-lymphocyte surface protein CD20, a transmembrane protein expressed on pre-B to mature B-cells and functions to regulate B-cells early in development [67]. RTX completely destroys this phase of B-lymphocyte growth and results in subsequent decline and depletion of pathogenic antibodies and minimizes pathogenic B-cell presentation of auto-antigens to T-cells. RTX has increasingly been reported to be effective in AIBD [68]. Heelan et al. [69] conducted a retrospective study of 92 patients (PV 84, PF 8) to assess the clinical response of patients with pemphigus to RTX using a modified fixed-dose rheumatoid arthritis protocol (1 g I.V. on days 1 and 15, followed by 500 mg if clinically warranted at 6-month intervals or repeated full dosing). Median time to relapse after the first treatment cycle was 15-months (95 % CI, 10.3–19.7). When comparing time to relapse for PV and PF, there was no statistically significant difference. The PV median time to relapse was 15-months (95 % CI, 8.6–21.4), and the PF median time to relapse was 12-months (1.5–22.5; $p=0.99$). All patients experienced improvement. Complete remission rates with or without adjuvant treatment at final follow-up were 89 % (56 patients complete remission without treatment, 26 patients complete remission with adjuvant treatment). No serious infectious adverse events occurred.

Reguiai et al. [70] showed that RTX appeared to be a durable, effective, and well-tolerated treatment for severe pemphigus. This retrospective study included 24 patients with severe pemphigus (9 PV, 4 PF), treated with RTX (n = 13) or systemic corticosteroids alone or combined with immunosuppressants (n = 11 control subjects). Of the 13 patients treated with RTX, 9 achieved complete remission 3-months after 1 RTX cycle. Thereafter, 7 patients (4 with maintenance therapy) relapsed within a mean of 18 months after the last RTX cycle and received 1 or 2 additional RTX cycles. Mean follow-up was 41-months after the first cycle and 28-months after the last. All 13 patients remained in complete remission (5 patients off therapy).

Cianchini et al. [71] demonstrated the efficacy of RTX in 42 patients (37 PV, 5 PF) with a median follow-up of 26.5-months. Leshem et al. [72] reported a total of 47 patients with pemphigus (42 PV, 3 PF) (2 discontinued due to infusion reactions but included in side-effect analysis) who were treated with RTX at a dosage of 1 g on day 1 and 15, most with concurrent immunosuppressive medications. The remission rates after the first treatment cycle reached 76 %. Repeating the treatment further increased the remission rates to 91 %. There was a 22 % relapse rate at a median time of 8-months, but 75 % of relapsing patients achieved remission again with additional cycles. Recently Kanwar et al. [73] sought to compare the efficacy, in terms of clinical and immunological outcomes in pemphigus patients of a high (2×1 g) versus a low dose (2×500 mg) of RTX. In this randomized, observer-blinded trial 22 patients were randomized into two-groups. Fifteen PV patients (7 in group A, 8 in group B); 7 PF patients (4 in group A, 3 in group B). Patients received either 1 g RTX or 500 mg RTX (day 1 and day 15) and were followed up for 48-weeks. There was no statistically significant difference in early and late clinical end points, and total cumulative dose of corticosteroids between the two groups. At week-40, the fall in Ikeda severity score was significantly more in the 2×1 g group than in 2×500 mg group (p=0.049). Patients in the 2×500 mg group received a significantly higher cumulative dose of azathioprine (p=0.018). The ELISA indices of dsg-1 and dsg-3 showed a statistically significant decline in the 2×1 g group only. B-cell repopulation occurred earlier in the 2×500 mg group by 8-weeks. The authors concluded that a few clinical and immunological study parameters suggest improved outcomes in patients receiving high-dose (2×1 g) RTX.

Miscellaneous

Gold is not a very commonly used agent in the treatment of PF. Pandya and Dyke [74] reviewed 26 pemphigus patients (21 PV, 3 PF, 2 PE) treated with intramuscular gold over a 10-year period. In 62 % of patients gold was an effective primary treatment or steroid-sparing agent. A mean of 3-months treatment was required in order to half the daily prednisolone dose. Four patients were disease free and treatment could be discontinued. Toxic effects developed in 42 % of patients, all of which resolved with discontinuation of therapy. The authors concluded that gold may be useful in patients unable to reduce corticosteroid requirement, however is limited by its toxic effects and slow onset of action.

There have been some reported cases of hydroxychloroquine used in PF as corticosteroid sparing agents [75–77]. This treatment modality may be especially pertinent in photosensitive individuals. Colchicine has also been successfully used in case reports [78]. Similarly, it is felt that for pemphigus patients with anything beyond very mild disease tetracycline antibiotics can be useful adjuncts but rarely successful as monotherapy [79–81].

More unusual treatments reported in the literature include the following. Two cases of milder localized PF have been reported to be treated with topical immunomodulators, tacrolimus and pimecrolmus [82, 83]. Etanercept was used to treat PF in a 57-year-old female unresponsive to oral corticosteroids [84]. The disease activity in this particular patient was closely related to high TNF-alpha serum levels.

Etanercept therapy produced a dramatic reduction in the serum level and a resolution of the clinical picture. Corticosteroids were tapered and discontinued after 2-months. Four-months later the patient was still receiving subcutaneous etanercept 25 mg twice-weekly and was symptom free.

Mizoribine is a newly developed immunosuppressive agent with pharmacological effects similar to MMF. A pilot study was performed to evaluate its effectiveness as an adjuvant therapy in the treatment of both PV and PF [85]. Eleven patients (8 PV, 3 PF) received a combination of prednisolone and mizoribine. Complete remission was observed in 3 of 8 PV patients and in 1 of 3 PF patients. These 4 patients had a rapid clinical response and achieved remission at a median of 11.8-months. Partial remission was achieved in 2 of the 3 PF patients with a median time to achieve partial remission of 16-months. Six (55.6 %) of the 11 patients with pemphigus had complete or partial remission and were able to taper their prednisolone. The authors concluded that the effectiveness of mizoribine therapy could be attributed to its corticosteroid-sparing properties as well as its immunosuppressive effects, and a larger series of patients with a longer follow-up are needed to fully assess the efficacy of this treatment.

Tocilizumab is a humanized monoclonal antibody, targeting IL6-receptor, used predominantly in the treatment of rheumatoid arthritis. Caso et al. [86] reported a female with both PF and Bechets. She had not responded to corticosteroids, immunosuppressants or biologic agents including adalimumab, anakinra, and infliximab. A complete, clinical, and serological remission was achieved with tocilizumab.

Evaluation and Treatment Algorithm

Early diagnosis and input by a dermatologist is important. The prognosis of PF can be very difficult to predict in the early stages. A treatment algorithm is presented in Fig. 2.8. Baseline investigations before embarking on therapy should include full blood count, renal and liver function, TPMT and G6PD. Initial treatment if inadequate can lead to early recurrences during corticosteroid tapering. In severe disease it is both necessary to halt disease progression and to maintain a remission. Treatment can therefore be divided into initial therapy and maintenance therapy. The initial treatment is the period until the disease is controlled and tapering of the corticosteroid dose has begun. During initial treatment, disease activity is evaluated primarily through clinical symptoms. Depending on the dose of the agent used, generally a 3-month trial is used prior to moving to the next agent, unless disease severity necessitates faster transfer to more aggressive therapies.

Following a diagnosis of PF, the authors have found for mild or localized cases topical corticosteroids, oral tetracyclines and/or topical tacrolimus can be commenced with close follow-up. These would be adjunctive therapy for more serious disease. Generally however oral corticosteroids are required. For severe or moderate conditions, the standard dose is 1 mg/kg per day, for milder cases 0.5 mg/kg may be enough. Corticosteroid sparing agents such as dapsone (1–2 mg/kg/day), colchicine

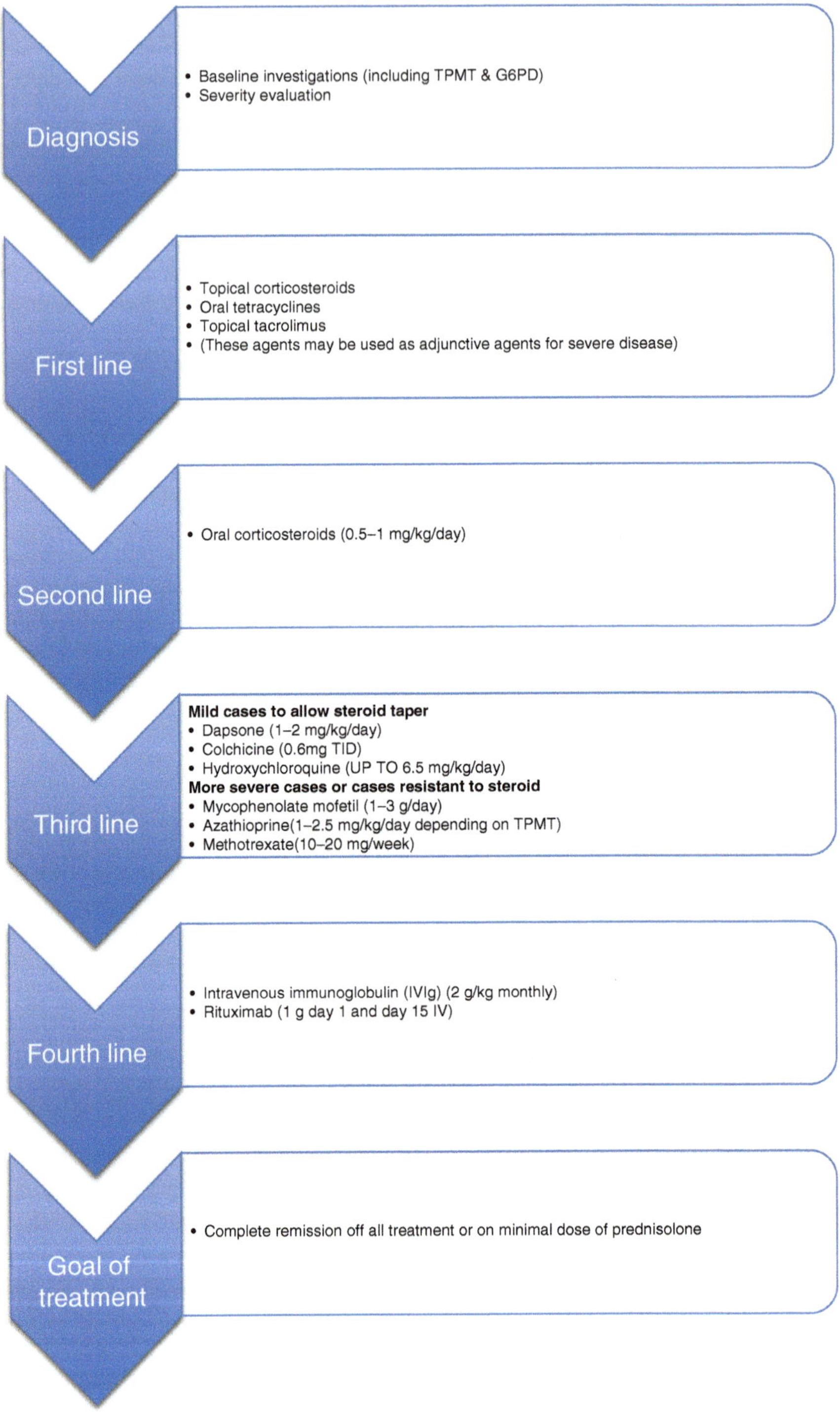

Fig. 2.8 Treatment algorithm

(0.6 mg TID) or hydroxychloroquine (up to 6.5 mg/kg/day) [especially if photo-distributed prominence of lesions] could be added at this point particularly for milder cases to allow a steroid taper. For more severe cases or cases resistant to steroid treatment, steroid-sparing immunosuppressant therapy can be commenced.

The order of preference is determined by multiple factors and is individualized to the patient. Generally the sequence of treatments according to tolerance and success of treatment is as follows: MMF (1–3 g/day), azathioprine (1–2.5 mg/kg/day depending on TPMT) and MTX (10–20 mg/week). When a patient is stable on a particular treatment modality a slow corticosteroid taper begins. If therapeutic effects remain inadequate with high indirect pemphigus titers, IVIg (2 g/kg monthly) can be commenced and subsequently RTX can be used for recalcitrant cases (1 g day 1 and day 15). Although initially thought of as a treatment for recalcitrant PF, RTX is proving to be the most effective agent in the treatment of diseases in the pemphigus grouping and is quickly becoming a first-line agent for PF. In our clinics, where insurer coverage or RTX is adequate, this is the first-line agent selected.

Each treatment modality is monitored for safety and efficacy. The goal of treatment although not always possible is a complete remission off all treatment or on minimal dose of prednisolone. The activity of disease is monitored by clinical examination (affected skin area, numbers of new blisters, Nikolsky's phenomenon) and circulating pemphigus autoantibodies.

Response to treatment is determined according to the definitions of an international consensus statement [87]. *Complete remission off therapy* (CR) is the absence of new or established lesions while the patient is not receiving any systemic therapy for at least 2-months. *Complete remission on therapy* (CROT) is the absence of new or established lesions while the patient is receiving minimal therapy. *Partial remission off therapy* (PR) is the presence of transient new lesions that heal within 1-week without treatment while the patient is not receiving any systemic therapy for at least 2-months. *Partial remission on minimal therapy* (PROT) is the presence of transient new lesions that heal within 1-week while the patient is receiving minimal therapy, including topical corticosteroids. *Relapse/flare* is the appearance of three or more new lesions each month that do not heal spontaneously within 1-week or the extension of established lesions in a patient who has achieved disease control. Complete and partial responses could be achieved without therapy or with minimal therapy (≤10 mg/day of prednisolone and/or minimal adjuvant therapy for ≥2 months).

Future Areas of Concentration; Therapeutic Questions and Deficiencies

The prognosis of untreated PF is better than that of PV, probably because lesions are more superficial and there is less risk of infection, fluid loss, and metabolic disturbance. However, unfortunately the treatment is no easier, since the doses of drugs needed to control PF can be similar to those used for PV.

Future research in this area should be more uniformly organized. Uniform diagnostic criteria and validated severity assessment scales for assessing response to treatment will make randomized control trials (RCTs) easier to compare. Studies with only one type of pemphigus also make comparisons easier. It may be difficult to do this in light of the much smaller numbers of diseases other than PV. More RCTs are required to compare the efficacy and safety of different doses of corticosteroids used with different steroid-sparing agents as are studies of long-term follow-up of patients to find out relapse rate after remission with different treatments. The subject of maintenance therapy to prevent relapse after remission also needs to be further addressed. The issue of RTX as a first line agent needs to be further elucidated and also its use as a maintenance therapy. Quality of life is increasingly becoming an important issue in pemphigus patients' treatment and this needs to be both clarified and incorporated into studies.

References

1. James KA, Culton DA, Diaz LA. Diagnosis and clinical features of pemphigus foliaceus. Dermatol Clin. 2011;29(3):405–12, viii. doi:10.1016/j.det.2011.03.012.
2. Joly P, Litrowski N. Pemphigus group (vulgaris, vegetans, foliaceus, herpetiformis, brasiliensis). Clin Dermatol. 2011;29(4):432–6. doi:10.1016/j.clindermatol.2011.01.013.
3. Bystryn J-C, Rudolph JL. Pemphigus. Lancet. 2005;366(9479):61–73. doi:10.1016/s0140-6736(05)66829-8.
4. Flores G, Qian Y, Diaz LA. The enigmatic autoimmune response in endemic pemphigus foliaceus. Actas Dermosifiliogr. 2009;100 Suppl 2:40–8.
5. Diaz LA, Sampaio SA, Rivitti EA, et al. Endemic pemphigus foliaceus (Fogo Selvagem): II. Current and historic epidemiologic studies. J Invest Dermatol. 1989;92(1):4–12.
6. Moraes ME, Fernandez-Vina M, Lazaro A, et al. An epitope in the third hypervariable region of the DRB1 gene is involved in the susceptibility to endemic pemphigus foliaceus (fogo selvagem) in three different Brazilian populations. Tissue Antigens. 1997;49(1):35–40.
7. Kouskoukis CE, Ackerman AB. What histologic finding distinguishes superficial pemphigus and bullous impetigo? Am J Dermatopathol. 1984;6(2):179–81.
8. Kouskoukis CE, Ackerman AB. Vacuoles in the upper part of the epidermis as a clue to eventuation of superficial pemphigus and bullous impetigo. Am J Dermatopathol. 1984;6(2):183–6.
9. Osteen FB, Wheeler Jr CE, Briggaman RA, et al. Pemphigus foliaceus. Early clinical appearance as dermatitis herpetiformis with eosinophilic spongiosis. Arch Dermatol. 1976;112(8):1148–52.
10. Hoss DM, Shea CR, Grant-Kels JM. Neutrophilic spongiosis in pemphigus. Arch Dermatol. 1996;132(3):315–8.
11. Gabbi TV, Bernardelli IM, Santi CG, et al. Pemphigus foliaceus with neutrophilic spongiosis evolving to an atypical pemphigus phenotype. J Am Acad Dermatol. 2004;51(6):1012–3. doi:10.1016/j.jaad.2004.07.038.
12. Matsuo K, Komai A, Ishii K, et al. Pemphigus foliaceus with prominent neutrophilic pustules. Br J Dermatol. 2001;145(1):132–6.
13. Furtado TA. Histopathology of pemphigus foliaceus. AMA Arch Derm. 1959;80(1):66–71.
14. Wilgram GF, Caulfield JB, Madgic EB. An electron microscopic study of acantholysis and dyskeratosis in pemphigus foliaceus: with a special note on peculiar intracytoplasmic bodies. J Invest Dermatol. 1964;43:287–99.
15. Rodriguez J, Bystryn JC. Pemphigus foliaceus associated with absence of intercellular antigens in lower layers of epidermis. Arch Dermatol. 1977;113(12):1696–9.

16. Bhogal B, Wojnarowska F, Black MM, et al. The distribution of immunoglobulins and the C3 component of complement in multiple biopsies from the uninvolved and perilesional skin in pemphigus. Clin Exp Dermatol. 1986;11(1):49–53.
17. Amerian ML, Ahmed AR. Pemphigus erythematosus. Presentation of four cases and review of literature. J Am Acad Dermatol. 1984;10(2 Pt 1):215–22.
18. Harrist TJ, Mihm MC. Cutaneous immunopathology. The diagnostic use of direct and indirect immunofluorescence techniques in dermatologic disease. Hum Pathol. 1979;10(6):625–53.
19. Feibelman C, Stolzner G, Provost TT. Pemphigus vulgaris. Superior sensitivity of monkey esophagus in the determination of pemphigus antibody. Arch Dermatol. 1981;117(9):561–2.
20. Shirakata Y, Amagai M, Hanakawa Y, et al. Lack of mucosal involvement in pemphigus foliaceus may be due to low expression of desmoglein 1. J Invest Dermatol. 1998;110(1):76–8. doi:10.1046/j.1523-1747.1998.00085.x.
21. Harman KE, Gratian MJ, Bhogal BS, et al. The use of two substrates to improve the sensitivity of indirect immunofluorescence in the diagnosis of pemphigus. Br J Dermatol. 2000;142(6):1135–9.
22. Bystryn JC, Abel E, DeFeo C. Pemphigus foliaceus. Subcorneal intercellular antibodies of unique specificity. Arch Dermatol. 1974;110(6):857–61.
23. Fitzpatrick RE, Newcomer VD. The correlation of disease activity and antibody titers in pemphigus. Arch Dermatol. 1980;116(3):285–90.
24. Ishii K, Amagai M, Hall RP, et al. Characterization of autoantibodies in pemphigus using antigen-specific enzyme-linked immunosorbent assays with baculovirus-expressed recombinant desmogleins. J Immunol. 1997;159(4):2010–7.
25. Crowther JR. ELISA. Theory and practice. Methods Mol Biol. 1995;42:1–218. doi:10.1385/0-89603-279-5:1.
26. Piette EW, Werth VP. Dapsone in the management of autoimmune bullous diseases. Dermatol Clin. 2011;29(4):561–4. doi:10.1016/j.det.2011.06.018.
27. Zhu YI, Stiller MJ. Dapsone and sulfones in dermatology: overview and update. J Am Acad Dermatol. 2001;45(3):420–34. doi:10.1067/mjd.2001.114733.
28. Gurcan HM, Ahmed AR. Efficacy of dapsone in the treatment of pemphigus and pemphigoid: analysis of current data. Am J Clin Dermatol. 2009;10(6):383–96. doi:10.2165/11310740-000000000-00000.
29. Basset N, Guillot B, Michel B, et al. Dapsone as initial treatment in superficial pemphigus. Report of nine cases. Arch Dermatol. 1987;123(6):783–5.
30. Chatterjee M, Meru S, Vasudevan B, et al. Pemphigus foliaceus masquerading as IgA pemphigus and responding to dapsone. Indian J Dermatol. 2012;57(6):495–7. doi:10.4103/0019-5154.103074.
31. Garcia-Melendez ME, Eichelmann K, Salas-Alanis JC, et al. Pemphigus foliaceus in an 11 year old mexican girl with response to oral dapsone. Case Rep Pediatr. 2013;2013:291256. doi:10.1155/2013/291256.
32. Maciejowska E, Jablonska S, Chorzelski T. Is pemphigus herpetiformis an entity? Int J Dermatol. 1987;26(9):571–7.
33. Genestier L, Paillot R, Quemeneur L, et al. Mechanisms of action of methotrexate. Immunopharmacology. 2000;47(2–3):247–57.
34. Peck SM, Osserman KE, Samuels AJ, et al. Studies in bullous diseases. Treatment of pemphigus vulgaris with immunosuppressives (steroids and methotrexate) and leucovorin calcium. Arch Dermatol. 1971;103(2):141–7.
35. Gurcan HM, Ahmed AR. Analysis of current data on the use of methotrexate in the treatment of pemphigus and pemphigoid. Br J Dermatol. 2009;161(4):723–31. doi:10.1111/j.1365-2133.2009.09246.x.
36. Rivitti EA, Camargo ME, Castro RM, et al. Use of methotrexate to treat pemphigus foliaceus. Int J Dermatol. 1973;12(2):119–22.
37. Jablonska S, Blaszczyk M. Treatment of pemphigus with methotrexate. Przegl Dermatol. 1970;57(3):331–6.

38. Piamphongsant T, Sivayathorn A. Pemphigus: combined treatment with methotrexate and prednisone. J Med Assoc Thai Chotmaihet Thangphaet. 1975;58(3):171–6.
39. Beissert S, Werfel T, Frieling U, et al. A comparison of oral methylprednisolone plus azathioprine or mycophenolate mofetil for the treatment of pemphigus. Arch Dermatol. 2006;142(11):1447–54. doi:10.1001/archderm.142.11.1447.
40. Rose E, Wever S, Zilliken D, et al. Intravenous dexamethasone-cyclophosphamide pulse therapy in comparison with oral methylprednisolone-azathioprine therapy in patients with pemphigus: results of a multicenter prospectively randomized study. J Dtsch Dermatol Ges. 2005;3(3):200–6.
41. van Dijk TJ, van Velde JL. Treatment of pemphigus and pemphigoid with azathioprine. Dermatologica. 1973;147(3):179–85.
42. Roenigk Jr HH, Deodhar S. Pemphigus treatment with azathioprine. Clinical and immunologic correlation. Arch Dermatol. 1973;107(3):353–7.
43. Allison AC, Almquist SJ, Muller CD, et al. In vitro immunosuppressive effects of mycophenolic acid and an ester pro-drug, RS-61443. Transplant Proc. 1991;23(2 Suppl 2):10–4.
44. Eugui EM, Mirkovich A, Allison AC. Lymphocyte-selective antiproliferative and immunosuppressive activity of mycophenolic acid and its morpholinoethyl ester (RS-61443) in rodents. Transplant Proc. 1991;23(2 Suppl 2):15–8.
45. Allison AC, Eugui EM. Immunosuppressive and other effects of mycophenolic acid and an ester prodrug, mycophenolate mofetil. Immunol Rev. 1993;136:5–28.
46. Allison AC, Eugui EM. Mycophenolate mofetil and its mechanisms of action. Immunopharmacology. 2000;47(2–3):85–118.
47. Powell AM, Albert S, Al Fares S, et al. An evaluation of the usefulness of mycophenolate mofetil in pemphigus. Br J Dermatol. 2003;149(1):138–45.
48. Mimouni D, Anhalt GJ, Cummins DL, et al. Treatment of pemphigus vulgaris and pemphigus foliaceus with mycophenolate mofetil. Arch Dermatol. 2003;139(6):739–42. doi:10.1001/archderm.139.6.739.
49. Nousari HC, Sragovich A, Kimyai-Asadi A, et al. Mycophenolate mofetil in autoimmune and inflammatory skin disorders. J Am Acad Dermatol. 1999;40(2 Pt 1):265–8.
50. Katz KH, Marks Jr JG, Helm KF. Pemphigus foliaceus successfully treated with mycophenolate mofetil as a steroid-sparing agent. J Am Acad Dermatol. 2000;42(3):514–5.
51. Bongiorno MR, Pistone G, Doukaki S, et al. Enteric-coated mycophenolate sodium in the treatment of refractory pemphigus. Int J Dermatol. 2010;49(6):693–9. doi:10.1111/j.1365-4632.2009.04291.x.
52. Chee SN, Murrell DF. The use of intravenous immunoglobulin in autoimmune bullous diseases. Dermatol Clin. 2011;29(4):565–70. doi:10.1016/j.det.2011.06.010.
53. Czernik A, Toosi S, Bystryn JC, et al. Intravenous immunoglobulin in the treatment of autoimmune bullous dermatoses: an update. Autoimmunity. 2012;45(1):111–8. doi:10.3109/08916934.2011.606452.
54. Ishii N, Hashimoto T, Zillikens D, et al. High-dose intravenous immunoglobulin (IVIG) therapy in autoimmune skin blistering diseases. Clin Rev Allergy Immunol. 2010;38(2–3):186–95. doi:10.1007/s12016-009-8153-y.
55. Amagai M, Ikeda S, Shimizu H, et al. A randomized double-blind trial of intravenous immunoglobulin for pemphigus. J Am Acad Dermatol. 2009;60(4):595–603. doi:10.1016/j.jaad.2008.09.052.
56. Ahmed AR, Dahl MV. Consensus statement on the use of intravenous immunoglobulin therapy in the treatment of autoimmune mucocutaneous blistering diseases. Arch Dermatol. 2003;139(8):1051–9. doi:10.1001/archderm.139.8.1051.
57. Jolles S. A review of high-dose intravenous immunoglobulin (hdIVIg) in the treatment of the autoimmune blistering disorders. Clin Exp Dermatol. 2001;26(2):127–31.
58. Pasricha JS, Khaitan BK, Raman RS, et al. Dexamethasone-cyclophosphamide pulse therapy for pemphigus. Int J Dermatol. 1995;34(12):875–82.
59. Pasricha JS, Thanzama J, Khan UK. Intermittent high-dose dexamethasone-cyclophosphamide therapy for pemphigus. Br J Dermatol. 1988;119(1):73–7.

60. Pasricha JS, Sood VD, Minocha Y. Treatment of pemphigus with cyclophosphamide. Br J Dermatol. 1975;93(5):573–6.
61. Pasricha JS, Poonam. Current regimen of pulse therapy for pemphigus: minor modifications, improved results. Indian J Dermatol Venereol Leprol. 2008;74(3):217–21.
62. Pasricha JS, Khaitan BK. Curative treatment for pemphigus. Arch Dermatol. 1996;132(12):1518–9.
63. Pasricha JS, Das SS. Curative effect of dexamethasone-cyclophosphamide pulse therapy for the treatment of pemphigus vulgaris. Int J Dermatol. 1992;31(12):875–7.
64. Pasricha JS. Pulse therapy as a cure for autoimmune diseases. Indian J Dermatol Venereol Leprol. 2003;69(5):323–8.
65. Saha M, Powell AM, Bhogal B, et al. Pulsed intravenous cyclophosphamide and methylprednisolone therapy in refractory pemphigus. Br J Dermatol. 2010;162(4):790–7. doi:10.1111/j.1365-2133.2009.09590.x.
66. Guillaume JC, Roujeau JC, Morel P, et al. Controlled study of plasma exchange in pemphigus. Arch Dermatol. 1988;124(11):1659–63.
67. Zakka LR, Shetty SS, Ahmed AR. Rituximab in the treatment of pemphigus vulgaris. Dermatol Ther (Heidelb). 2012;2(1):17. doi:10.1007/s13555-012-0017-3. 17 [pii].
68. Gurcan HM, Keskin DB, Stern JN, et al. A review of the current use of rituximab in autoimmune diseases. Int Immunopharmacol. 2009;9(1):10–25. doi:10.1016/j.intimp.2008.10.004. S1567-5769(08)00319-6 [pii].
69. Heelan K, Al-Mohammedi F, Smith MJ, et al. Durable remission of pemphigus with a fixed-dose rituximab protocol. JAMA Dermatol. 2014. doi:10.1001/jamadermatol.2013.6739 [published Online First: Epub Date].
70. Reguiai Z, Tabary T, Maizières M, et al. Rituximab treatment of severe pemphigus: long-term results including immunologic follow-up. J Am Acad Dermatol. 2012;67(4):623–9. doi:10.1016/j.jaad.2011.12.019.
71. Cianchini G, Lupi F, Masini C, et al. Therapy with rituximab for autoimmune pemphigus: results from a single-center observational study on 42 cases with long-term follow-up. J Am Acad Dermatol. 2012;67(4):617–22. doi:10.1016/j.jaad.2011.11.007.
72. Leshem YA, Hodak E, David M, et al. Successful treatment of pemphigus with biweekly 1-g infusions of rituximab: a retrospective study of 47 patients. J Am Acad Dermatol. 2012. doi:10.1016/j.jaad.2012.08.010.
73. Kanwar AJ, Vinay K, Sawatkar GU, et al. Clinical and immunological outcomes of high- and low-dose rituximab treatments in patients with pemphigus: a randomized, comparative, observer-blinded study. Br J Dermatol. 2014;170(6):1341–9. doi:10.1111/bjd.12972.
74. Pandya AG, Dyke C. Treatment of pemphigus with gold. Arch Dermatol. 1998;134(9):1104–7.
75. Hymes SR, Jordon RE. Pemphigus foliaceus. Use of antimalarial agents as adjuvant therapy. Arch Dermatol. 1992;128(11):1462–4.
76. Perry HO, Brunsting LA. Pemphigus foliaceus. Further observations. Arch Dermatol. 1965;91:10–23.
77. Schiff M. Jamarsan therapy of pemphigus erythematosus. Observations on 2 patients treated with Brazilian regimen. Arch Dermatol. 1961;84:103–8.
78. Takahashi A, Nishijima C, Umehara K, et al. Pemphigus foliaceus successfully treated with colchicine and topical corticosteroid. Eur J Dermatol. 2010;20(6):825–6. doi:10.1684/ejd.2010.1064.
79. Alpsoy E, Yilmaz E, Basaran E, et al. Is the combination of tetracycline and nicotinamide therapy alone effective in pemphigus? Arch Dermatol. 1995;131(11):1339–40.
80. Gaspar ZS, Walkden V, Wojnarowska F. Minocycline is a useful adjuvant therapy for pemphigus. Australas J Dermatol. 1996;37(2):93–5.
81. Chen S, Lu X, Zhou G. Mild pemphigus foliaceus responding to combination therapy with niacinamide and tetracycline. Int J Dermatol. 2003;42(12):981–2.
82. Termeer CC, Technau K, Augustin M, et al. Topical tacrolimus (protopic) for the treatment of a localized pemphigus foliaceus. J Eur Acad Dermatol Venereol. 2004;18(5):636–7. doi:10.1111/j.1468-3083.2004.00980.x.

83. Tyros G, Kalapothakou K, Christofidou E, et al. Successful treatment of localized pemphigus foliaceus with topical pimecrolimus. Case Rep Dermatol Med. 2013;2013:489618. doi:10.1155/2013/489618.
84. Gubinelli E, Bergamo F, Didona B, et al. Pemphigus foliaceus treated with etanercept. J Am Acad Dermatol. 2006;55(6):1107–8. doi:10.1016/j.jaad.2006.08.041.
85. Hashimoto T, Kawakami T, Koga H, et al. Therapeutic effect of mizoribine on pemphigus vulgaris and pemphigus foliaceus. Dermatol Ther. 2012;25(4):382–5. doi:10.1111/j.1529-8019.2012.01469.x.
86. Caso F, Iaccarino L, Bettio S, et al. Refractory pemphigus foliaceus and Behcet's disease successfully treated with tocilizumab. Immunol Res. 2013;56(2–3):390–7. doi:10.1007/s12026-013-8411-1.
87. Murrell DF, Dick S, Ahmed AR, et al. Consensus statement on definitions of disease, end points, and therapeutic response for pemphigus. J Am Acad Dermatol. 2008;58(6):1043–6. doi:10.1016/j.jaad.2008.01.012.

Chapter 3
Pemphigus Herpetiformis

Phillip Laws and Neil H. Shear

Abstract Pemphigus herpetiformis is a rare variant of pemphigus first described almost 40 years ago. Clinical features overlapping with dermatitis herpetiformis but histopathologically and immunologically consistent with pemphigus are typical. Diagnosis is often delayed due to the unusual presentation and absence of blisters. Initial reports implicated antibodies to desmoglein-1 (Dsg1) as key in pathogenesis. It is increasingly clear this is not universally the case and may include Dsg-3 and/or desmocollin antibodies. Although treatment is based on small case series reports suggest a combination approach of corticosteroid and dapsone may be most appropriate with other options including azathioprine, methotrexate or mycophenolate mofetil. The response to rituximab remains to be established. This chapter provides an overview of pemphigus herpetiformis, summarises treatment options and provides a proposed strategy for management.

Keywords Pemphigus Herpetiformis • Immunobullous disease • Autoantibody • Desmoglein

Introduction

Pemphigus forms a heterogeneous group of autoimmune blistering skin disorders of which pemphigus vulgaris (PV) and pemphigus foliaceus (PF) are the most common. Over the last 20–30 years an increasing awareness of other subtypes has emerged including: pemphigus herpetiformis (PH), pemphigus vegetans, paraneoplastic pemphigus (PNP) and pemphigus erythematosus. PH was first described by Jablonska et al. in 1975 as a distinct entity notable due to clinical features similar to

P. Laws, MBChB (✉)
Department of Dermatology, Chapel Allerton Hospital, University of Leeds, Leeds, West Yorkshire, UK
e-mail: phillaws@yahoo.com

N.H. Shear, MD, FRCPC
Division of Dermatology, Department of Medicine (Clinical Pharmacology), Sunnybrook Health Sciences Centre/University of Toronto, Toronto, ON, Canada

N. Sami (ed.), *Autoimmune Bullous Diseases: Approach and Management*,
DOI 10.1007/978-3-319-26728-9_3

dermatitis herpetiformis but histopathology consistent with pemphigus [1]. A number of diagnostic terms had previously been applied to the disease including dermatitis herpetiformis with acantholysis, mixed bullous disease and sulfonamide-responsive pemphigus. Earlier reports suggested the existence of such an entity but with a reluctance to identify it as a distinct entity, preferring to classify it as a subtype of PF. Specific examples of this include a case series of seven patients with pemphigus who initially presented with eosinophilic spongiosis but no blistering [2]. Review of these cases suggests that at least two of these patients could be classified as PH. While there is undoubtedly some overlap with PF it is now generally accepted to represent a distinct disease entity; in part due to the unusual clinical presentation and different approach to management. This chapter provides an overview of clinical presentation, diagnosis, pathogenesis and management of PH.

Demographics and Epidemiology

Patients with PH typically present in the fifth or sixth decade of life although a wide range of ages have been reported including several pediatric cases, the youngest of which presented at 5-years-old [3, 4]. The oldest reported patient was 92-years-old [5]. There would appear to be no gender or ethnic bias. One exception to the above description includes areas of endemic PF where the average age and female predominance are marked [6]. Case series reported from larger centres indicate PH represents approximately 5–8 % of pemphigus cohorts [7, 8].

Clinical Presentation

Clinical presentation is variable but may appear similar to dermatitis herpetiformis. Urticated, annular, erythematous plaques are observed over the trunk and limbs and may be grouped (Fig. 3.1). Vesiculobullous or pseudovesicular erythematous plaques are also frequently reported and probably represent later stage disease (Fig. 3.2). Lesions may have a herpetiform appearance. The rash is characteristically associated with severe pruritus. Oral lesions are rare. Peripheral blood eosinophilia is seen in approximately 40 % of patients and may be fivefold greater than the upper limit of normal (authors' experience).

Histopathology

The histopathological features of PH are variable over time and multiple biopsies may be required, particularly when the diagnosis is not considered and immunofluorescence studies are not performed. Typical histological findings include an

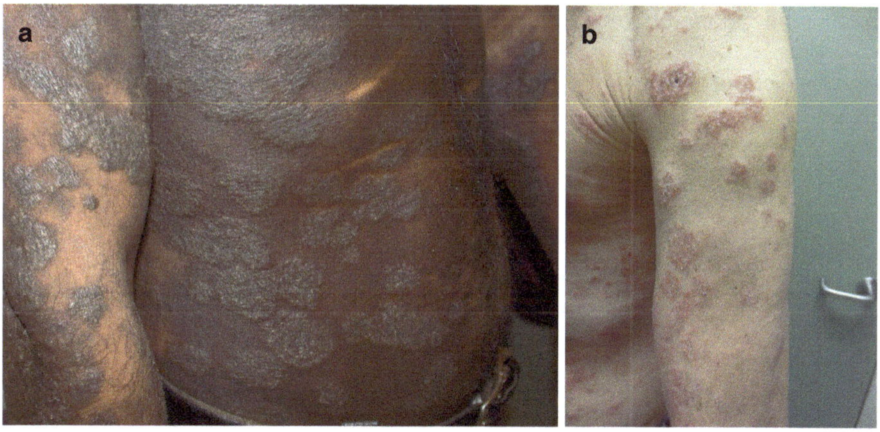

Fig. 3.1 (**a**, **b**) Clinical appearance of pemphigus herpetiformis with annular, urticated, erythematous plaques over the trunk, arms and legs (From Laws et al. [49]. Reprinted with permission from John Wiley and Sons)

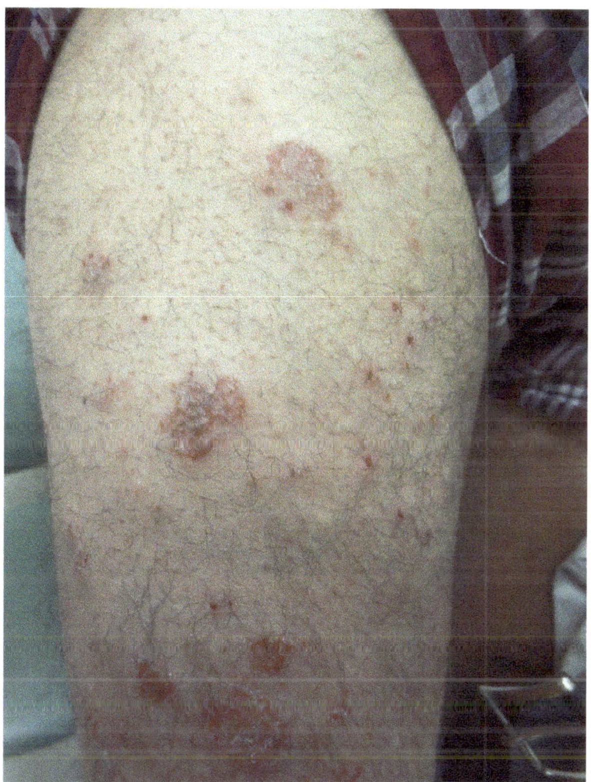

Fig. 3.2 Clinical appearance of pemphigus herpetiformis with vesiculobullous erythematous plaques (From Laws et al. [49]. Reprinted with permission from John Wiley and Sons)

eosinophilic spongiosis and intraepithelial blisters (subcorneal or suprabasal) that may include eosinophils or neutrophils [9]. Studies report eosinophilic spongiosis in 20 %, neutrophilic spongiosis in 20 % and a mixed neutrophilic and eosinophilic spongiosis in 60 % (Figs. 3.3 and 3.4) [9]. Acantholysis may be absent or only detectable after multiple biopsies or a protracted disease course.

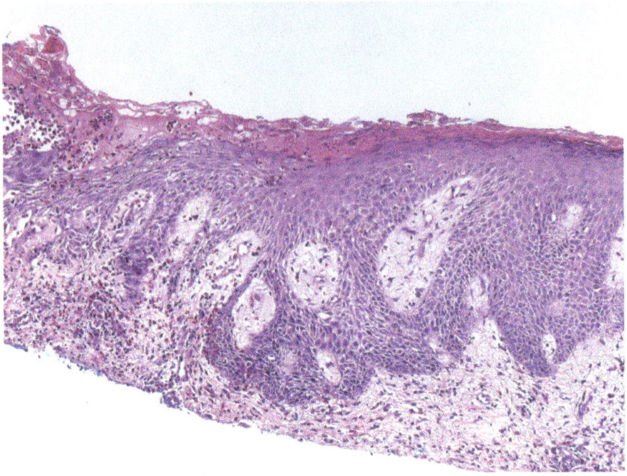

Fig. 3.3 Skin biopsy (×100, HE) demonstrating eosinophilic and neutrophilic spongiosis with focal suprabasal acantholysis (From Laws et al. [49]. Reprinted with permission from John Wiley and Sons)

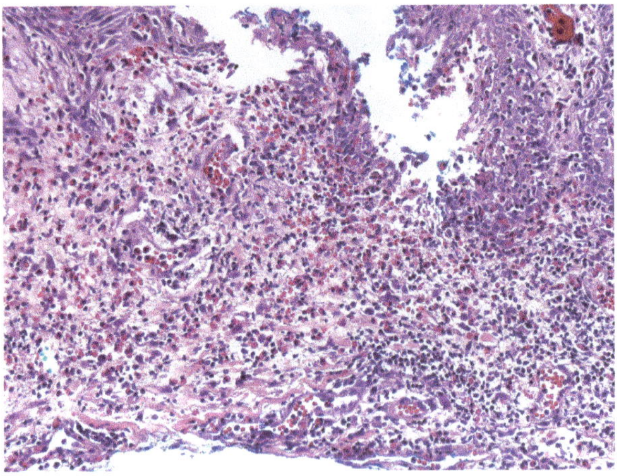

Fig. 3.4 Skin biopsy (×200, HE) demonstrating eosinophilic and neutrophilic spongiosis with focal suprabasal acantholysis (From Laws et al. [49]. Reprinted with permission from John Wiley and Sons)

Immunopathology

Direct Immunofluorescence (DIF)

DIF findings for PH typically overlap with both PF and/or PV. Intercellular deposits of immunoglobulin (Ig) G and/or complement (C3) is typical and may be suprabasal or subcorneal [9]. Increasing numbers of case reports have been published detailing unusual additional findings in patients with PH including the presence of IgA antibodies within the intercellular space and IgG binding to the basement membrane [10]. The significance of this remains to be determined and is discussed in more detail below.

Indirect Immunofluorescence

PF is characteristically associated with antibodies to Desmoglein (Dsg)1 while PV is associated with antibodies to Dsg3. The majority of patients with PH reported to date have antibodies to Dsg1 or Dsg3 [11]. Ishii et al. have reported on sera of 20 patients with PH demonstrating reactivity to Dsg1 and Dsg3 in 80 % (n = 16/20) and 20 % (n = 4/20) respectively [11]. Of note in this study no patients demonstrated reactivity to both Dsg1 and Dsg3. A smaller study of 7 patients reported in Brazil (endemic for PF) reported antibodies only to Dsg1 [12]. Recent studies have suggested that PH may have a broader autoantibody profile and that in some patients antibodies may be directed at desmocollin glycoproteins [13, 14].

Disease Association

Due to the small number of cases reported in the literature it is unclear if there is any disease association with PH. Case reports detailing an association with malignancy include lung cancer [15–17], esophageal cancer [18], and prostate cancer [19]. Of note PNP is generally an aggressive, treatment resistant form of pemphigus with striking mucosal involvement. If an association with PH and malignancy was established, the diagnostic criteria for PNP may need to be adapted to ensure clear distinction between pemphigus subtypes.

Other diseases reported in association with PH include psoriasis [20, 21], systemic lupus erythematosus [22], autoimmune haemolytic anaemia [23], and Human Immunodeficiency Virus [24]. In one patient with psoriasis it would seem that PH may have been precipitated by ultraviolet light therapy prescribed as treatment for psoriasis [21]

Drug induced PH has been reported following administration of thiopronine [25] and penicillamine [26].

Diagnosis

Differential Diagnosis of Pemphigus Herpetiformis
Pemphigus vulgaris
Pemphigus foliaceus
Bullous pemphigoid
Linear IgA Bullous Dermatosis
IgA pemphigus
IgG/IgA pemphigus
Atopic dermatitis
Allergic contact dermatitis
Drug-induced eruption
Dermatitis herpetiformis

The differential diagnosis of PH is broad and frequently the diagnosis is overlooked. The differential diagnosis includes PV, PF, bullous pemphigoid, linear IgA bullous dermatosis, dermatitis, drug rashes, IgG/IgA pemphigus and allergic contact dermatitis. Table 3.1 provides a summary of key findings of some of these diseases. IgG/IgA pemphigus is a newly described disease that requires further investigation. Research to date would indicate that this entity overlaps with PH but may be distinguished from PH due to the presence of IgG and IgA antibodies to Dsg1 [27].

The first description of PH by Jablonska et al. in 1975 proposed diagnostic criteria including clinical features of dermatitis herpetiformis and direct immunofluorescence findings of pemphigus [1]. Since then diagnostic criteria have been developed to include urticated erythema and/or vesiculobullous lesions in the context of pruritus. Current proposed diagnostic criteria are summarized below. While this is typical it should be emphasized that these criteria are not definitive and reports of PH in the absence of Dsg1 or Dsg3 have been reported [28].

Pemphigus Herpetiformis: Diagnostic Criteria

Clinical
Pruritus
Urticated erythema (± blister or erosion)

Histopathology
Eosinophilic/neutrophilic spongiosis
Variable acantholysis

Immunofluorescence
Epidermal intercellular deposits of IgG

NB. These criteria are not exclusive to pemphigus herpetiformis and should be interpreted in light of clinical scenario

Table 3.1 Differential diagnosis of pemphigus herpetiformis and distinguishing features

	Clinical presentation	Oral involvement	Histopathology	IMF	Autoantigen	Peripheral blood eosinophilia
Pemphigus herpetiformis	Pruritic urticated erythema, vesiculobullous	Rarely	Eosinophilic spongiosis, intraepidermal neutrophils, acantholysis (may be absent), intraepithelial blisters,	IgG	Dsg1, Dsg3	++
Pemphigus vulgaris	Flaccid blisters, erosions	Yes, may be dominant feature of disease	Suprabasal acantholysis	IgG	Dsg3 ± Dsg1	+
Pemphigus foliaceus	Superficial blisters, crusted erosions (may be seborrheic in distribution)	No	Subcorneal acantholysis	IgG	Dsg1	+
Linear IgA Bullous dermatosis	Vesiculobullous ("string of pearls" pattern)	No	Subepidermal blister with predominant neutrophilic infiltrate	Linear IgA BMZ	LAD-1, BP180	–
Bullous pemphigoid	Pruritic urticated erythema, tense blisters	No	Subepidermal blister with eosinophilic infiltrate	IgG BMZ	BP180, BP230	++

IMF immunofluorescence, *Dsg* desmoglein, *BMZ* basement membrane zone, *LAD* Linear IgA dermatosis autoantigen, *BP* bullous pemphigoid

Pathogenesis

Pemphigus is an autoimmune disease of epidermal cell adhesion with antibodies directed at components of the desmosome. In the majority of patients with pemphigus antibodies to desmoglein, a protein of the cadherin superfamily drives this. Cadherins are broadly categorized as classical cadherins or desomosomal cadherins. The desomosomal cadherins include desmogleins and desmocollins.

Epidermal cell adhesion is maintained through adherin and desomosomal junctions. Adherin junctions typically form weak associations while desmosomes provide structural integrity. Transmembrane desmogleins and desmocollins form the extracellular component of the desmosomal plaque and interact with intracellular desmoplakins, plakoglobins and plakophilins (Fig. 3.5). These latter proteins provide a point of binding for intracellular keratin.

There are four isoforms of desmoglein (Dsg1-4) and three isoforms of desmocollins (Dsc1-3). Dsg1 and Dsg3 are essential to epidermal function. Dsg1 is found predominantly within the upper epidermis (stratum granulosum) while Dsg3 is located within the lower levels of the epidermis (stratum basale and spinosum). As discussed in previous chapters PV is typically caused by antibodies directed at Dsg1 and Dsg3. Mucosal desmosomes are predominantly mediated by Dsg3 and antibodies directed at Dsg3 are therefore key in the development of mucosal disease. It is therefore interesting to note that despite Dsg3 antibodies in PH mucosal lesions are

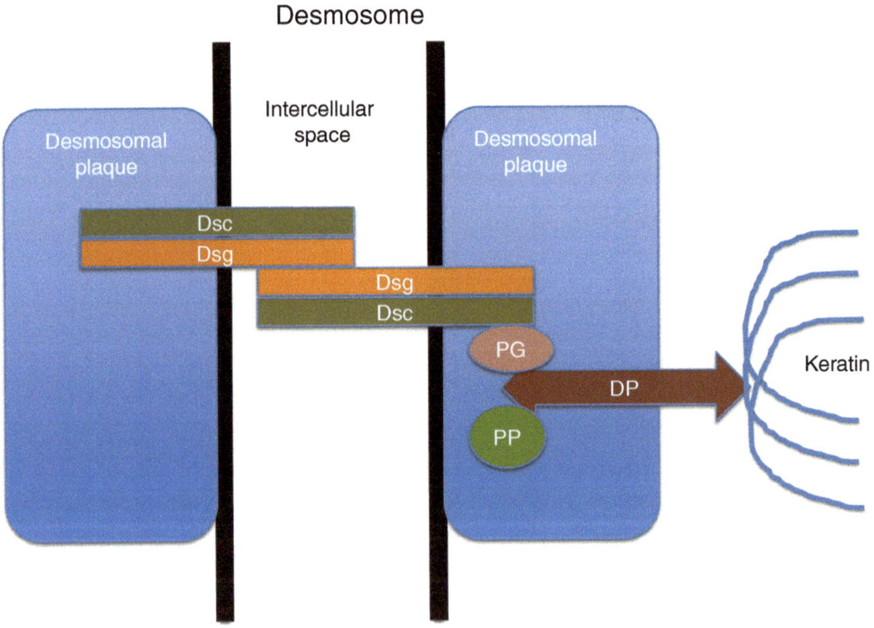

Fig. 3.5 Diagrammatic representation of desmosome. *Dsc* desmocollin, *Dsg* desmoglein, *PG* plakoglobin, *PP* plakophilin, *DP* desmoplakin

rare. Patients with PF develop antibodies to Dsg1, which are largely absent from the mouth, and consequently experience skin limited disease.

Recent studies have provided evidence that antibodies other than Dsg1 or Dsg3 may induce PH. A case report by Tateishi et al. describe a case of PH with antibodies to Dsc1 only [29]. The role of Dsc in pemphigus disease is increasingly being examined in greater detail and appears to be significant. Spindler et al. have reported that desmocollins are important in the pathology of pemphigus through interactions with Dsg1 but not Dsg3 [30].

Classical pemphigus disease (both PF and PV) results in acantholysis, blister formation and clinical disease. Despite the presence of Dsg 1 or Dsg3 in PH the relative lack of acantholysis and blistering is notable. The underlying mechanism behind acantholysis and blistering remains to be fully explained but several mechanisms have been proposed. These include:

1. Steric hindrance – Antibodies directed at anchoring proteins disrupt cell adhesion and prevent attachment [31]. Antibodies in PH may be different and therefore not induce acantholysis to the same extent.
2. Activation of plasmin – Antibody binding initiates signal transduction which induces plasminogen activator (PA). PA then activates plasmin and consequently disruption of the desmosome. This theory is now considered unlikely [32, 33].
3. Acantholysis would appear to be dependent on pemphigus gamma-globulins and it has been suggested that this protein may not be elevated in PH [34].
4. Epitope recognition – Specific antigenic epitopes may be influential in determining disease expression. Epitope recognition perhaps offers the best explanation for differential expression of acantholysis in patients with apparently the same antibody profile [35].

It is increasingly clear that pemphigus subtypes may change over time in some patients. This occurs to such an extent that PF may develop in to PV or vice versa [36, 37]. This is also supported by Maciejowska et al. who reported 33 % (n=5/15) of patients with PH progressed to classical PF later in the disease course [7]. It has been proposed that this occurs through epitope spreading [38].

The mechanism of epitope spreading remains unclear. One explanation would be that the inflammatory milieu in pemphigus disease enhances further epitope recognition and cellular damage results in exposure of previously unexposed epitopes. With an enhanced spectrum of antibodies recognising multiple epitopes clinical expression of disease may change. This is the source of significant research in the literature with intramolecular and intermolecular epitope spread hypothesized [39, 40]. The theory of intramolecular epitope spreading is supported by Lebeau et al. who report a patient with PH who initially developed Dsg3 antibodies to ectodomain 1 of the protein which changed over the duration of disease to ectodomain four predominant expression [41]. This change in antibody profile was accompanied by development of mucosal disease. It would appear that PH has a broader epitope distribution than PV and perhaps provides evidence that PH may represent an undifferentiated pemphigus phenotype which in some patients later progress to PV or PF [38].

The complexity of immunobullous disease is further evident in a recent report of PH and mucous membrane pemphigoid in the same patient [13]. Direct immunofluorescence (DIF) demonstrated strong IgG and weak IgA to keratinocyte surface with C3 at the basement membrane zone. Further studies demonstrated IgG antibodies to Dsc-1 and IgG antibodies to BP180 and laminin 332. The authors hypothesized that intermolecular epitope spreading between Dsc1 and BMZ antigens may explain the dual pathology evident in their patient.

Previous research has proposed a role for complement in PH disease phenotype. Complement has a role in immune activation and acantholysis and the relative presence or absence may determine the extent of acantholysis. This has been largely discredited as it would seem that IgG4 is predominant in PH disease and this subtype of IgG does not activate complement [11]. However, while IgG4 appears to be to be present in the majority of patients Santi et al. demonstrated that IgG1 and/or IgG3 is present in 57 % (n=4/7) patients [12]. IgG1 and IgG3 have been demonstrated to induce eosinophilic degranulation and may play a role in disease expression in some patients [42].

Interleukin (IL)-8 would also appear to play an important role in the pathogenesis of PH. O'Toole et al. have previously reported marked deposition of IL-8 within the epidermis and demonstrated that this accumulation plays an important role in accumulation of neutrophils [43].

Management

PH was described nearly 40 years ago and is a rare and challenging disease to recognise. The evidence to guide treatment is therefore limited to small case series and case reports. Following a diagnosis of PH most patients will require systemic therapy. Topical corticosteroid may complement this therapy but is rarely sufficient to control disease in isolation. Evidence to date supports the role of corticosteroids and sulphonamide derivatives. Corticosteroids play an important role in therapy and have been reported in numerous case reports and series. Ingber et al. report use of corticosteroid as single agent therapy at doses up to 2 mg/kg [44]. This approach to management is likely to be limited by side effects of high dose corticosteroids, and in our opinion should be reserved for resistant disease or used at lower doses (≤1 mg/kg) combined with other agents in an attempt to limit corticosteroid exposure.

A case series reported by Maciejowska et al. of 15 patients reported good responses to combination dapsone (100–200 mg daily) and prednisone (25–60 mg daily) in 7 patients [7]. Three patients treated with dapsone alone did not respond. Five patients required high dose corticosteroid for disease control. The rationale for dapsone is based on clinical features overlapping with dermatitis herpetiformis and the presence of neutrophils in some cases. Our own experience suggests that most patients will experience at least a partial response to a sulfonamide drug such as dapsone (approximately 100 mg daily) or sulfasalazine (3 g daily).

In the event that corticosteroids and dapsone (or similar) fail to provide adequate control treatment, options should be broadly similar to PV or PF. This may include: azathioprine (up to 2.5 mg/kg daily), mycophenolate mofetil (MMF; up to 3 g daily), mycophenolate sodium (up to 1440 mg daily), cyclophosphamide (100 mg daily in one patient) [7, 45], methotrexate (up to 25 mg weekly) [46], rituximab (1 g intravenously day 1 and 15) and intravenous immunoglobulin (1 g/kg/month in one patient) [47]. Other reported therapies include sulfapyridine [44] and plasmapheresis [7, 47].

Rituximab, a CD20 chimeric monoclonal antibody, has transformed the management of PV and PF with dramatic and sustained treatment response in the majority of patients while maintaining a favourable safety profile [48]. However, in our experience two patients treated with rituximab for PH did not dramatically improve. This is also supported by a case report of a 9-year-old male diagnosed with PH who did not respond to rituximab [46]. This latter patient received extensive treatment including corticosteroid, dapsone, MMF, azathioprine, doxycycline, and rituximab before responding to a combination of corticosteroids and methotrexate. It is important to note that this is a very small number of patients on which to establish a response and the authors feel rituximab should still be considered as a useful treatment option for PH. If it was established that rituximab was ineffective in treating PH disease this would raise significant questions regarding disease pathogenesis.

Authors' Opinion

PH should be considered a discrete entity on account of distinct clinical presentation in the context of immunofluorescence findings typical for pemphigus. While some patients will progress and develop more typical PF, this is not universal. A fluid concept of pemphigus disease is perhaps best adopted to highlight the overlapping clinical, histological and immunofluorescence findings.

Disease severity is best assessed on percentage body surface area (BSA) affected as conventional tools frequently rely on blister counts and mucosal involvement that is unlikely to be relevant in the majority of patients. This should be complemented by an assessment of impact on quality of life (e.g., Dermatology Life Quality Index). We would describe mild disease as BSA < 5 %, moderate disease 5–10 % BSA and severe disease BSA > 10 %.

Following a diagnosis of PH treatment is typically commenced as per the algorithm in Fig. 3.6. For moderate to severe disease corticosteroids should be considered at a dose of 1 mg/kg generally alongside dapsone (typically up to 150 mg daily although may increase to max dose 300 mg). We suggest corticosteroids should be maintained for a minimum of 2 weeks after disease control (absence of new lesions and/or symptoms). The onset of action of dapsone may be rapid although treatment should be continued for a minimum of 6 weeks before assessing treatment response.

In the event of treatment failure with dapsone and/or corticosteroid we recommend azathioprine (1–2 mg/kg), methotrexate (up to 25 mg weekly) or MMF (up to

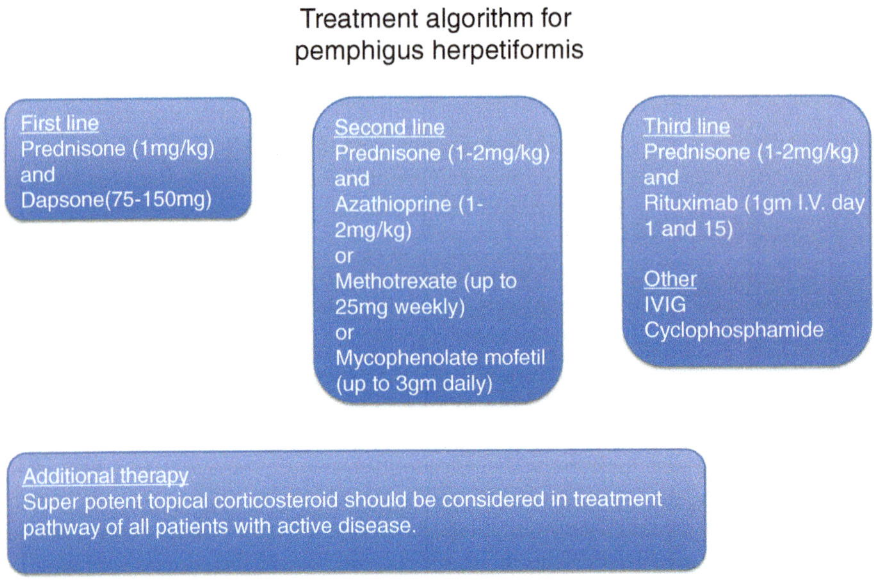

Fig. 3.6 Recommended algorithm for the treatment of pemphigus herpetiformis. *IVIG* intravenous immunoglobulin

3 g daily) as third line agents. Treatment is likely to be delivered alongside corticosteroids and therefore response is best assessed by the ability to effectively reduce corticosteroid dose. These agents may take greater than 8 weeks to impact upon disease and should be managed accordingly.

Rituximab should be considered in any patient who is unresponsive to corticosteroid and at least one systemic agent (preferably dapsone). We adopt a dosing strategy of 1 g intravenously at day 1 and day 15. Response to treatment should be assessed after approximately 8 weeks.

For patients resistant to the above agents cyclophosphamide or intravenous immunoglobulin (IVIG) should be considered.

It is important to address side effects of long-term corticosteroid usage in a timely manner and consideration of vitamin D, calcium and a bisphosphonate (or similar) should be discussed with the patient. We also recommend regular blood pressure and blood sugar monitoring.

Future Direction

Increasingly complex immunological pemphigus profiles are reported in the literature detailing features of overlapping disease phenotypes. This fascinating area of dermatology presents a significant diagnostic challenge and an opportunity to develop our understanding of immune regulation and skin function. Increasing evidence suggests that epitope spreading is a dynamic process that is clinically relevant and may be open to manipulation through therapeutic intervention. In developing our understanding of this complex area of dermatopathology it is anticipated that more accurate diagnostic concepts may be developed which allow greater understanding of disease and more rational treatment strategies. This is perhaps most prominent in the field of biologic therapies which afford a targeted approach to manipulation of the immune system and have transformed management of pemphigus reducing both mortality and morbidity in this patient group.

Acknowledgements

Funding Sources None

Conflict of Interest
P.M.L. None declared
N.H.S. None declared

References

1. Jablonska S, Chorzelski TP, Beutner EH, Chorzelska J. Herpetiform pemphigus, a variable pattern of pemphigus. Int J Dermatol. 1975;14(5):353–9.
2. Emmerson RW, Wilson-Jones E. Eosinophilic spongiosis in pemphigus. A report of an unusual histological change in pemphigus. Arch Dermatol. 1968;97(3):252–7.
3. Hocar O, Ait Sab I, Akhdari N, Hakkou M, Amal S. A case of pemphigus herpetiformis in a 12-year-old male. ISRN Pediatr. 2011;2011:712560.
4. Duarte IB, Bastazini Jr I, Barreto JA, Carvalho CV, Nunes AJ. Pemphigus herpetiformis in childhood. Ped Dermatol. 2010;27(5):488–91.
5. Isogai R, Kawada A, Aragane Y, Amagai M, Tezuka T. A case of herpetiform pemphigus with anti-desmoglein 3 IgG autoantibodies. J Dermatol. 2004;31(5):407–10.
6. Morini JP, Jomaa B, Gorgi Y, Saguem MH, Nouira R, Roujeau JC, et al. Pemphigus foliaceus in young women. An endemic focus in the Sousse area of Tunisia. Arch Dermatol. 1993;129(1):69–73.
7. Maciejowska E, Jablonska S, Chorzelski T. Is pemphigus herpetiformis an entity? Int J Dermatol. 1987;26(9):571–7.
8. Micali G, Musumeci ML, Nasca MR. Epidemiologic analysis and clinical course of 84 consecutive cases of pemphigus in eastern Sicily. Int J Dermatol. 1998;37(3):197–200.
9. Kasperkiewicz M, Kowalewski C, Jablonska S. Pemphigus herpetiformis: from first description until now. J Am Acad Dermatol. 2014;70(4):780–7.
10. Ohata C, Koga H, Teye K, Ishii N, Hamada T, Dainichi T, et al. Concurrence of bullous pemphigoid and herpetiform pemphigus with IgG antibodies to desmogleins 1/3 and desmocollins 1–3. Br J Dermatol. 2013;168(4):879–81.
11. Ishii K, Amagai M, Komai A, Ebihara T, Chorzelski TP, Jablonska S, et al. Desmoglein 1 and desmoglein 3 are the target autoantigens in herpetiform pemphigus. Arch Dermatol. 1999;135(8):943–7.
12. Santi CG, Maruta CW, Aoki V, Sotto MN, Rivitti EA, Diaz LA. Pemphigus herpetiformis is a rare clinical expression of nonendemic pemphigus foliaceus, fogo selvagem, and pemphigus vulgaris. Cooperative Group on Fogo Selvagem Research. J Am Acad Dermatol. 1996;34(1):40–6.
13. Ohata C, Higashi Y, Yamagami J, Koga H, Ishii N, Kanekura T, et al. Coexistence of pemphigus herpetiformis with IgG antibodies to desmocollin 1 and pemphigoid with IgG antibodies to BP180 C-terminal domain and laminin gamma2. JAMA Dermatol. 2013;149(4):502–4.

14. Nakamura Y, Takahata H, Teye K, Ishii N, Hashimoto T, Muto M. A case of pemphigus herpetiformis-like atypical pemphigus with IgG anti-desmocollin 3 antibodies. Br J Dermatol. 2014;171(6):1588–90.
15. Vicente MA, Iranzo P, Castell T, Baradad M, Palou J, Mascaro JM. Pemphigus herpetiformis associated with neoplasm of the lung. Med Cutan Ibero Lat Am. 1989;17(6):373–8.
16. Kubota Y, Yoshino Y, Mizoguchi M. A case of herpetiform pemphigus associated with lung cancer. J Dermatol. 1994;21(8):609–11.
17. Palleschi GM, Giomi B. Herpetiformis pemphigus and lung carcinoma: a case of paraneoplastic pemphigus. Acta Derm Venereol. 2002;82(4):304–5.
18. Arranz D, Corral M, Prats I, Lopez-Ayala E, Castillo C, Vidaurrazaga C, et al. Herpetiform pemphigus associated with esophageal carcinoma. Acta Dermosifiliogr. 2005;96(2):119–21.
19. Marzano AV, Tourlaki A, Cozzani E, Gianotti R, Caputo R. Pemphigus herpetiformis associated with prostate cancer. J Eur Acad Dermatol Venereol. 2007;21(5):696–8.
20. Morita E, Amagai M, Tanaka T, Horiuchi K, Yamamoto S. A case of herpetiform pemphigus coexisting with psoriasis vulgaris. Br J Dermatol. 1999;141(4):754–5.
21. Sanchez-Palacios C, Chan LS. Development of pemphigus herpetiformis in a patient with psoriasis receiving UV-light treatment. J Cut Path. 2004;31(4):346–9.
22. Marinovic B, Basta-Juzbasic A, Bukvic-Mokos Z, Leovic R, Loncaric D. Coexistence of pemphigus herpetiformis and systemic lupus erythematosus. J Eur Acad Dermatol Venereol. 2003;17(3):316–9.
23. Shimizu K, Hashimoto T, Wang N, Watanabe K, Ohata Y, Kikuchi A, et al. A case of herpetiform pemphigus associated with autoimmune hemolytic anemia: detection of autoantibodies against multiple epidermal antigens. Dermatology. 1996;192(2):179–82.
24. Bull RH, Fallowfield ME, Marsden RA. Autoimmune blistering diseases associated with HIV infection. Clin Exp Dermatol. 1994;19(1):47–50.
25. Verdier-Sevrain S, Joly P, Thomine E, Belanyi P, Gilbert D, Tron F, et al. Thiopronine-induced herpetiform pemphigus: report of a case studied by immunoelectron microscopy and immunoblot analysis. Br J Dermatol. 1994;130(2):238–40.
26. Marsden RA, Dawber RP, Millard PR, Mowat AG. Herpetiform pemphigus induced by penicillamine. Br J Dermatol. 1977;97(4):451–2.
27. Kowalewski C, Hashimoto T, Amagai M, Jablonska S, Mackiewicz W, Wozniak K. IgA/IgG pemphigus: a new atypical subset of pemphigus? Acta Derm Venereol. 2006;86(4):357–8.
28. Miura T, Kawakami Y, Oyama N, Ohtsuka M, Suzuki Y, Ohyama B, et al. A case of pemphigus herpetiformis with absence of antibodies to desmogleins 1 and 3. J Eur Acad Dermatol Venereol. 2010;24(1):101–3.
29. Tateishi C, Tsuruta D, Nakanishi T, Uehara S, Kobayashi H, Ishii M, et al. Antidesmocollin-1 antibody-positive, antidesmoglein antibody-negative pemphigus herpetiformis. J Am Acad Dermatol. 2010;63(1):e8–10.
30. Spindler V, Heupel WM, Efthymiadis A, Schmidt E, Eming R, Rankl C, et al. Desmocollin 3-mediated binding is crucial for keratinocyte cohesion and is impaired in pemphigus. J Biol Chem. 2009;284(44):30556–64.
31. Koch PJ, Mahoney MG, Ishikawa H, Pulkkinen L, Uitto J, Shultz L, et al. Targeted disruption of the pemphigus vulgaris antigen (desmoglein 3) gene in mice causes loss of keratinocyte cell adhesion with a phenotype similar to pemphigus vulgaris. J Cell Biol. 1997;137(5):1091–102.
32. Singer KH, Sawka NJ, Samowitz HR, Lazarus GS. Proteinase activation: a mechanism for cellular dyshesion in pemphigus. J Invest Dermatol. 1980;74(5):363–7.
33. Hashimoto K, Shafran KM, Webber PS, Lazarus GS, Singer KH. Anti-cell surface pemphigus autoantibody stimulates plasminogen activator activity of human epidermal cells. A mechanism for the loss of epidermal cohesion and blister formation. J Exp Med. 1983;157(1):259–72.
34. Morioka S, Naito K, Ogawa H. The pathogenic role of pemphigus antibodies and proteinase in epidermal acantholysis. J Invest Dermatol. 1981;76(5):337–41.
35. Kubo A, Amagai M, Hashimoto T, Doi T, Higashiyama M, Hashimoto K, et al. Herpetiform pemphigus showing reactivity with pemphigus vulgaris antigen (desmoglein 3). Br J Dermatol. 1997;137(1):109–13.

36. Kawana S, Hashimoto T, Nishikawa T, Nishiyama S. Changes in clinical features, histologic findings, and antigen profiles with development of pemphigus foliaceus from pemphigus vulgaris. Arch Dermatol. 1994;130(12):1534–8.
37. Ishii K, Amagai M, Ohata Y, Shimizu H, Hashimoto T, Ohya K, et al. Development of pemphigus vulgaris in a patient with pemphigus foliaceus: antidesmoglein antibody profile shift confirmed by enzyme-linked immunosorbent assay. J Am Acad Dermatol. 2000;42(5 Pt 2):859–61.
38. Ohyama B, Nishifuji K, Chan PT, Kawaguchi A, Yamashita T, Ishii N, et al. Epitope spreading is rarely found in pemphigus vulgaris by large-scale longitudinal study using desmoglein 2-based swapped molecules. J Invest Dermatol. 2012;132(4):1158–68.
39. Lehmann PV, Forsthuber T, Miller A, Sercarz EE. Spreading of T-cell autoimmunity to cryptic determinants of an autoantigen. Nature. 1992;358(6382):155–7.
40. Steinman L, Conlon P. Viral damage and the breakdown of self-tolerance. Nat Med. 1997;3(10):1085–7.
41. Lebeau S, Muller R, Masouye I, Hertl M, Borradori L. Pemphigus herpetiformis: analysis of the autoantibody profile during the disease course with changes in the clinical phenotype. Clin Exp Dermatol. 2010;35(4):366–72.
42. Kaneko F, Mori M, Tsukinaga I, Miura Y. Pemphigus vulgaris of esophageal mucosa. Arch Dermatol. 1985;121(2):272–3.
43. O'Toole EA, Mak LL, Guitart J, Woodley DT, Hashimoto T, Amagai M, et al. Induction of keratinocyte IL-8 expression and secretion by IgG autoantibodies as a novel mechanism of epidermal neutrophil recruitment in a pemphigus variant. Clin Exp Dermatol. 2000;119(1):217–24.
44. Ingber A, Feuerman EJ. Pemphigus with characteristics of dermatitis herpetiformis. A long-term follow-up of five patients. Int J Dermatol. 1986;25(9):575–9.
45. Seitz CS, Staegemeir E, Amagai M, Rose C, Brocker EB, Zillikens D. Pemphigus herpetiformis with an autoimmune response to recombinant desmoglein 1. Br J Dermatol. 1999;141(2):354–5.
46. Leithauser LA, Mutasim DF. A case of pemphigus herpetiformis occurring in a 9-year-old boy. Ped Dermatol. 2013;30(6):760–2.
47. Matsukura S, Takahashi K, Hirokado M, Ikezawa Y, Nakamura K, Fukuda S, et al. Recalcitrant pemphigus herpetiformis with high titer of immunoglobulin G antibody to desmoglein 1 and positive IgG antibody to desmocollin 3, elevating thymus and activation-regulated chemokine. Int J Dermatol. 2014;53(8):1023–6.
48. Heelan K, Al-Mohammedi F, Smith MJ, Knowles S, Lansang P, Walsh S, et al. Durable remission of Pemphigus with a fixed-dose Rituximab protocol. JAMA Dermatol. 2014;50(7):703–8.
49. Laws PM, et al. Pemphigus Herpetiformis: a case series and review of the literature. Int J Dermatol. 2015;54(9):1014–22.

Chapter 4
Bullous Pemphigoid

Megan H. Noe and Janet A. Fairley

Abstract Bullous pemphigoid is the most common cutaneous autoimmune blistering diseases with an estimated incidence in the United States of 24 cases per million person-years. It is a chronic disease of the elderly that can cause significant morbidity secondary to pruritus and open wounds. High potency topical corticosteroids are effective for patients with limited disease and in treating disease flares. Oral corticosteroids are the main stay of early treatment for more extensive disease because of their fast onset of action, but should not be used for long-term management at high doses because of the significant risk of potentially serious side effects. Steroid-sparing agents such as azathioprine, mycophenolate mofetil and methotrexate have shown to be effective in decreasing the dose of systemic corticosteroids required. For more recalcitrant cases, IVIG and rituximab can also be considered. The choice of an appropriate treatment must also balance the risks of systemic immunosuppression in this elderly population with other medical comorbidities.

Keywords Bullous pemphigoid • Autoimmune blistering disease • Treatment • Topical steroids • Systemic steroids • Tetracycline • Minocycline • Niacinamide • Dapsone • Methotrexate • Azathioprine • Mycophenolate mofetil • Cyclosporine • Plasmapheresis • IVIG • Rituximab • Cyclophosphamide • Omalizumab

Abbreviations

ABD	Autoimmune bullous disease
BP	Bullous pemphigoid
BSA	Body surface area
IF	Immunofluorescence
IVIG	Intravenous immunoglobulin
mg/m^2	milligrams per square meter

M.H. Noe, MD, MPH • J.A. Fairley, MD (✉)
Department of Dermatology, The University of Iowa,
200 Hawkins Drive, Iowa City, IA 52242, USA
e-mail: janet-fairley@uiowa.edu

N. Sami (ed.), *Autoimmune Bullous Diseases: Approach and Management*,
DOI 10.1007/978-3-319-26728-9_4

Introduction

Bullous pemphigoid (BP) is the most common autoimmune bullous disease (ABD) of the skin, characterized by the development of autoantibodies against BP antigen 180 (BPAG2, collagen XVII) and BP antigen 230 (BPAG1), proteins found within the hemidesmosome [1]. Older reports from Europe suggest an incidence of 6–7 cases per million person-years [2, 3]; however, more recent reports suggest the incidence may be increasing to between 13 and 43 cases per million person-years [4–6]. A recent study in the United States estimates an incidence of 24 per million person-years [7]. BP is almost exclusively a disease of the elderly and is rarely seen in people under the age of 60 [8].

BP is characterized by pruritus, urticarial plaques and tense blisters (Fig. 4.1) that develop on the trunk and extremities; however, some patients present with only pruritus. Symptomatic mucosal involvement is rare and lesions heal without scarring. A skin biopsy shows a sub-epidermal blister with eosinophils and superficial dermal edema (Fig. 4.2a). The gold standard for diagnosis is direct immunofluorescence (IF) which shows linear deposition of IgG and C3 along the dermal-epidermal junction (Fig. 4.2b). Indirect IF can be performed to look for the presence of circulating antibodies and the substrate of choice is salt-split skin. On salt-split skin, the fluorescence appears on the roof of the blister, which differentiates BP from other ABDs such as epidermolysis bullosa acquisita, where the binding occurs at the base of the blister. An ELISA is commercially available to test for IgG antibodies to BP230 and immunodominant NC16A portion of BP180 in patient sera.

In the United States, the 1-year mortality rate has been estimated to be between 11 and 23 % [7, 9, 10]. A recent study showed the mortality of BP patients was no different to that of age-matched controls, suggesting the mortality of BP patients may

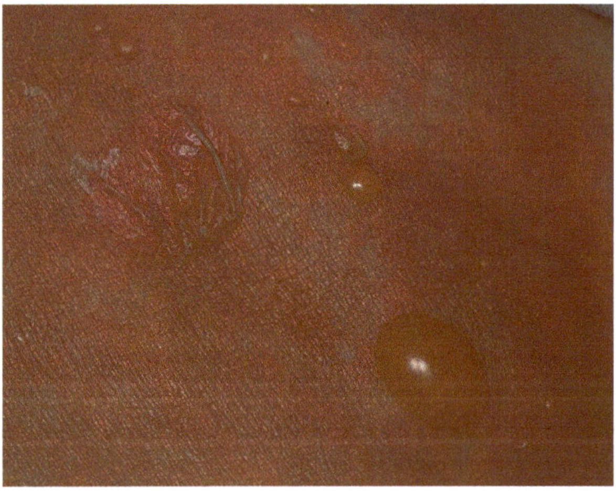

Fig. 4.1 Bullous pemphigoid. Typical clinical findings of tense bullae on an erythematous/urticarial base are seen on the upper back of this patient

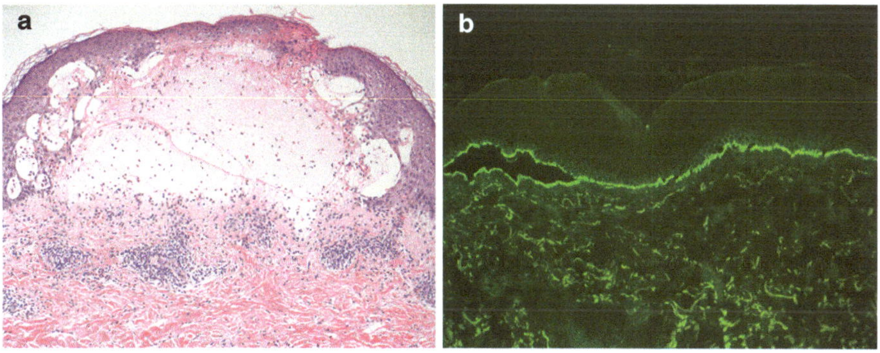

Fig. 4.2 Histology of bullous pemphigoid. (**a**). Hematoxylin and eosin staining showing a subepidermal blister with an inflammatory infiltrate demonstrating a predominance of eosinophils. (**b**). Direct immunofluorescence demonstrating C3 deposition along the dermal-epidermal junction (Images courtesy of Brian Swick, MD)

be secondary to advanced age and comorbid medical conditions, rather than disease-specific issues [9]. However, these results conflict with other studies showing a higher mortality than expected with an age-matched population [7]. Overall, the major concern for patients is the significant morbidity secondary to pruritus and open wounds from blisters. Hence, the treatment is aimed at decreasing these symptoms along with facilitating healing to prevent secondary complications including infections.

There are currently no FDA-approved drugs for the treatment of bullous pemphigoid. The treatment of bullous pemphigoid is mainly based on case reports and physician experience. The most recent Cochrane Review, completed in 2010, identified ten randomized control trials with a total of 1049 patients [11]. All studies had different criteria for comparison with no placebo group. The evidence available in the literature regarding the effectiveness of steroid-sparing therapy will be examined below.

Topical Therapy

The evidence for high potency topical corticosteroids is favorable, although time intensive, and may be associated with poor patient compliance. The best evidence comes from a randomized, non-blinded multi-center trial of 341 patients with moderate to severe bullous pemphigoid that showed treatment with a potent topical corticosteroid (clobetasol propionate) was as effective and, in the "severe-disease" group, superior to treatment with oral prednisone (0.5 mg/kg/day for those with moderate disease and 1.0 mg/kg/day for those with severe disease) [12]. Among the patients with moderate disease, there were no significant differences between the overall survival, rate of control at 3 weeks, or incidence of severe complications between the two groups. However for those with severe disease, and treated with 1.0 mg/kg/day oral prednisone versus clobetasol propionate, the topical clobetasol was superior to oral prednisone with an overall increased survival and better disease control at 3 weeks.

Severe complications were also higher in the group that received oral prednisone. It is important to keep in mind that this study was performed in an in-patient setting with nurses performing the application of topical steroids twice daily. These results may not be transferrable to those treated in an out-patient setting, and the time associated with the application of topical steroids to a large area would likely lead to poor patient compliance.

A follow up to this study, looking only at topical therapy regimens, was performed in 312 moderate to extensive BP patients. This study showed the standard regimen of 40 g daily of topical clobetasol tapered over 12 months was no better in controlling disease than the mild regimen of 10–30 g daily (depending on weight and disease extent) tapered over 4 months [13], suggesting that lower starting doses and faster tapers are appropriate.

A retrospective report of 96 patients, treated with clobetasol propionate found that 62 % were controlled with topical corticosteroids alone and only 25 % required adjunctive systemic treatment [14]. Other studies show rapid epithelization (4–17 days) in hospitalized patients with the use of high potency topical corticosteroids (clobetasol propionate) only, without any local or systemic side effects [15].

A single case series examined the use of topical tacrolimus for the treatment of BP and described two patients, on multiple oral medications, including oral prednisone. When topical tacrolimus was added, the oral prednisone was tapered, which was not possible before the addition of topical tacrolimus. However, the authors do note that topical tacrolimus is significantly more expensive than potent topical corticosteroids [16].

Systemic Corticosteroids

The evidence available for treatment with systemic corticosteroids suggests the type of steroid does not matter and a starting dose between 0.5 and 0.75 mg/kg of prednisone-equivalents is adequate to achieve control and remission. The randomized-controlled trial comparing topical and oral corticosteroids discussed above, showed prednisone dosed at 1.0 mg/kg/day did not have better efficacy and was associated with increased morbidity when compared with 0.5 mg/kg/day [12]. A randomized control trial looking at the initial starting dose of prednisolone 0.75 mg/kg/day vs 1.25 mg/kg/day did not show a statistically significantly difference in similar parameters between the two groups at 21 days. However, when a taper was initiated at half the initial starting dose, more patients in the high-dose group (55 % vs 33 %) were still free from all skin lesions [17]. A randomized control trial of 57 patients treated with methylprednisolone vs prednisolone at 1.0–1.5 mg/kg showed no difference in pruritus or number of bullae between the two systemic corticosteroids [18]. A retrospective review of patients treated with prednisone 1 mg/kg showed the time to suppression of blister formation was directly proportional to the number of blisters [19], suggesting that initial disease severity and the length of treatment with oral steroids, including the dosage taper schedule, may be more important than the starting dose.

Antibiotics & Niacinamide (Nicotinamide)

Looking at antibiotics alone, the evidence is limited. A retrospective review of 22 patients with BP treated with minocycline as adjuvant therapy showed a major response in six patients, a minor response in 11 and no response in five patients [20]. Thornfeldt and Menkes report two cases of men where their disease was resistant to potent topical steroids but cleared with tetracycline (250–1000 mg daily), one in conjunction with oral steroids. Remission was maintained on once daily oral tetracycline (250–500 mg) [21].

A single open-label study examined the use of oral erythromycin in fifteen patients with BP. All patients had contraindications to systemic corticosteroids or immunosuppressive therapy and were treated with 1 g erythromycin three times daily for 10–15 days [22]. Ten out of 15 patients responded to the erythromycin monotherapy in the initial phase of treatment and were continued on 1 g twice daily.

While there are no reports of niacinamide as monotherapy, there is evidence for niacinamide, used in conjunction with tetracycline antibiotics. There is one randomized, open-labeled trial comparing the combination of 500 mg of niacinamide three times daily, and 500 mg of tetracycline four times daily, versus prednisone therapy in 20 patients with bullous pemphigoid [23]. There were no statistically significant differences in response parameters between the two groups, although the numbers were quite small. The literature shows two additional case series and two case reports, encompassing a total of 13 patients successfully treated with tetracycline (500–2000 mg/day) in addition to niacinamide (1500–2500 mg/day) [24–27].

Dapsone

Venning et al. looked at 15 newly diagnosed BP patients treated with dapsone at a starting dose of 50 mg daily, increasing to 100 mg daily if no response was appreciated after 5–7 days. Five patients showed a complete response to treatment within 2 weeks, four showed no response and six were considered to be partial responders [28]. Bouscarat et al. retrospectively studied 36 BP patients treated with dapsone and 15 of those received dapsone as monotherapy (50–200 mg daily). Of those treated with dapsone only, 7 % of patients were considered complete responders and 20 % partial responders. Patients treated with dapsone in conjunction with topical or oral steroids showed a higher response rate [29]. As this study suggests, dapsone may have a role as adjuvant therapy in difficult to treat BP, but not as monotherapy. There is a single study of 13 patients with recalcitrant BP, requiring high doses of prednisone and azathioprine, treated with dapsone as adjuvant therapy (150–300 mg daily) with complete remission in 12 patients. Patients were more easily tapered off prednisone and maintained with statistically lower doses of prednisone, as compared to before dapsone was started [30]. These studies suggest that while dapsone could potentially be a non-immune suppressing alternative, it does not seem to be very effective, especially as monotherapy.

Azathioprine

Three randomized control trials, one cohort study and three cases series are available in the literature, examining the use of azathioprine to treat BP. Guillaume et al. took 100 patients with active BP and randomly assigned them to one of three groups: prednisolone alone (1 mg/kg/day), prednisolone + azathioprine (100–150 mg/day), or prednisolone + 4 large volume plasma exchanges. There was no difference in the number of patients in complete remission at 28 days or at 6 months and severe complications were highest in the group on azathioprine [31]. However, Burton et al. compared azathioprine plus prednisone with prednisone alone in 25 patients. This study concluded that azathioprine (2.5 mg/kg/day) reduced the maintenance dose of prednisone by 45 % without increased serious side effects or mortality [32]. Similarly, in a randomized control trial comparing oral methylprednisolone (0.5 mg/kg/d) plus azathioprine (2 mg/kg/day) with methylprednisolone plus mycophenolate mofetil (1 g BID), complete resolution and severe or life threatening events were observed to be similar in both groups. Time to resolution was quicker in the azathioprine group, although not statistically significant [33].

In smaller cohort studies and cases series, Ahmed et al. concluded combined therapy with azathioprine plus prednisone appears to be superior to prednisone alone in the treatment of BP in a series of 36 patients because the dose of prednisone was reduced by 50 % in people treated with azathioprine [34]. Greaves et al. used azathioprine in 11 patients on long-term prednisone and the prednisone was decreased or discontinued in all 11 patients; however he cautioned that corticosteroids should be used together with azathioprine during the acute stage since it has a slow onset of action [35]. A 4-year follow up of these patients showed 44 % remained in remission on azathioprine alone [36]. A small series (n = 5) of azathioprine as monotherapy showed a good response in four of five patients [37].

A systematic review published in 2011 reviewed the above seven published studies in which patients with bullous pemphigoid were treated with azathioprine and concluded that a level 2A recommendation was given to the use of azathioprine in combination with oral corticosteroids. No significant benefit of azathioprine with oral corticosteroids has been proven compared to monotherapy with oral corticosteroids, but combination therapy may be considered when the need exists for a corticosteroid-sparing effect [38].

Methotrexate

Most of the data available for methotrexate is as an adjuvant to either topical or oral corticosteroids. There is a single case report of a 90 year-old man successfully treated with low dose methotrexate as monotherapy that cleared his psoriasis and BP [39]. Further evidence from a single prospective study where 16 patients were treated with methotrexate as a first line therapy, showed 14/16 patients who did not discontinue methotrexate due to side effects achieved clinical remission by the end of the study period; in ten patients (62.5 %), topical clobetasol was added for severe pruritus [40]. The other evidence available is from case series. Dereure et al. studied 18 patients treated with high potency topical steroids for 2–3 weeks and an initial methotrexate dose of 7.5–10 mg/week with a maximum dose of 12.5 mg weekly. All patients showed a complete remission at 2 months, and all but one was maintained on methotrexate alone [41]. Heilborn reviewed 11 cases of patients over 70 years of age whose BP was not well controlled on potent topical steroids. Low dose methotrexate (5 mg/week) was initiated and increased to a maximum of 12.5 mg/week. All patients responded with decreased disease activity [42]. Bohm et al. reported on three successful cases using methotrexate as maintenance therapy after remission was achieved with topical or oral steroids [43]. A retrospective chart review found that five of eight elderly patients (average age 73.5 years) with treatment resistant BP, still active on oral prednisone, had clearance one month after adding low-dose methotrexate (5–10 mg/week), and all patients on methotrexate required lower doses of prednisone [44]. Another retrospective review reported 138 consecutive patients with a new diagnosis of BP. Ninety-eight patients were started on methotrexate 5 mg/week and 61 (62 %) were able to continue methotrexate monotherapy while 37 patients (38 %) benefited from the addition of prednisone. Only five of the patients treated with methotrexate had to discontinue the medication secondary to side effects, including gastrointestinal track irritation, anemia, increased liver enzymes and transient alveolitis [45].

Mycophenolate Mofetil

With the exception of the randomized control trial listed above comparing azathioprine and mycophenolate mofetil as steroid sparing agents, all other available data for mycophenolate mofetil in the treatment of BP is from case reports, including a total of five patients treated successfully with a dose of 2 g/day. In three of these patients, mycophenolate mofetil was used in conjunction with oral steroids as a steroid sparing agent. The systemic steroids were discontinued or tapered to physiological dosages over a period of 1–3 months without disease recurrence [46–48]. One report also described two patients treated successfully with mycophenolate mofetil as monotherapy without the usage of any systemic steroids [48]. In doses of 2 g/day, mycophenolate mofetil is generally well tolerated with gastrointestinal irritation being the most common side effect. A slightly increased risk of bacterial and viral infections and reversible myelosuppression have also been less commonly reported.

Cyclosporine

There are two published reports using cyclosporine for the treatment of bullous pemphigoid. Barthelme et al. retrospectively studied seven patients treated with cyclosporine dosed 6–8 mg/kg/day [49]. Four patients were treated with cyclosporine alone and two of these were considered treatment failures. Treatment was successful in all patients treated with corticosteroids in addition to cyclosporine during flares, but 2/3 patients relapsed after cyclosporine was discontinued. The main side effects were increased creatinine, which was reversible, and hypertension. Another case series reports successful treatment of two patients with cyclosporine (6 mg/kg/day) with a short clinical follow up. One was also on prednisone 20 mg daily which was tapered and discontinued 2 months after starting cyclosporine. The second patient was treated with 3 months of cyclosporine with disease remission for 2 months after discontinuation of the cyclosporine [50].

Plasmapheresis

Plasmapheresis has been a long-standing therapeutic option for the acute treatment of BP, usually in conjunction with systemic steroids with the first report of its success published in the French literature in 1979 [51]. This study described 12 patients treated with oral prednisolone (0.5 mg/kg) and four large volume (1.5 × theoretical plasma volumes) plasma exchanges over 2 weeks. Eight of twelve patients achieved disease control by 1 month. Five of these eight patients were able to successfully taper their steroids without a disease flare. Among the four patients who were not controlled on the initial treatment, all required an increase in prednisone up to 0.75 mg/kg (three patients) and up to 1 mg/kg/day with four additional plasma exchanges in a single patient [52]. After this initial study, a multi-center randomized trial was initiated. All patients received prednisolone (0.3 mg/kg), increased weekly if the disease remained active and 24/41 patients also received eight large-volume plasma exchanges over 4 weeks. The initial dose of prednisolone was effective in 13 of 22 patients receiving plasma exchange but in none of 15 patients receiving prednisolone only. Control of the disease was obtained with a mean daily prednisolone dose of 0.52 mg/kg in the plasma exchange group and 0.97 mg/kg in the other group [53]. As discussed previously, Guillaume et al. studied 100 patients with active BP who were randomly assigned to one of three groups: prednisolone alone (1 mg/kg/day), prednisone + azathioprine (100–150 mg/day), or prednisolone + 4 large volume plasma exchanges, and found no difference by adding plasma exchange to systemic steroids [31].

Despite these conflicting results, there are smaller case reports and case series that support the use of plasmapheresis to treat BP [54–61]. One study of 21 patients comparing steroids in conjunction with plasmapheresis versus steroids alone observed that adding plasma exchange had a lower rate of relapse at 6 months and required lower doses of steroids [61]. Egan et al. found plasmapheresis to be an effective steroid sparing therapy in their series of 10 patients. However, they did point out that due to its high cost and potential morbidity, plasmapheresis should not be recommended as first line therapy for bullous pemphigoid, and reserved for recalcitrant cases [55].

Immunoadsorption

Immunoadsorption (also termed immunoapheresis) is similar to plasmapheresis but specifically removes only immunoglobulin and immune complexes from patients' circulation. While used in other parts of the world when an immediate decrease in circulating antibodies is desired, it is not currently approved for use in autoimmune blistering disease in the United States. Case reports show it can be used successfully in conjunction with oral steroids and other immunosuppressive medications with less treatment-limiting side effects than plasmapheresis [62].

Intravenous Immunoglobulin (IVIG)

Initial studies examining the use of IVIG for the treatment of BP showed unsuccessful results. Godard et al. reported a study of 11 patients with BP after previous treatment with oral prednisone who then received IVIG infusion [63]. Nine patients received 400 mg/kg/day × 5 days as monotherapy and two received 100 mg/kg/day and then 300 mg/kg/day for a total of 5 days. Two patients were also being treated with low dose prednisolone (0.2–1.0 mg/kg/day). One patient in the monotherapy group and both in the low dose IVIG group saw no improvement. The other eight patients saw rapid improvement in pruritus and reduction in development of new blisters.

Another case series of 15 patients with BP who experienced significant side effects on conventional therapy reported more successful results after treatment with IVIG [64]. All patients received clinical remission in 2–4 months of IVIG monotherapy, dosed at 2 g/kg given over 3 days every 4 weeks until no new lesions appeared. Then the interval between subsequent infusions was increased as tolerated. No serious side effects were reported. A case series looking at ELISA titers of ten patients treated with IVIG (2 g/kg given over 3 days every 4 weeks until healed) showed that treatment with IVIG caused gradual decline in BP180 and BP230 titers [65].

The rest of the available data comes from case reports totaling nine patients [66–71]. There is no uniform protocol or long term follow-up in these reports. However, three patients were considered treatment failures. The six patients who did respond to IVIg showed a steroid sparing effect in dosages ranging between 1 and 2 g/kg/cycle of IVIg administered every 2–4 weeks. Hence, it seems that IVIg can be an alternative treatment if oral conventional treatment is contraindicated or not tolerated, but needs to be administered every 4 weeks to maintain control of the bullous pemphigoid.

Rituximab

There are currently reports of 20 cases of BP treated with rituximab. Lourari et al. present five cases treated with rituximab 375 mg/m^2 weekly × 4 weeks [66]. All five were being treated with topical steroids and two were also being treated with oral steroids (20 mg daily and 40 mg daily) and one with a second immunosuppressive agent (azathioprine). Three patients had complete remission of the BP. One had partial remission, and one patient with a history of ischemic cardiac disease died 10 days after the first infusion. One patient required a second course of rituximab 11 months later. Hall et al. treated seven patients with persistent disease activity on 17.5 mg or more daily prednisone, with rituximab dosed 1000 mg on days 0 and 14 [67]. All patients showed cessation of disease activity and tolerated the infusions without serious adverse effects. Six months after treatment, all patients were tapered to 25 % of their starting prednisone dose or 10 mg daily. Two patients did experience a flare of their disease at 7 and 11.5 months.

Of the other case reports, there were eight adults [68–73] treated with rituximab. Six were initially treated with oncology dosing of 375 mg/m^2 weekly × 4 weeks, while two were treated with the rheumatology dosing of 1000 mg on days 0 and 14. Six of the eight patients were treated with concomitant systemic therapy. Four required a second cycle. One patient developed clostridium difficile enteropathy 4 weeks after the last rituximab infusion and subsequently died after developing hospital acquired pneumonia [73]. The other seven patients achieved complete remission with an average follow up time of 23 months.

Cyclophosphamide

There are concerns regarding treatment of bullous pemphigoid with cyclophosphamide, given the serious side effects of cyclophosphamide. In a retrospective study of ten patients treated with cyclophosphamide 100 mg/day, in addition to oral steroids, three patients died in the first 3 months attributable to side effects of the cyclophosphamide [74]. Four patients developed non-lethal bone marrow suppression and septicemia. However at the end of follow up, five patients did achieve clinical remission without additional treatment. Gaul et al. published a retrospective study of 20 patients with refractory BP treated with oral cyclophosphamide (50–100 mg/day) [75]. Eleven patients achieved complete clinical remission: eight patients on 50 mg/day and three on 100 mg/day. Four patients failed treatment and another patient self-discontinued treatment secondary to poor compliance. Twelve of 20 patients developed bone marrow suppression, but only three required discontinuation of therapy. One patient had intolerable gastrointestinal side effects and another died from heart failure that was not attributable to cyclophosphamide. A final case report of a woman with BP unresponsive to all other therapies reported success with pulsed IV dexamethasone (100 mg daily × 3 days) monthly and 50 mg daily of cyclophosphamide, without any treatment limiting side effects in 9 months of treatment [76].

Omalizumab

There is emerging evidence that specifically targeting IgE can provide symptomatic relief for patients with BP without the risk of side effects from broad immunosuppression. Omalizumab is a humanized monoclonal antibody which binds to IgE, preventing its binding to both the high and low affinity IgE receptors. It was originally FDA approved for moderate to severe asthma, but recently was approved in chronic urticaria, and studies suggest it may also be effective in the treatment of BP. Yu et al. published a case series of six patients with recalcitrant BP, unable to discontinue high-dose corticosteroids, treated with omalizumab. It was dosed using the asthma dosing nomogram, which is based on weight and serum IgE levels. Five of six patients responded to treatment with omalizumab without any serious adverse effects. Three used omalizumab as monotherapy and two others used it as a steroid-sparing agent in the induction and maintenance of remission [77]. Dufour and colleagues reported treatment of a 5 month old infant with severe, recalcitrant juvenile BP with omalizumab as monotherapy. New blister formation stopped after the initial injection and complete clinical clearing was achieved [78]. Another recently published case report of a 28 year-old male with BP who failed treatment with systemic steroids and daily cyclophosphamide, was significantly improved after two doses of omalizumab [79]. While initial reports are promising, further studies are needed with a larger cohort of BP patients to examine the long term response and compare omalizumab to other steroid sparing agents.

Treatment Recommendations

The treatment of BP can be divided into three phases: baseline, consolidation and tapering, as proposed by the international panel of experts in 2008 [80]. Baseline is defined as the point in which treatment is initiated, with a goal of obtaining disease control as quickly as possible. Consolidation, or control of disease activity, begins when no new blisters develop and older lesions have started to heal. The end of the consolidation phase is when no new lesions have developed for at least 2 weeks and the patient has healed approximately 80 % of older lesions. At this time, the patient is transitioned to maintenance therapy. Characterizing the extent of disease can help guide treatment; however, there is currently no validated measure of disease stratification. For the purpose of this discussion, mild disease is characterized as the presence of urticarial plaques and/or tense bullae and erosions covering less than 5 % BSA. Moderate disease is the presence of bullae and erosions on 5–25 % BSA, and severe disease is the presence of bullae or erosions on >25 % BSA. A summary of our treatment recommendations can be seen in Fig. 4.3.

Systemic steroids are the initial mainstay of treatment to achieve baseline control. Prednisone, the most common systemic steroid prescribed, can be initiated at 0.5–0.75 mg/kg/day and can be divided twice daily, if necessary for better tolerance. Since many patients may be on systemic steroids for greater than 3 months, precautions should be taken to minimize the risk of osteoporosis [81]. Although the literature does not support routine prophylaxis of dermatology patients for pneumocystis pneumonia, it can be considered on an individual basis, particularly in those at higher risk such as patients with underlying lung disease or immunosuppression from HIV or cancer [82]. When treatment with prednisone is initiated, the patient should also have an initial laboratory evaluation in possible anticipation of starting

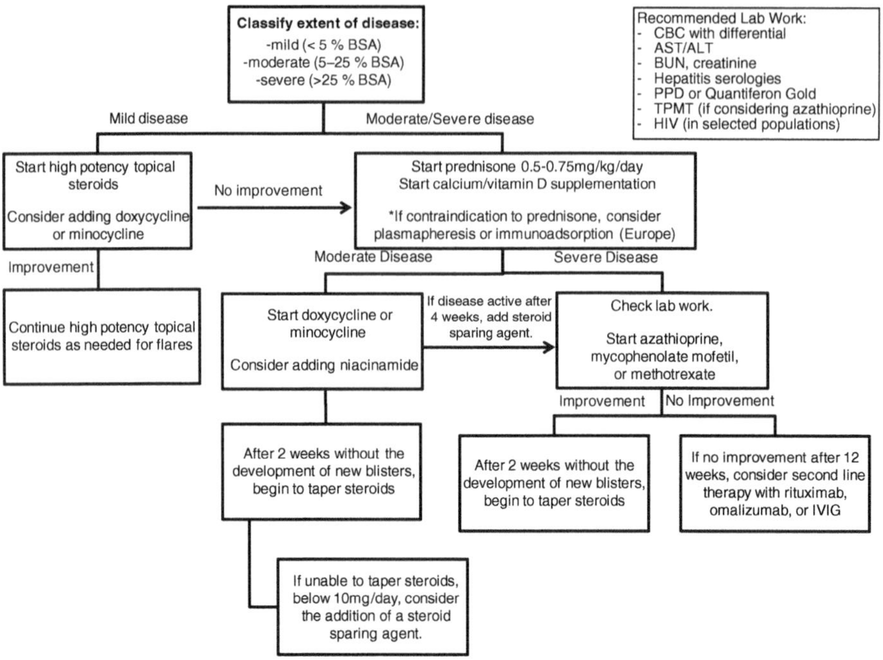

Fig. 4.3 Proposed treatment algorithm for bullous pemphigoid. Recommendations for mild and moderate/severe disease are given

an immune suppressing steroid sparing treatment. These baseline labs include a complete blood count with a differential, liver and kidney function tests, and screening for infections (hepatitis and tuberculosis). HIV testing can be considered in select populations and thiopurine methyltransferase should be checked if treatment with azathioprine is being considered. The patient's vaccination status should also be ascertained and updated if possible prior to initiation of immunosuppressive therapy. If there is a serious contraindication to systemic steroids, plasmapheresis or immunoadsorption (in Europe) can be used in the baseline and consolidation phase. However both these treatment modalities should be used in conjunction with one of the secondary immunosuppressive agents discussed below.

Patients with moderate to severe disease, who are unable to taper steroids to below 10 mg/day, can also be started on a steroid sparing agent. For moderate disease, initiation of a tetracycline class antibiotic, such as minocycline or doxycycline 100 mg twice daily can often control the disease without the risks of systemic immunosuppression. For patients with moderate to severe disease, azathioprine (starting at 50 mg twice daily and titrating based on the TPMT levels to a maximum dose of 2.5 mg/kg/day), mycophenolate mofetil (starting at 500 mg twice daily and titrating to a maximum dose of 3 g/day) or methotrexate (starting at 10 mg/week and titrating to 15 mg/week) can be considered depending on the patients other medical co-morbidities and medications. Therapy should be maintained for 12 weeks, with dose escalation as appropriate, to determine the full response before considering the patient to be a treatment failure. If the patient is a true treatment failure, switching to an alternative first-line medication is recommended.

For patients who fail to respond to oral steroid-sparing agents, other treatment options include rituximab, omalizumab and IVIG. For rituximab, initial studies show a benefit with the oncology protocol: 375 mg/m^2 weekly × 4 weeks. However more evidence for dosing 1 g on days 0 and 14 is emerging with other cutaneous autoimmune blistering diseases so this schedule can also be considered [67]. Omalizumab is dosed using a nomogram based on serum IgE and weight and injections are given every 2 or 4 weeks depending on the dose. IVIG infusions are typically given 2 g/kg/cycle divided over several days, every 4 weeks until the disease is no longer active, at which point the frequency of the infusions is decreased. Rituximab is the preferred treatment due to both being cost effective and more anecdotal reported experience in BP.

As the patient enters the end of the consolidation phase, and new lesions have not developed in more than 2 weeks and pruritus is under control, the dosage of systemic steroids should be tapered by decreasing the dosage by half the previous dose every 2–3 weeks until reaching a dose of 10 mg/day. At that point, to prevent adrenal crisis, steroids should be tapered slowly, decreasing the dose by 1–2.5 mg every 2–3 weeks. Some patients may require low-dose prednisone in conjunction with a steroid-sparing agent for disease control and doses less than 10 mg/day are reasonable for long-term treatment.

The average case of bullous pemphigoid lasts about 5–6 years [83], although this can be highly variable on an individual level. When patients remain symptom free for greater than 6 months, it can be reasonable to slowly taper immunosuppressive therapy. The development of new blisters or pruritus suggests the disease is still active and maintenance dose of immunosuppressive therapy should be continued. Periodic monitoring of serum IgG autoantibody titers to BP180 with the help of ELISA, if available, can also be helpful to determine if a patient could potentially clinically relapse if all medications are discontinued.

Future Directions

As stated earlier, the treatment of BP is mainly based on case reports and physician experience, with only ten previously published randomized control trials. Further comparative research is necessary to determine the most appropriate steroid sparing agents, taking into account the side effect profile and possible complications of long-term treatment with immunosuppressive medications. Research focused on cost-effective treatment is also currently lacking in the literature. Comparing the treatment cost of older immunosuppressive medications, associated laboratory monitoring and complications to newer, more targeted, and expensive drugs is important for making treatment decisions in the changing environment of cost-conscious healthcare. Since almost all current therapy still relies on broad-based immunosuppression, continued studies aimed at understanding the pathogenesis of disease development and progression are essential to the search for better therapy and a real "cure" for autoimmune blistering diseases.

References

1. Bernard P, Borradori L. Pemphigoid group. In: Bolognia J, Jorizzo J, Rapini R, editors. Dermatology (Basel, Switzerland). 3rd ed. Philadelphia: Elsevier; 2012. p. 475–90.
2. Bernard P, Vaillant L, Labeille B, Bedane C, Arbeille B, Denoeux JP, et al. Incidence and distribution of subepidermal autoimmune bullous skin diseases in three French regions. Bullous Diseases French Study Group. Arch Dermatol. 1995;131(1):48–52.
3. Zillikens D, Wever S, Roth A, Weidenthaler-Barth B, Hashimoto T, Brocker EB. Incidence of autoimmune subepidermal blistering dermatoses in a region of central Germany. Arch Dermatol. 1995;131(8):957–8.
4. Joly P, Baricault S, Sparsa A, Bernard P, Bedane C, Duvert-Lehembre S, et al. Incidence and mortality of bullous pemphigoid in France. J Invest Dermatol. 2012;132(8):1998–2004.
5. Langan SM, Smeeth L, Hubbard R, Fleming KM, Smith CJ, West J. Bullous pemphigoid and pemphigus vulgaris--incidence and mortality in the UK: population based cohort study. BMJ (Clin Res Ed). 2008;337:a180.
6. Bertram F, Brocker EB, Zillikens D, Schmidt E. Prospective analysis of the incidence of autoimmune bullous disorders in Lower Franconia, Germany. J Dtsch Dermatol Ges. 2009;7(5):434–40.
7. Brick KE, Weaver CH, Lohse CM, Pittelkow MR, Lehman JS, Camilleri MJ, et al. Incidence of bullous pemphigoid and mortality of patients with bullous pemphigoid in Olmsted County, Minnesota, 1960 through 2009. J Am Acad Dermatol. 2014;71(1):92–9.
8. Jung M, Kippes W, Messer G, Zillikens D, Rzany B. Increased risk of bullous pemphigoid in male and very old patients: a population-based study on incidence. J Am Acad Dermatol. 1999;41(2 Pt 1):266–8.
9. Parker SR, Dyson S, Brisman S, Pennie M, Swerlick RA, Khan R, et al. Mortality of bullous pemphigoid: an evaluation of 223 patients and comparison with the mortality in the general population in the United States. J Am Acad Dermatol. 2008;59(4):582–8.
10. Colbert RL, Allen DM, Eastwood D, Fairley JA. Mortality rate of bullous pemphigoid in a US medical center. J Invest Dermatol. 2004;122(5):1091–5.
11. Kirtschig G, Middleton P, Bennett C, Murrell DF, Wojnarowska F, Khumalo NP. Interventions for bullous pemphigoid. Cochrane Database Syst Rev. 2010(10):CD002292.
12. Joly P, Roujeau JC, Benichou J, Picard C, Dreno B, Delaporte E, et al. A comparison of oral and topical corticosteroids in patients with bullous pemphigoid. N Engl J Med. 2002;346(5):321–7.
13. Joly P, Roujeau JC, Benichou J, Delaporte E, D'Incan M, Dreno B, et al. A comparison of two regimens of topical corticosteroids in the treatment of patients with bullous pemphigoid: a multicenter randomized study. J Invest Dermatol. 2009;129(7):1681–7.
14. Ingen-Housz-Oro S, Valeyrie-Allanore L, Ortonne N, Roujeau JC, Wolkenstein P, Chosidow O. Management of bullous pemphigoid with topical steroids in the clinical practice of a single center: outcome at 6 and 12 months. Dermatol (Basel Switzerland). 2011;222(2):176–9.
15. Westerhof W. Treatment of bullous pemphigoid with topical clobetasol propionate. J Am Acad Dermatol. 1989;20(3):458–61.
16. Chu J, Bradley M, Marinkovich MP. Topical tacrolimus is a useful adjunctive therapy for bullous pemphigoid. Arch Dermatol. 2003;139(6):813–5.
17. Morel P, Guillaume JC. Treatment of bullous pemphigoid with prednisolone only: 0.75 mg/kg/day versus 1.25 mg/kg/day. A multicenter randomized study. Ann Dermatol Venereol. 1984;111(10):925–8.
18. Dreno B, Sassolas B, Lacour P, Montpoint S, Lota I, Giordano F, et al. Methylprednisolone versus prednisolone methylsulfobenzoate in pemphigoid: a comparative multicenter study. Ann Dermatol Venereol. 1993;120(8):518–21.
19. Chosidow O, Saada V, Diquet B, Roujeau JC, Revuz J. Correlation between the pretreatment number of blisters and the time to control bullous pemphigoid with prednisone 1 mg/kg/day. Br J Dermatol. 1992;127(2):185–6.

20. Loo WJ, Kirtschig G, Wojnarowska F. Minocycline as a therapeutic option in bullous pemphigoid. Clin Exp Dermatol. 2001;26(5):376–9.
21. Thornfeldt CR, Menkes AW. Bullous pemphigoid controlled by tetracycline. J Am Acad Dermatol. 1987;16(2 Pt 1):305–10.
22. Altomare G, Capella GL, Fracchiolla C, Frigerio E. Treatment of bullous pemphigoid with erythromycin: a reappraisal. Eur J Dermatol. 1999;9(7):583–5.
23. Fivenson DP, Breneman DL, Rosen GB, Hersh CS, Cardone S, Mutasim D. Nicotinamide and tetracycline therapy of bullous pemphigoid. Arch Dermatol. 1994;130(6):753–8.
24. Berk MA, Lorincz AL. The treatment of bullous pemphigoid with tetracycline and niacinamide. A preliminary report. Arch Dermatol. 1986;122(6):670–4.
25. Kolbach DN, Remme JJ, Bos WH, Jonkman MF, De Jong MC, Pas HH, et al. Bullous pemphigoid successfully controlled by tetracycline and nicotinamide. Br J Dermatol. 1995;133(1):88–90.
26. Shiohara J, Yoshida K, Hasegawa J, Uhara H, Takata M, Saida T, et al. Tetracycline and niacinamide control bullous pemphigoid but not pemphigus foliaceus when these conditions coexist. J Dermatol. 2010;37(7):657–61.
27. Honl BA, Elston DM. Autoimmune bullous eruption localized to a breast reconstruction site: response to niacinamide. Cutis. 1998;62(2):85–6.
28. Venning VA, Millard PR, Wojnarowska F. Dapsone as first line therapy for bullous pemphigoid. Br J Dermatol. 1989;120(1):83–92.
29. Bouscarat F, Chosidow O, Picard-Dahan C, Sakiz V, Crickx B, Prost C, et al. Treatment of bullous pemphigoid with dapsone: retrospective study of thirty-six cases. J Am Acad Dermatol. 1996;34(4):683–4.
30. Jeffes 3rd EW, Ahmed AR. Adjuvant therapy of bullous pemphigoid with dapsone. Clin Exp Dermatol. 1989;14(2):132–6.
31. Guillaume JC, Vaillant L, Bernard P, Picard C, Prost C, Labeille B, et al. Controlled trial of azathioprine and plasma exchange in addition to prednisolone in the treatment of bullous pemphigoid. Arch Dermatol. 1993;129(1):49–53.
32. Burton JL, Harman RR, Peachey RD, Warin RP. Azathioprine plus prednisone in treatment of pemphigoid. Br Med J. 1978;2(6146):1190–1.
33. Beissert S, Werfel T, Frieling U, Bohm M, Sticherling M, Stadler R, et al. A comparison of oral methylprednisolone plus azathioprine or mycophenolate mofetil for the treatment of bullous pemphigoid. Arch Dermatol. 2007;143(12):1536–42.
34. Ahmed AR, Maize JC, Provost TT. Bullous pemphigoid. Clinical and immunologic follow-up after successful therapy. Arch Dermatol. 1977;113(8):1043–6.
35. Greaves MW, Burton JL, Marks J, Dawber RP. Azathioprine in treatment of bullous pemphigoid. Br Med J. 1971;1(5741):144–5.
36. Burton JL, Greaves MW. Azathioprine for pemphigus and pemphigoid a 4 year follow up. Br J Dermatol. 1974;91(1):103–9.
37. van Dijk TJ, van Velde JL. Treatment of pemphigus and pemphigoid with azathioprine. Dermatologica. 1973;147(3):179–85.
38. Schram ME, Borgonjen RJ, Bik CM, van der Schroeff JG, van Everdingen JJ, Spuls PI. Off-label use of azathioprine in dermatology: a systematic review. Arch Dermatol. 2011;147(4):474–88.
39. Gunay U, Gunduz K, Ermertcan AT, Kandiloglu AR. Coexistence of psoriasis and bullous pemphigoid: remission with low-dose methotrexate. Cutan Ocul Toxicol. 2013;32(2):168–9.
40. Bara C, Maillard H, Briand N, Celerier P. Methotrexate for bullous pemphigoid: preliminary study. Arch Dermatol. 2003;139(11):1506–7.
41. Dereure O, Bessis D, Guillot B, Guilhou JJ. Treatment of bullous pemphigoid by low-dose methotrexate associated with short-term potent topical steroids: an open prospective study of 18 cases. Arch Dermatol. 2002;138(9):1255–6.
42. Heilborn JD, Stahle-Backdahl M, Albertioni F, Vassilaki I, Peterson C, Stephansson E. Low-dose oral pulse methotrexate as monotherapy in elderly patients with bullous pemphigoid. J Am Acad Dermatol. 1999;40(5 Pt 1):741–9.

43. Bohm I, Bauer R. Treatment of bullous pemphigoid with low-dose methotrexate. Der Hautarzt Zeitschrift fur Dermatologie Venerologie und verwandte Gebiete. 1997;48(12):910–4.
44. Paul MA, Jorizzo JL, Fleischer Jr AB, White WL. Low-dose methotrexate treatment in elderly patients with bullous pemphigoid. J Am Acad Dermatol. 1994;31(4):620–5.
45. Kjellman P, Eriksson H, Berg P. A retrospective analysis of patients with bullous pemphigoid treated with methotrexate. Arch Dermatol. 2008;144(5):612–6.
46. Bohm M, Beissert S, Schwarz T, Metze D, Luger T. Bullous pemphigoid treated with mycophenolate mofetil. Lancet. 1997;349(9051):541.
47. Nousari HC, Griffin WA, Anhalt GJ. Successful therapy for bullous pemphigoid with mycophenolate mofetil. J Am Acad Dermatol. 1998;39(3):497–8.
48. Grundmann-Kollmann M, Korting HC, Behrens S, Kaskel P, Leiter U, Krahn G, et al. Mycophenolate mofetil: a new therapeutic option in the treatment of blistering autoimmune diseases. J Am Acad Dermatol. 1999;40(6 Pt 1):957–60.
49. Barthelemy H, Thivolet J, Cambazard F, Bendelac A, Mauduit G, Granier F, et al. Cyclosporin in the treatment of bullous pemphigoid: preliminary study. Ann Dermatol Venereol. 1986;113(4):309–13.
50. Thivolet J, Barthelemy H, Rigot-Muller G, Bendelac A. Effects of cyclosporin on bullous pemphigoid and pemphigus. Lancet. 1985;1(8424):334–5.
51. Roujeau JC, Revuz J, Touraine R, Joneau-Fabre M, Mannoni P. Cortico-resistant bullous pemphigoid. Favorable results with plasmapheresis. Nouv Presse Med. 1979;8(41):3362.
52. Guillaume JC, Roujeau JC, Touzet C, Revuz J, Touraine R. [Treatment of bullous pemphigoid by plasma exchange and prednisolone]. Presse Med (Paris France: 1983). 1985;14(20):1139–42.
53. Roujeau JC, Guillaume JC, Morel P, Crickx B, Dalle E, Doutre MS, et al. Plasma exchange in bullous pemphigoid. Lancet. 1984;2(8401):486–8.
54. Yamada H, Yaguchi H, Takamori K, Ogawa H. Plasmapheresis for the treatment of pemphigus vulgaris and bullous pemphigoid. Therap A. 1997;1(2):178–82.
55. Egan CA, Meadows KP, Zone JJ. Plasmapheresis as a steroid saving procedure in bullous pemphigoid. Int J Dermatol. 2000;39(3):230–5.
56. Mazzi G, Raineri A, Zanolli FA, Da Ponte C, De Roia D, Santarossa L, et al. Plasmapheresis therapy in pemphigus vulgaris and bullous pemphigoid. Transfus A Sci. 2003;28(1):13–8.
57. Chang B, Tholpady A, Huang RS, Nedelcu E, Bai Y. Clinical and serological responses following plasmapheresis in bullous pemphigoid: two case reports and a review of the literature. Blood Transfus. 2014;12(2):269–75.
58. Kitabata Y, Sakurane M, Orita H, Kamimura M, Siizaki K, Narukawa N, et al. Double filtration plasmapheresis for the treatment of bullous pemphigoid: a three case report. Ther A. 2001;5(6):484–90.
59. Lee MW, Lee WS, Choi JH, Sung KJ, Moon KC, Koh JK. A case of severe bullous pemphigoid treated with plasmapheresis. J Dermatolog Treat. 2001;12(1):59–60.
60. Konstadt JW, Remlinger K, Schild J, Aronson I, Bennin B, Solomon L. Refractory bullous pemphigoid leading to respiratory arrest and successfully treated with plasmapheresis. Arch Dermatol. 1990;126(9):1241–2.
61. Guillot B, Donadio D, Guilhou JJ, Meynadier J. Long term plasma exchange therapy in bullous pemphigoid. Acta Derm Venereol. 1986;66(1):73–5.
62. Muller PA, Brocker EB, Klinker E, Stoevesandt J, Benoit S. Adjuvant treatment of recalcitrant bullous pemphigoid with immunoadsorption. Dermatol (Basel Switzerland). 2012;224(3):224–7.
63. Godard W, Roujeau JC, Guillot B, Andre C, Rifle G. Bullous pemphigoid and intravenous gammaglobulin. Ann Int Med. 1985;103(6 (Pt 1)):964–5.
64. Ahmed AR. Intravenous immunoglobulin therapy for patients with bullous pemphigoid unresponsive to conventional immunosuppressive treatment. J Am Acad Dermatol. 2001;45(6):825–35.
65. Sami N, Ali S, Bhol KC, Ahmed AR. Influence of intravenous immunoglobulin therapy on autoantibody titres to BP Ag1 and BP Ag2 in patients with bullous pemphigoid. J Eur Acad Dermatol Venereo. 2003;17(6):641–5.

66. Lourari S, Herve C, Doffoel-Hantz V, Meyer N, Bulai-Livideanu C, Viraben R, et al. Bullous and mucous membrane pemphigoid show a mixed response to rituximab: experience in seven patients. J Eur Acad Dermatol Venereo. 2011;25(10):1238–40.
67. Hall 3rd RP, Streilein RD, Hannah DL, McNair PD, Fairley JA, Ronaghy A, et al. Association of serum B-cell activating factor level and proportion of memory and transitional B cells with clinical response after rituximab treatment of bullous pemphigoid patients. J Invest Dermatol. 2013;133(12):2786–8.
68. Saouli Z, Papadopoulos A, Kaiafa G, Girtovitis F, Kontoninas Z. A new approach on bullous pemphigoid therapy. Ann Oncol. 2008;19(4):825–6.
69. Reguiai Z, Tchen T, Perceau G, Bernard P. Efficacy of rituximab in a case of refractory bullous pemphigoid. Ann Dermatol Venereol. 2009;136(5):431–4.
70. Saraceno R, Citarella L, Spallone G, Chimenti S. A biological approach in a patient with psoriasis and bullous pemphigoid associated with losartan therapy. Clin Exp Dermatol. 2008;33(2):154–5.
71. Kasperkiewicz M, Shimanovich I, Ludwig RJ, Rose C, Zillikens D, Schmidt E. Rituximab for treatment-refractory pemphigus and pemphigoid: a case series of 17 patients. J Am Acad Dermatol. 2011;65(3):552–8.
72. Wang TS, Tsai TF. Remission of bullous pemphigoid after rituximab treatment in a psoriasis patient on regular low-dose methotrexate. Acta Derm Venereol. 2014;94(1):108–9.
73. Schmidt E, Seitz CS, Benoit S, Brocker EB, Goebeler M. Rituximab in autoimmune bullous diseases: mixed responses and adverse effects. Br J Dermatol. 2007;156(2):352–6.
74. Taieb A, Klene C, Maleville J. Immediate treatment of bullous pemphigus with a corticosteroid-cyclophosphamide combination. Ann Dermatol Venereol. 1986;113(12):1223–9.
75. Gual A, Iranzo P, Mascaro Jr JM. Treatment of bullous pemphigoid with low-dose oral cyclophosphamide: a case series of 20 patients. J Eur Acad Dermatol Venereo. 2014;28(6):814–8.
76. Dawe RS, Naidoo DK, Ferguson J. Severe bullous pemphigoid responsive to pulsed intravenous dexamethasone and oral cyclophosphamide. Br J Dermatol. 1997;137(5):826–7.
77. Yu KK, Crew AB, Messingham KA, Fairley JA, Woodley DT. Omalizumab therapy for bullous pemphigoid. J Am Acad Dermatol. 2014;71(3):468–74.
78. Dufour C, Souillet AL, Chaneliere C, Jouen F, Bodemer C, Jullien D, et al. Successful management of severe infant bullous pemphigoid with omalizumab. Br J Dermatol. 2012;166(5):1140–2.
79. Yalcin AD, Genc GE, Celik B, Gumuslu S. Anti-IgE monoclonal antibody (omalizumab) is effective in treating bullous pemphigoid and its effects on soluble CD200. Clin Lab. 2014;60(3):523–4.
80. Murrell DF, Daniel BS, Joly P, Borradori L, Amagai M, Hashimoto T, et al. Definitions and outcome measures for bullous pemphigoid: recommendations by an international panel of experts. J Am Acad Dermatol. 2012;66(3):479–85.
81. Saag KG. Bone safety of low-dose glucocorticoids in rheumatic diseases. Ann N Y Acad Sci. 2014;1318:55–64.
82. Lehman JS, Kalaaji AN. Role of primary prophylaxis for pneumocystis pneumonia in patients treated with systemic corticosteroids or other immunosuppressive agents for immune-mediated dermatologic conditions. J Am Acad Dermatol. 2010;63(5):815–23.
83. Brennan JG, Montgomery H. Pemphigus and other bullous dermatoses: correlation of clinical and pathologic findings. J Invest Dermatol. 1953;21(6):349–61; discussion 61–3.

Chapter 5
Ocular Cicatricial Pemphigoid

Swetha Dhanireddy, Armin Maghsoudlou, Janine M. Preble, Malinga D. Ratwatte, and C. Stephen Foster

Abstract Ocular cicatricial pemphigoid is a result of immune dysfunction leading to deposition of immunoglobulins and complement at the conjunctival basement membrane zone. This can lead to irreversible scarring. Patients are treated with suitable systemic immunomodulatory treatments which are usually individualized to the patient depending on the patient's age, disease stage, and presence of non-ocular symptoms. The approach to choosing the proper chemotherapy is through a stepladder algorithm. The ultimate goal of therapy is to treat the patient with corticosteroid-sparing systemic agent. The focus of this chapter will be the medical treatment strategies available for OCP based upon clinical severity, extent and progression of the disease.

Keywords Ocular cicatricial pemphigoid • Dapsone • Azathioprine • Mycophenolate mofetil • Cyclophosphamide • Methotrexate • Plasmapheresis • Rituximab • Intravenous Immunoglobulin

Introduction

Mucous membrane pemphigoid (MMP) encompasses a group of autoimmune inflammatory subepithelial blistering diseases affecting primarily various mucous membranes. Ocular complications seen in 60 % of MMP cases, known as ocular

S. Dhanireddy, MD, BS • A. Maghsoudlou, MD • J.M. Preble, MS
Massachusetts Eye Research and Surgery Institution, Ocular Immunology and Uveitis Foundation, Cambridge, MA, USA

M.D. Ratwatte, BA (Cantab)
Massachusetts Eye Research and Surgery Institution, Ocular Immunology and Uveitis Foundation, Cambridge, MA, USA

School of Clinical Medicine, University of Cambridge, Cambridge, Cambridgeshire, UK

C.S. Foster, MD, FACS, FACR (✉)
Massachusetts Eye Research and Surgery Institution; Ocular Immunology and Uveitis Foundation, Cambridge, MA, USA

Department of Ophthalmology, Harvard Medical School,
Boston, MA, USA
e-mail: sfoster@mersi.com

N. Sami (ed.), *Autoimmune Bullous Diseases: Approach and Management*,
DOI 10.1007/978-3-319-26728-9_5

cicatricial pemphigoid (OCP), is the second most-commonly involved mucous membrane affecting conjunctival tissue [1, 2]. OCP is a rare, vision-threatening disorder, affecting approximately 1 in 12,000–1 in 60,000, with an average age of 65 years. It is more commonly seen in females, with a ratio of 2–3:1 [3].

OCP is a result of immune dysfunction leading to deposition of immunoglobulins and complement at the conjunctival basement membrane zone (BMZ). The most commonly identified immunoreactants are IgG, IgA and C3, deposited in a linear fashion unique to OCP [4]. The disease can initially present unilaterally or bilaterally; in patients with unilateral involvement, the other eye is typically affected within 2 years [4, 5]. The typical sequence of OCP progression begins with subepithelial fibrosis leading to foreshortening of fornices, followed by the formation of symblepharon from palpebral to the bulbar conjunctiva. Later stages of the disease present with extensive conjunctival scarring, ankyloblepharon, trichiasis, and distichiasis. The disease also causes loss of goblet cells, along with the occlusion of lacrimal and accessory lacrimal glands leading to dry eye and ocular surface pathology [1, 4]. Combination of clinical findings and immunohistopathology of biopsied conjunctiva leads to the diagnosis of OCP.

The First International Consensus on MMP categorized patients into "low-risk" and "high-risk" groups based upon the site(s) of involvement. Ocular involvement falls into the "high-risk" group, therefore requiring aggressive systemic therapy [1, 2]. The focus of this chapter will be the medical treatment strategies available for OCP based upon clinical severity, extent and progression of the disease.

Staging

OCP may present as symmetric or asymmetric disease; therefore each eye must be graded separately. The Foster classification categorizes OCP into four stages, depending on clinical features. Stage 1 findings consist of conjunctival inflammation, mucous discharge, small-patched rose bengal-staining conjunctival epithelium, and conjunctival subepithelial fibrosis (Fig. 5.1). Stage 2 exhibits foreshortening of the conjunctival fornix . Stage 2 is further subdivided (a) through (d) depending on the degree of fornix shortening: (a) 0–25 % (b) 25–50 % (c) 50–75 % (d) >75 % fornix shortening (Fig. 5.3b). Stage 3 includes symblepharon formation and is also further subdivided (a) through (d) depending on the percentage of horizontal involvement of symblephara, (a) 0–25 % (b) 25–50 % (c) 50–75 % (d) >75 % involvement of symblephra (Fig. 5.2a,b, and 5.3a. Stage 4 or end-stage OCP is characterized by severe sicca syndrome, ocular surface keratinization, and ankyloblepharon [4–6] (Figs. 5.1, 5.2, and 5.3).

OCP is a systemic autoimmune disease as a result of dysregulation of the immune system [7, 8]; therefore, the treatment is targeted towards both systemic and local immune processes and their subsequent sequelae. The goal of therapy is to abolish inflammation, prevent further cicatrization and promote healing.

It is important to emphasize that systemic, not topical treatment is required to adequately control OCP. Previous attempts of controlling OCP's activity with

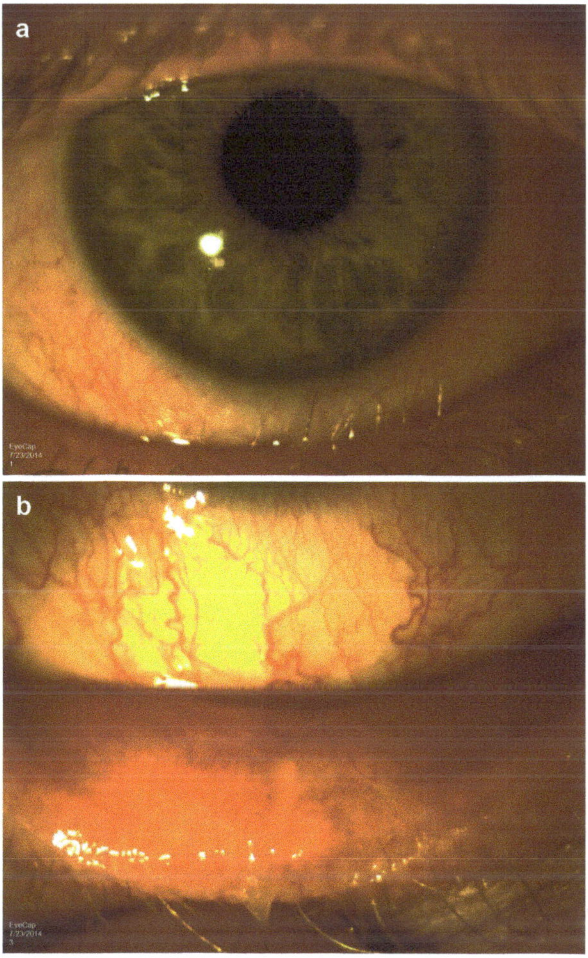

Fig. 5.1 (**a**, **b**) External photos of the same patient with biopsy proven OCP, showing extensive blepharitis, fornix foreshortening, lash-cornea touch, cicatricial changes to lower eyelid

topical corticosteroids, cyclosporine, mitomycin-C, and retinoids have failed. Furthermore, although oral prednisone may control ocular inflammation acutely, it does not suffice for long-term immunosuppression to control disease activity and therefore it is an inappropriate treatment regimen to accomplish sustainable remission [4, 5, 9, 10].

Deciding on the most suitable systemic immunomodulatory treatment is dependent on the patient's age, disease stage, and presence of non-ocular symptoms. Prior to initiating therapy, the patient should undergo a formal assessment of disease stage. Checking the following is crucial to allow for proper drug monitoring: baseline renal and liver function tests, and complete blood count (CBC). Discussion about various treatment options, potential side effects and

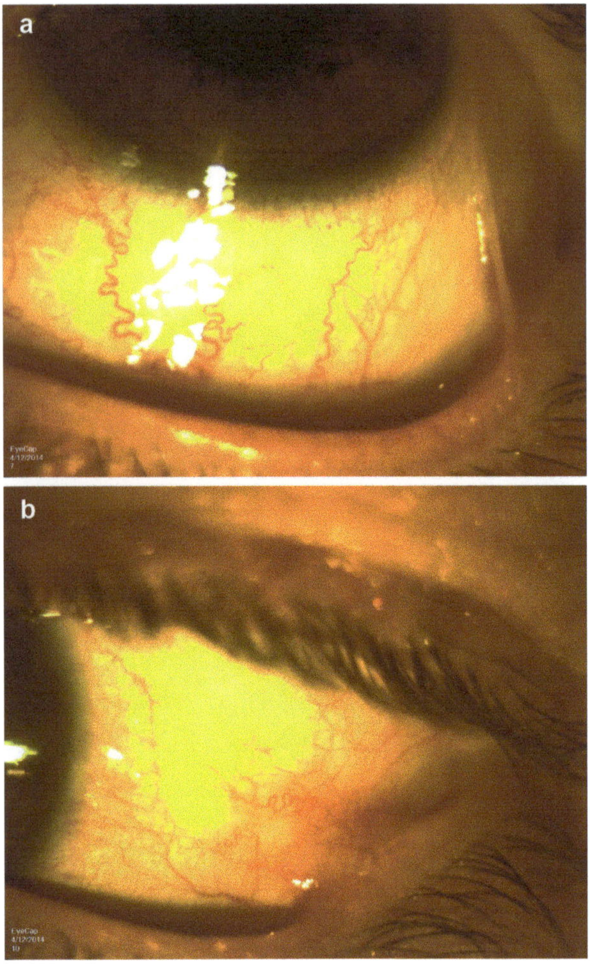

Fig. 5.2 (**a**, **b**) External photos of the same patient depicting stage 3 OCP. Patient is currently on immunomodulatory therapy, in remission

the willingness to commit to frequent follow-up visits is important for patient awareness and compliance [3, 4]. Systemic immunosuppressive therapy is appropriate in patients with active, progressive OCP (not in end-stage "burned out" disease); therapy can prevent further scarring, but cannot reverse previous damage [4]. The approach to choosing the proper chemotherapy is through a stepladder algorithm. Patients with mild to moderate disease are started on the least potent therapeutic options and if they fail to respond, continue to progress or are intolerant to side effects, patients are treated with addition of or

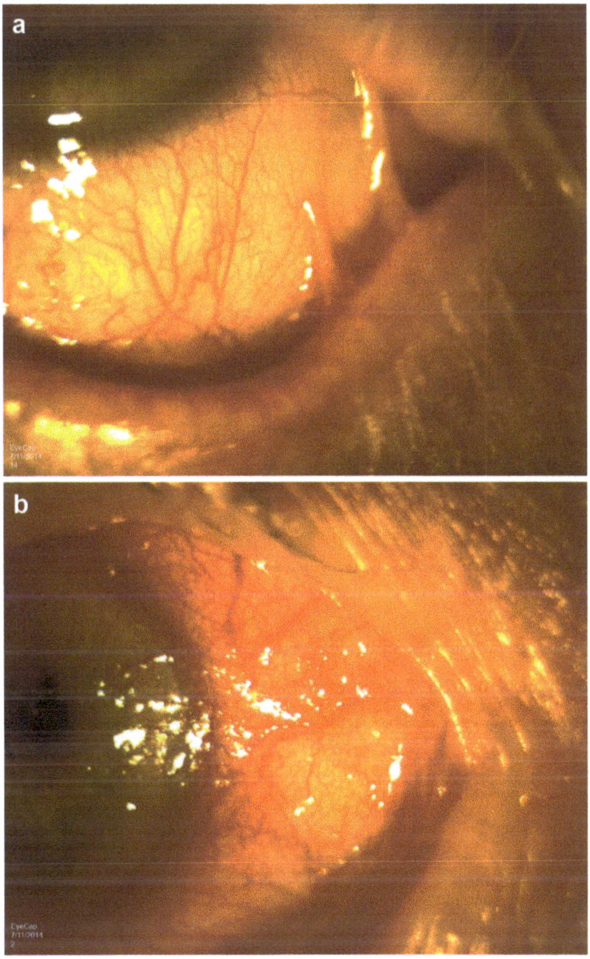

Fig. 5.3 (**a**, **b**) Photos of actively inflamed, rapidly progressing OCP. Patient failed methotrexate and is awaiting insurance approval for IV-Ig and rituximab infusions

substitution with more potent therapeutic options. The ultimate goal of therapy is to treat the patient with corticosteroid-sparing systemic therapy successfully keeping them in steroid-free remission for 2 years. Once the patient has reached the 2-year milestone, medication is slowly tapered. During tapering of medication, close monitoring is continued to observe for relapses [4]. After discontinuing medication, patients have a 30 % risk of recurrence; therefore, lifelong follow-up is recommended [5, 11]. The specific immunomodulatory therapies in the treatment of OCP are discussed in detail in the following sections.

OCP Stepladder Immunosuppressive Therapy Algorithm

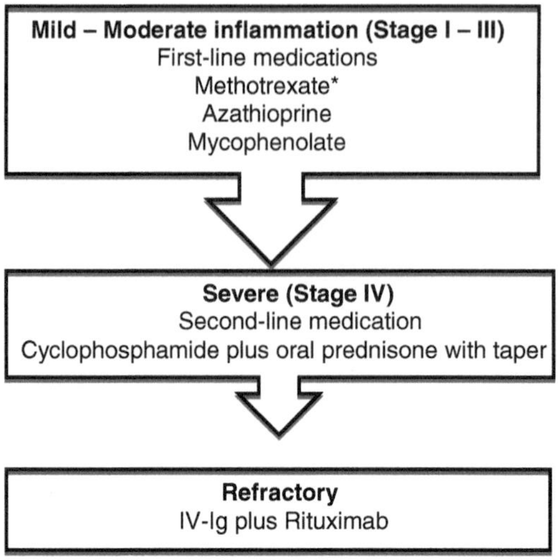

*Most commonly used first-line medication because of the long track record of its application among ocular diseases for over four decades and well-known side effect profile.

Tetracycline

Tetracyclines were discovered as the natural fermentation product of the soil bacterium Streptomyces aureofaciens in 1948 and were chemically purified for the first time in 1952 [12]. They have shown efficacy on inflammation, immunomodulation, cell proliferation, angiogenesis, metal chelation, ionophoresis, and bone metabolism [13].

Tetracycline has a direct and indirect anti-inflammatory effect [14, 15]. Tetracycline or minocycline, alone or in combination with nicotinamide, were shown to be effective in cicatricial pemphigoid diseases [16, 17]. Kohler et al., in 1980, showed the synergic anti-neutrophil effect of tetracycline and nicotinamide combination in treatment of erythema elevatum diutinum [18]. Tetracycline (500–2000 mg/day) therapy alone as monotherapy or in combination with nicotinamide (500–2500 mg/day) is also effective in treating pemphigoid [19–21]. Tetracyclines are usually well-tolerated drugs. Common side effects include cutaneous side effects and gastrointestinal upset. Rash, purpura and photosensitivity are reported with both minocycline and doxycycline. Dizziness is reported in almost 10 % of the patients [22].

However, tetracycline's efficacy to achieve durable remission in OCP has not shown encouraging results. Therefore, the use of tetracycline as monotherapy or in combination with immunosuppressive agents is not administered in the treatment of OCP.

Dapsone

Dapsone is a sulfone derivative (4–4′ diaminodiphenylsulfone) [5] with antibacterial and anti-inflammatory properties. In the early twentieth century, theories on selective toxicity based on the ability of certain dyes to kill microbes developed, eventually leading to the discovery of dapsone by Ernest Fourneau and Gladwin Buttle [23]. Dapsone was originally utilized in the treatment of leprosy. Later, in 1953, Rook et al. reported 11 of 17 patients with bullous pemphigoid responded to treatment with sulfapyridine [24]. Person et al. in 1977 and Foster et al. in 1986 confirmed these results, noting the efficacy of dapsone in treating dermatitis herpetiformis and bullous pemphigoid [5, 25].

Dapsone's applicability in OCP is due to its anti-inflammatory (immunomodulating) effects [26]. The anti-inflammatory mode of action of dapsone is through inhibiting the migration of neutrophilic polymorphonuclear leukocytes [27] and suppressing effects on peroxidase enzyme systems present in monocytes, neutrophils, eosinophils, and mast cells. However, the specific cellular and molecular events involved in the anti-inflammatory effect of dapsone are unknown [5].

Foster et al. studied the efficacy of dapsone in patients with OCP, finding 88 % (14 out of 16) with mild-to-modest inflammatory activity responded to dapsone. Treatment failures in this study were in patients with 3–4+ conjunctival inflammation prior to therapy [5] indicating that dapsone is one drug of choice as first line therapy in mild to moderate OCP [5, 26].

The initial dose of dapsone employed is 2 mg/kg/day with a maximum dose of 200 mg/day. Dosage adjustments are based on therapeutic response and drug tolerance. Patients are monitored every 4–6 weeks; monitoring parameters include CBC emphasized attention on hemoglobin, hematocrit, and reticulocyte count [5].

The most common potential side effects are hemolysis and methaemoglobinemia [5, 27]. Doses greater than 50 mg/day inevitably produce some degree of hemolysis, usually well tolerated [27]. Low-grade hemolysis is acceptable under the circumstances of desired therapeutic response and adequate compensation by reticulocytosis. However, a progressive drop in hematocrit may require discontinuation [5, 26]. Wetheim et al. reported up to 33 % of patients treated with dapsone for OCP with a daily dose of 50 mg twice daily taken orally with clinically significant hemolytic anemia and a persistent fall in hemoglobin from baseline [26]. Previously published reports note approximately 10 % of patients with hemolysis required discontinuation of therapy [5, 28]. Glucose-6-phosphate hydrogenase deficient patients are at a higher risk of developing hemolytic anemia when treated with dapsone [26].

Fern et al. also confirmed dapsone was effective in treating mild to moderate OCP, however, all the patients relapsed after discontinuing therapy [27]. Foster et al. reported 41 % of patients treated with dapsone relapsed within 6 months of discontinuing therapy. Relapsed inflammation responds to either restarting dapsone or starting immunosuppressive agent: azathioprine, 2 mg/kg initial dose [5, 27].

Although dapsone is a relatively safe medication [27], its primary deficiencies are the high rate of recurrence after discontinuation and its inability to control the disease as a monotherapy [5, 27]. Thus, dapsone is not commonly utilized in the treatment of OCP.

Methotrexate

In 1948, methotrexate (MTX) was introduced as an anti-neoplastic agent [29]. In 1965, MTX was employed in the treatment of ocular diseases [30], and since then, multiple series have reported its effectiveness in managing ocular inflammation [31–36]. MTX, an anti-metabolite, functions as an immunosuppressive agent through lowering cell proliferation, increasing CD95 sensitivity of activated T-cells leading to an accelerated rate of T-cell apoptosis, inhibiting enzymes involved in purine metabolism and subsequently increasing endogenous adenosine concentrations, and altering cytokine production and humoral responses [37].

Gangaputra et al. retrospectively studied the outcome of noninfectious ocular inflammation when treated with methotrexate as a single, non-corticosteroid immunosuppressive agent. A total of 639 eyes were assessed, affected by multiple etiologies of ocular inflammation and 109 of the included eyes were diagnosed with OCP. Results demonstrated 39.5 % of patients with OCP reached complete suppression of inflammation sustained for ≥28 days within 6 months of treatment. Furthermore, 65 % of the patients with complete control of OCP continued to improve between 6 and 12 months of therapy and reached complete control of inflammation by 12 months of MTX therapy. Corticosteroid-sparing success defined as completely inactive inflammation at ≥2 visits spanning ≥28 days after tapering oral prednisone dose to ≤10 mg/day was observed in 36.5 % of patients with OCP within 6 months of treatment. Moreover, corticosteroid-sparing success continued to improve to 66.9 % within 12 months of treatment. Durable control of inflammation after tapering oral prednisone to ≤5 mg/day was achieved in 60.7 % of patients with OCP [38].

MTX is indicated for mild to moderate OCP; it is administered as one of the first-line medications. Although MTX is available in oral, subcutaneous (SC) and intravenous routes, it is initially employed orally and at once a week dosage, which reduces the potential risk of occult side effects [4, 39]. Patients are observed closely, monitoring CBC, renal panel, and liver function testing every 6 weeks. MTX is initiated at a dose of 15 mg once a week and increased according to the patients' response and tolerability to treatment, with maximum dose of 40 mg weekly. Folic acid is administered concomitantly at a dose of 1 mg daily.

Patients may develop side effects within the first year of therapy. Gangaputra et al. reported up to 18 % of patients discontinued MTX due to side effects within the first year [38]. The commonly reported side effects are fatigue, GI related: nausea, vomiting and anorexia, and transaminitis [1, 4, 32, 34, 38, 40]. Switching to subcutaneous administration may alleviate gastrointestinal side effect. Other potential side effects include cytopenia, stomatitis [41–44], and pneumonitis [1, 45–48]. Serious and rare adverse effects are bone marrow suppression (0.02 cases/person-year), liver cirrhosis (0.002 cases/person-year), and malignancy [1, 38, 49]. Miserocchi et al. reviewed treatment related side effects in 61 patients with MMP and concluded that MTX exhibited the fewest number of adverse effects, as compared to azathioprine, cyclophosphamide, and dapsone [50]. Baker et al. had similar findings, stating that within the first year of therapy, the portion of patients discontinuing treatment because of side effects was the same among MTX and mycophenolate mofetil (0.09) and significantly higher for azathioprine (0.24) [51]. MTX is a non-dose dependent teratogen, exposure leading to miscarriages and fetal malformations [52, 53]. Therefore, prior to initiating therapy, proper birth control measures should be discussed and recommended, and substitution of therapy should occur ≥3 months before attempting conception [38].

Overall, systemic use of MTX therapy for ocular inflammation is moderately effective in adequately controlling inflammation and decreasing dependency on corticosteroids MTX is tolerated relatively well and carries low risk of serious side effects when patients are closely monitored [38].

Azathioprine

In 1957, George Herbert Hitching and Gertrude Elion developed an anti-metabolite medication, azathioprine (Imuran®), which interferes with DNA and RNA synthesis [54], thus acting as an immunosuppressive drug. The first usage of azathioprine was in combination with glucocorticoids to immune suppress post kidney allotransplantation recipients [54–59].

Azathioprine's first use in the treatment of OCP came after a study by Dantzig in 1974, publishing results of azathioprine in the treatment of OCP [9]. The efficacy of azathioprine in treating OCP was further confirmed by Dave et al., who reported success in the treatment of four patients with mucous membrane pemphigoid with ocular involvement [60]. Currently, azathioprine holds the US Food and Drug Administration approval for the treatment of rheumatoid arthritis [61], organ transplantation [62] and various dermatologic [63], gastrointestinal [64] and rheumatologic diseases [65]. Azathioprine's pertinence among ophthalmalmic diseases is preventing corneal graft rejections and treating non-infectious ocular inflammatory conditions.

Pasadhika et al. evaluated outcomes of ocular inflammation patients managed on azathioprine as the sole immunosuppressive agent. One hundred forty-five patients were included in the data analysis and of the 145 patients, 33 patients

(23 %) had MMP. Each patient was followed from the initiation of azathioprine until therapy was discontinued. Treatment success was evaluated by the time-to-successful tapering of prednisone to ≤10 mg, ≤5 mg, and 0 mg daily while maintaining control of inflammation over at least two visits spanning at least 28 days. Approximately 43 % of MMP patients had control of their ocular inflammation within 6 months of treatment. Corticosteroid-sparing success by 6 months was second highest in MMP (39 %). Patients with intermediate uveitis and mucous membrane pemphigoid (MMP) were most likely to achieve both control of inflammation and corticosteroid-tapering success compared to other ocular inflammatory sites involved in this study [54].

Azathioprine is one of the first-line medications in treating OCP. The recommended dose based on TPMT levels up to 3 mg/kg/day, as the maximum dose [4]. The most common adverse effects leading to discontinuation of azathioprine are gastrointestinal upset, followed by bone marrow suppression, elevated liver enzymes, infection, allergic reaction and arthralgia [4, 54]. Pasadhika et al. estimated 24 % of patients would discontinue azathioprine due to side effects within 1 year [54]. Its main advantages are a lower cost compared to most alternative agents and some evidence of safety during pregnancy [66, 67]. Also, this medication has been used for ocular inflammatory diseases for the past forty decades, thus unknown long-term toxicities of therapy are less likely [54]. Similar to MTX monitoring, patients are evaluated every 6 weeks, each time with a complete examination and blood work to assess CBC with differential, aspartate transaminase, alanine transaminase, blood urea nitrogen (BUN) and creatinine.

Mycophenolate Mofetil

Mycophenolate mofetil (MMF; CellCept®) was originally introduced in the 1950s as an antifungal medication and in the process was discovered to have antineoplastic and immunosuppressive properties [68]. In 1995, the U.S. Food and Drug Administration approved MMF as an immunosuppressive agent to reduce acute renal graft rejection and prolonging renal graft survival [69]. Since then, it has been utilized as a corticosteroid-sparing therapy for solid organ transplant rejection and multiple autoimmune diseases and systemic disorders [70–76]. Ocular application of MMF was first conducted in rats with experimental autoimmune uveitis showing encouraging results [77] and then preliminary studies were performed in humans with OCP [70]. Results revealed MMF to be effective in 9 of 10 eyes (five patients) during 1-year follow-up.

MMF is a morpholinoethyl ester of mycophenolic acid, with an immunosuppressive action by reversible inhibition of inosine-5′ monophosphate dehydrogenase in the de novo pathway of purine synthesis without affecting the salvage pathway of purine synthesis. Therefore, MMF selectively inhibits T- and B- lymphocyte replication [78, 79] and may be the reason for fewer side effects compared to other antimetabolites [75, 78].

Thorne et al. retrospectively evaluated treatment outcomes of MMF in 84 patients with various inflammatory eye diseases, 11 % of these patients were diagnosed with OCP. Treatment success was based on ability to control ocular inflammation and taper oral prednisone to ≤10 mg daily. Treatment success was achieved in 82 % of the patients with median time of 3.5 months with majority of the patients reaching this goal in the first 6 months of treatment. Of the patients to reach treatment success, 70 % were able to taper to ≤5 mg oral prednisone daily successfully, and 40 % were able to discontinue oral prednisone without relapse of their disease. The rate of treatment success among patients who previously had not received IMT was 0.27 per person-month with median time to treatment success of 2.4 months. The rate of treatment success among patients who received IMT previously was 0.09 per person-month with median time to treatment success of 4.7 months. Even then, treatment success was >60 % among patients previously treated with IMT. In conclusion, MMF is not only an effective corticosteroid-sparing agent to treat OCP but also among patients resistant to other IMTs [80].

Doycheva et al. were the first to report long-term efficacy and tolerability of MMF in the therapy of OCP. The study consisted of retrospectively assessing 19 eyes with OCP diagnosis that were treated with MMF with follow-up of at least 4 years. At the time of MMF treatment initiation, 17 of 19 eyes (89 %) had active inflammation. During the therapy, 11 eyes (58 %) had complete resolution of inflammation and 8 eyes (11 %) had mild inflammation. Rate of relapse was 0.09 per patient-year with a mean time of 42 months after the initiation of MMP. Also during treatment, progression of conjunctival cicatrization was prevented in 9 eyes (47 %), mild progression of cicatrization was reported in 8 eyes (42 %) and conjunctival cicatrization progressed to stage IV in 2 eyes (11 %). Overall, the results from this study suggest MMF is an adequate immunosuppressive agent with the capacity to maintain long-term inflammatory control and recommending it as first-line therapy for patients with OCP [81].

Nottage et al. retrospectively studied the outcomes of inflammatory control and rate of discontinuation of MMF in the treatment of OCP. The study consisted of 23 OCP patients that were treated with MMF. All of the patients had disease process of Foster stage 2 or greater. Eight out of the 23 patients (34.8 %) had failed IMT previously. Fifteen of the 23 patients (65.2 %) were treated with MMF as initial therapy. Overall, 19 patients achieved control of inflammation, and 16 out of the 19 patients (82.4 %) were treated with MMF as monotherapy. Of all the patients who achieved inflammatory suppression (19 patients), 3.27 months was the median length of time to disease control. The patients who had failed IMT previously, 4.10 months was the median length of time to disease control and 3.85 months for those who were IMT naïve prior to starting MMF. In 5 of the total 23 patients, MMF was discontinued due to response failure (4 patients) and allergic reaction (1 patient). Based on these observations, MMF was concluded to be an appropriate monotherapy and initial systemic immunosuppressive agent for controlling active OCP [82].

Side effect profile of MMF is found to be minimal and overall well tolerated [68, 70, 80, 83–86]. Nottage et al. observed 3 out of 23 patients to have developed side effects. One of the three patients (4.3 %) developed a rash leading to cessation of

MMF. Another patient had mild thrombocytopenia, which resolved with a decrease in MMF dose. Third patient had hypokalemia, myalgia, insomnia, and anorexia, which also resolved with lowering the dose and switching to mycophenolate sodium [82]. Saw et al. and Doycheva et al. both reported mild and transient side effects of MMF while evaluating the effectiveness and toxicity of different IMT in OCP management [81, 84]. Saw et al. went on to conclude MMF having the lowest risk of side effects when compared to other IMT [84]. The most common potential side effects observed with the use of MMF are gastrointestinal upset (diarrhea, vomiting), increased liver enzymes, and fatigue [68, 71, 80, 81] which are typically reversible and resolve with dose reduction. MMF has not been associated with causing any major organ toxicity, infection or malignancy [71, 81, 82].

MMF is employed as an orally administered medication, initially at a dose of 500 mg twice a day and titrated depending on disease control and tolerability with a maximum dose of 3 g/day. Similar to other IMT monitoring, patients are evaluated every 6 weeks and blood work is obtained to assess CBC with differential, renal panel, and liver function testing. The most appropriate application of MMF is to utilize it as a corticosteroid-sparing, first-line, monotherapy or as an adjunctive immunosuppressive agent for active OCP [68, 70, 80–82, 87].

Cyclophosphamide

Cyclophosphamide (Cytoxan®), a nitrogen mustard derived alkylating agent, became the eighth cytotoxic anticancer medication to be approved by the United States Food and Drug Administration [88, 89]. The first use of cyclophosphamide in ocular conditions was in 1952 to treat idiopathic uveitis [90] and since then it has been used to treat various ocular inflammatory diseases [91, 92]. Cyclophosphamide generates immunomodulatory effects on rapidly proliferating cells, by alkylating nucleophilic groups on DNA bases leading to cross-linking of DNA bases, abnormal base pairing, or DNA strand breakage. The end result is damage to cells undergoing mitosis and consequently suppression of lymphocyte function (B cells more than T cells) [1, 92, 93].

Pujari et al. assessed the outcomes of cyclophosphamide therapy as a single immunosuppressive agent during follow-up, with or without local or systemic corticosteroids and non-steroidal anti-inflammatory drugs (NSAIDs), for treating non-infectious ocular inflammation. Of the 215 patients in this study, 45.6 % had OCP, being the most common diagnosis in affected eyes. Results revealed that within 6 months, 43 % of patients with OCP had complete control of inflammation, sustained over at least two visits spanning at least 28 days. Success continued to improve, complete inactivity was observed in 68.7 % patients with OCP by 12 months. Disease remission leading to discontinuation of the medication occurred at the rate of 0.32/person-year and 63.1 % of patients achieved remission at or prior to 2 years [92]. Overall, cyclophosphamide achieved beneficial effects with sustained control of inflammation among non-infectious ocular inflammatory cases in 49 and 76 % by 6 and 12 months respectively [92].

Elder et al. conducted a prospective study among 19 eyes of ten patients diagnosed with either severe OCP or marked OCP who previously failed other systemic immunosuppressive therapy. They were treated with cyclophosphamide and short-term high dose oral prednisolone. All patients were treated with oral cyclophosphamide at an initial dose of 1.5–2.0 mg/kg/day and oral prednisolone 60 mg/day or 80 mg/day and other oral immunosuppressive agents were discontinued. All but one patient were treated with cyclophosphamide for longer than 6 months. The reason for discontinuing treatment in one patient was due to unpleasant feelings of being distant from the world, 'like being on [recreational] drugs'. The goal lymphocyte count was 0.5–1.0 × 10^9/l, which was accomplished on a maintenance dose ranging from 50 to 150 mg/day. When clinical response was observed, prednisolone was reduced and when ocular and systemic features were clinically stable, prednisolone was stopped completely. The duration of prednisolone ranged from 4 to 8 months. The results of this study revealed ocular inflammation resolved in 15 eyes in a mean time of 2.4 months. During this study two eyes perforated; one from acute microbial keratitis and the other from progressive corneal thinning. Throughout the study, systemic infections requiring antibiotics did not develop in any of the patients. Progressive cicatrization was observed in 21 % of inflamed eyes (4 out of 19 eyes). Overall, these results suggest cyclophosphamide plus short term high dose oral prednisolone effectively controls severe ocular inflammation seen in OCP, although progression of ocular cicatrization might be inevitable in some cases [89]. Mondino et al. [10, 94] and Foster et al. [5, 95] reported findings confirming Elder et al.'s work, describing oral cyclophosphamide and short-term high dose prednisolone to be the most reasonable therapeutic regimen for adequate control of ocular inflammation and prevention of cicatrization among OCP patients.

Intravenously (IV) administered cyclophosphamide is used for rapid ocular inflammatory arrest, specifically prior to ocular surface surgery. High dose oral prednisone is also initiated simultaneously; dosed 1 mg/kg/day with a maximum dose of 60 mg/day and tapered weekly. Inflammation that has failed to respond to less potent immunomodulatory therapy is also treated with pulse IV cyclophosphamide therapy [96, 97]. IV cyclophosphamide is dosed at 1 g/m^2 body surface area every 2 weeks. The dose is adjusted depending on the patients' response and tolerability to treatment, and white blood count (WBC) with an optimal range of 3.0 ×10^3/μL to 4.5 ×10^3/μL. Oral dosing given in 100–150 mg/day range ("full" doses) appear more likely to succeed (controlling inflammation compared to doses of <100 mg but more likely to lead to dose-limiting toxicity) than lower doses [92]. Good hydration is encouraged, 8–10 cups of non-caffeinated fluid daily to prevent bladder toxicity especially with oral cyclophosphamide and hydration is supplemented with infusions for IV cyclophosphamide [91].

Careful consideration is exercised before starting cyclophosphamide, it is reserved for vision-threatening ocular diseases which have previously failed less potent immunomodulatory therapy or non-infectious ocular inflammatory cases associated with systemic disease. After treatment with cyclophosphamide, a higher rate of medication-free remission has been reported compared to methotrexate [38], azathioprine [54], mycophenolate mofetil [83] and cyclosporine [98]. However, given the side effect profile of the medication, diligent monitoring by an ophthalmologist and commitment to compliance by the patient are fundamental to achieve optimal results.

Pujari et al. found that the most common side effects leading to discontinuation of cyclophosphamide are leukopenia and cystitis/blood in the urine, seen in 18.1 and 7.7 % respectively within the first year of therapy. The most common opportunistic infection leading to discontinuation is *Pneumocystis carinii*, reported in 3.0 % of the patients in the first year [92]. Cyclophosphamide increases the risk of malignancy, especially bladder carcinoma [9, 89, 99] and increases overall cancer mortality [49, 100–103]. Therefore, the use of cylcophosphamide is limited to 1 year due to the increased risk of developing cancer [91]. Also, it crosses the placental blood barrier and is excreted in breast milk, thus is classified as a teratogenic medication and contraindicated if a patient is breastfeeding [104, 105]. Although the potential side effects of cyclophosphamide are greater than alternative immunosuppressive agents, its application should not be deferred or delayed under appropriate circumstances when this medication is indicated given its success rates of remission and vision-saving capacity [92].

Close monitoring is especially emphasized with the use of cyclophosphamide. CBC with differential is required every other week for IV cyclophosphamide to ensure the WBC is within the optimal range. For both IV and oral cyclophosphamide, monitoring CBC, renal panel, liver function enzymes, and urine analysis every 6 weeks is endorsed. Being that cyclophosphamide is recommended to be employed for no longer than 1 year, patients are transitioned to other IMT (i.e., MTX, azathioprine, mycophenolate) to achieve 2 full years of corticosteroid-free remission.

Plasmapheresis

Plasmapheresis refers to extracorporeal separation of blood components resulting in filtered plasma. Methods used in plasmapheresis to achieve filtered plasma are centrifugation, double filtration plasmapheresis (DFPF) and a combination of both techniques [106, 107]. It has been proven to be effective in the variety of the diseases, especially in those in which circulating antibodies are the main pathogenesis factor. Clinical indications are broad and include more than 60 diseases [108]. Although there is no formal recommendation in using plasmapheresis in treatment of bolus pemphigoid, several reports advocated its beneficial application in conjunction with immunosuppressive therapy in controlling severe or refractory cases, specifically with persistent ocular involvement [109–112].

Clinical indications of plasmapheresis in mucus membrane pemphigoid include rapid control of severe active disease when corticosteroids and immunosuppressive dosage reduction is needed, especially in patients with multiple comorbidities such as diabetes, or when above treatments are contraindicated and in resistant drug therapy diseases [113, 114].

The most effective method is 40–60 ml/kg plasma exchanges as often as every other day. In each cycle, five to ten plasma exchanges usually are performed. Automated centrifuge-based technology is the simplest, easiest and most used technique in the U.S. [115]. However, due to subsequent FFP or human albumin infusion, the risk of disease contraction such as hepatitis and AIDS is present. Other adverse complications include allergic reaction with fever, chills, hypotension and procedure complications including vein puncture, thrombosis and pneumothorax [116].

To avoid rebound phenomena, plasmapheresis should be accompanied by an immunosuppressive therapy. Turner et al. reported complete remission in four out of seven patients with pemphigus vulgaris with five series of plasma exchanges over an average of 8 days. In all cases, intravenous cyclophosphamide was administered immediately after plasmapheresis to prevent rebound flare [117]. There are also two reports on combination apheresis and cyclophosphamide in patients with mucus membrane pemphigoid [118, 119]. Hashimoto reported a 73-year-old man with anti-epiligrin cicatricial pemphigoid and ocular lesions resistant to conventional therapy successfully controlled with plasmapheresis. These cases suggested a possible role of plasma exchange treatment of otherwise refractory cases.

However, clinical trials evaluating plasmapheresis' efficacy among OCP patients are absent. The current data available is based on case reports or its effectiveness in other autoimmune diseases. Therefore, given the life threatening side effect profile and lack of evidence of its efficacy in OCP, plasmapheresis is not a recommended therapy to treat OCP.

Intravenous Immunoglobulins and Rituximab

Intravenous immunoglobulins' (IV-Ig) applicability among ocular autoimmune diseases originates from its efficacy in re-regulation of the immune system through, among other mechanisms, idiotypic anti-idiotypic regulatory network manipulations. IV-Igs are retrieved from pooled human plasma from multiple donors [120]. The precise mechanism of action of IV-Ig as an anti-inflammatory and immunomodulating agent is yet to be elucidated. However, some of the proposed effects it has on the immune system are the following: (1) modulation and blockage of Fc receptors on the surface of macrophages; (2) modulation of the complement system; (3) reduction in titers of pathogenic autoantibody; (4) induction or suppression of the production of cytokines; (5) neutralization of toxins; (6) modulation of cell proliferation, apoptosis, and demyelination; (7) alteration in sensitivity to corticosteroids [121–123].

Systemic immunosuppressive therapy is the mainstay treatment for OCP. Nonetheless, multiple studies have shown some cases progressing while treated with IMT [50, 95, 124, 125] and a risk of advancing to end-stage OCP [126]. Therefore, when conventional approach fails to adequately control disease activity, achieve clinical remission or is intolerable to IMT side effects, IV-Ig is an appropriate alternative treatment option.

Foster et al. in a preliminary, uncontrolled study were the first to assess the safety and effectiveness of IV-Ig for treating OCP among ten patients, who were otherwise resistant to conventional IMT. IV-Ig infusions were administered at a dose of 2–3 g/kg/cycle, divided over 3 days and repeated every 2–6 weeks. The duration of therapy ranged from 16 to 23 months (mean of 19.3 months) without medication induced side effects. Results revealed termination of clinical progression and resolution of chronic conjunctivitis in all of the ten patients [127].

Letko et al. evaluated the clinical outcomes of IV-Ig therapy to conventional IMT among patients with OCP. Patients were enrolled in the study when ocular involvement of MMP was noted and confirmed by biopsy. At the time of enrollment into this study, all patients were diagnosed with stage 2 OCP. They were placed into two groups, group A and group B, each consisted of eight patients. Both of these groups were studied at the same time. Group A patients were treated with IV-Ig as monotherapy while group B patients were treated with conventional IMT or in combination with systemic corticosteroids. All of the patients were followed for a minimum of 18 months after diagnosis of OCP. The mean length of therapy was 24 months (range 16–30) for group A and 45 months (range 21–90) for group B. The median time from initiation of therapy to achieving clinical remission was 4 and 8.5 months in group A and B, respectively, with a statistically significant difference ($P<0.01$). Recurrence of ocular inflammation was not observed in any of the patients in group A. On the other hand, in group B, recurrence was noted in five patients. All of the eight patients in group A, at the last follow up visit, revealed no progression of their ocular inflammation and both eyes in each patient were quiescent. On the contrary, at the last follow up visit, four of the eight patients in group B progressed from stage 2 to stage 3 and some level of conjunctival inflammation was observed in five patients. The findings of this study demonstrate encouraging outcomes for IV-Ig application to halt disease progression and achieve remission, making it a favorable alternative to conventional IMT among patients with OCP [126].

Sami et al. studied 15 patients with severe MMP refractory to systemic corticosteroids and IMT who then were treated with IV-Ig therapy. These patients' quality of life during this study was evaluated: first, before starting IV-Ig therapy, and second, at the last visit. A numeric scoring system was used, assigning a score based on the symptoms of the disease and the side effects of treatment affecting their lifestyle. The scoring system was as follows: (1), poor; (2), unsatisfactory; (3), livable; (4), reasonably good; (5), high quality of life. Among the 15 patients, the average score at the last visit was 4.7 [128].

RTX is a monoclonal antibody against CD20 protein, mainly targeting B-cells [129]. Combination treatment regimen with rituximab (RTX) plus IV-Ig is an effective modality to treat OCP, stage 3 or 4, moderate to severe inflammation, rapidly progressive, or recalcitrant to conventional IMT. Foster et al. conducted a preliminary report studying the efficacy and safety of combination therapy of RTX and IV-Ig compared to other IMT among OCP patients. A total of 12 OCP patients were evaluated. Six patients were in study group and six patients were in control group. The study group patients received RTX plus IV-Ig while control group received more aggressive IMT but not RTX and IV-Ig. Prior to each infusion, complete blood count and complete metabolic profile were checked. Dosing for IV-Ig was 2 g/kg divided over three consecutive days and this is repeated at a monthly interval. Rituximab dosing is 375 mg/m^2 body surface area once a week for 8 weeks and then switched to once a month interval. The average follow up was 57.5 and 55.5 months in the control group and the study group, respectively. Results showed all patients in the study group did not have progression of their OCP and visual acuity was stable. Patients in the control group all had progression of their OCP and deterioration of their vision. Immediate or delayed side effects were not observed in any of the patients in the study group. Employing combination regimen of RTX and IV-Ig successfully arrested progression of the disease and as a result restored the patients' quality of life [129]. The combination therapy of IV-Ig plus rituximab has shown to be very effective in attaining durable remission. Therefore, this combination therapy is favored for refractory cases of OCP.

Prior to the study conducted by Foster et al., reports of RTX application in treating OCP were based on case reports. Ross et al. reported a patient with severe OCP who failed oral prednisone, dapsone, and cyclophosphamide but showed response to RTX infusions. However, adjuvant therapy with oral prednisone and MMF was required to achieve remission [130]. Schumann et al. described a patient with OCP who was unresponsive to dapsone and cyclophosphamide who then showed positive outcomes after receiving four RTX infusions [131]. Concomitant therapy was administered in this patient with intravenous and oral corticosteroids. Schmidt et al. observed partial response in a MMP patient after four infusions of RTX with accompanying therapy of pulse dexamethasone and cyclophosphamide therapy. When RTX is utilized as monotherapy or in combination with other immunosuppressive therapy, the primary concern is a high risk of systemic infections potentially leading to lethal septicemia [132, 133]. Employing RTX in combination with IV-Ig, an immunomodulating agent without immunosuppressing, as adjuvant therapy, has shown to be an appropriate and safe therapeutic regimen under indicated circumstances. The study conducted by Foster et al. reported no deaths or infections in any of the patients treated with RTX.

Conclusions and Future Directions

The treatment of OCP has certainly evolved over several decades when ophthalmologists have encountered refractory disease. The majority of patients will initially require conventional immune suppression for control of their OCP. However, biologic treatments are more target specific, and treatments such as rituximab and IVIg have the potential to improve clinical outcomes and quality of life. These results could provide a basis for the earlier usage of targeted therapies in the treatment algorithm of OCP.

References

1. Neff AG, Turner M, Mutasim DF. Treatment strategies in mucous membrane pemphigoid. Ther Clin Risk Manag. 2008;4(3):617–26.
2. Higgins GT, Allan RB, Hall R, et al. Development of ocular disease in patients with mucous membrane pemphigoid involving the oral mucosa. Br J Ophthalmol. 2006;90:964–7.
3. Kirzhner M, Jakobiec FA. Ocular cicatricial pemphigoid: a review of clinical features, immunopathology, differential diagnosis and current management. Semin Ophthalmol. 2011;26(4–5):270–7.
4. Ahmed M, Zein G, Khawaja F, Foster CS. Ocular cicatricial pemphigoid: pathogenesis, diagnosis and treatment. Prog Retin Eye Res. 2004;23(6):579–92.
5. Foster CS. Cicatricial pemphigoid. Trans Am Ophthalmol Soc. 1986;84:527–663.
6. Foster CS, Wilson LA, Ekins MB. Immunosuppressive therapy for progressive ocular cicatricial pemphigoid. Ophthalmology. 1982;89:340–53.
7. Chan RY, Bhol K, Tesavibul N, et al. The role of antibody to human beta 4 integrin in conjunctival basement membrane separation: possible in vitro model for ocular cicatricial pemphigoid. Invest Ophthamol Vis Sci. 1999;40:2283–90.
8. Foster CS, Ahmed AR. Intravenous immunoglobulin therapy for ocular cicatricial pemphigoid: a preliminary study. Ophthalmology. 1999;106:2136–43.
9. Dantzig PI. Immunosuppressive and cytotoxic drugs in dermatology. Arch Dermatol. 1974;110:393–406.
10. Mondino BJ, Brown SI. Ocular cicatricial pemphigoid. Ophthalmology. 1981;88:95–100.
11. Foster CS, Neumann R, Tauber J. Long-term results of systemic chemotherapy for ocular cicatricial pemphigoid. Doc Ophthalmol. 1992;82:223–9.
12. Stephens CR. The structure of aureomycin. J Am Chem Soc. 1954;76:3568–75.
13. Sapadin AN, Fleischmajer R. Tetracyclines: nonantibiotic properties and their clinical implications. J Am Acad Dermatol. 2006;54:258–65.
14. Webster GF, Leyden JJ, McGinley KJ, et al. Suppression of polymorphonuclear leukocyte chemotactic factor production in Propionibacterium acnes by sub-minimal inhibitory concentrations of tetracyclines and erythromycin. Antimicrob Agents Chemother. 1982;21:770–2.
15. Webster G, Del Rosso JQ. Anti-inflammatory activity of tetracyclines. Dermatol Clin. 2007;25:133–5.
16. Poskitt L, Wojnarowska F. Treatment of cicatricial pemphigoid with tetracycline and nicotinamide. Clin Exp Dermatol. 1995;20:258–9.
17. Mallon E, Wojnarowska F. Cicatricial pemphigoid presenting with unusual palmar involvement, successfully treated with a combination of nicotinamide and tetracycline. Clin Exp Dermatol. 1994;19:526–30.
18. Kohler IK, Lorincz AL. Erythema elevatum diutinum treated with niacinamide and tetracycline. Arch Dermatol. 1980;116:693–5.
19. Berk MA, Lorincz AL. The treatment of bullous pemphigoid with tetracycline and niacinamide a preliminary report. Arch Dermatol. 1986;122:670–4.
20. Thornfeldt CR, Menkes AW. Bullous pemphigoid controlled by tetracycline. J Am Acad Dermatol. 1987;16:305–10.
21. Pereyo NG, Davis LS. Generalized bullous pemphigoid controlled by tetracycline therapy alone. J Am Acad Dermatol. 1995;32(1):138–9.
22. Smith CJ, Sayles H, Mikuls TR, Michaud K. Minocycline and doxycycline therapy in community patients with rheumatoid arthritis: prescribing patterns, patient-level determinants of use, and patient-reported side effects. Arthritis Res Ther. 2011;13:2–8.
23. Fourneau E. Action antistreptococcique des dérivés sulfurés organiques. CE Acad Sci. 1937;204:1763.
24. Rook A, Waddington E. Pemphigus and pemphigoid. Br J Dermatol. 1953;65:425–31.
25. Persons JR, Rogers RS. Bullous pemphigoid responding to sulfapyridine and the sulfones. Arch Dermatol. 1977;113:610–5.

26. Wertheim MS, Males JJ, Cook SD, et al. Dapsone induced haemolytic anaemia in patients treated for ocular cicatricial pemphigoid. Br J Ophthalmol. 2006;90:516.
27. Fern AI, Jay JL, Young H, et al. Dapsone therapy for the acute inflammatory phase of ocular pemphigoid. Br J Ophthalmology. 1992;76:332–5.
28. Doan S, Lerouic JF, Robin H, et al. Treatment of ocular cicatricial pemphigoid with sulfasalazine. Ophthalmology. 2001;108:1565–8.
29. Farber S, Diamond LK. Temporary remissions in acute leukemia in children produced by folic antagonist 4-aminopteroglutamic acid (aminopterin). N Engl J Med. 1948;238:787–93.
30. Wong VG. Methotrexate in the therapy of cyclitis. Trans Am Acad Ophthalmol Otolaryngol. 1965;69:279–93.
31. Okada AA. Immunomodulatory therapy for ocular inflammatory disease: a basic manual and review of the literature. Ocul Immunol Inflamm. 2005;13:335–51.
32. Kaplan-Messas A, Barkana Y, Avni I, et al. Methotrexate as a first-line corticosteroid-sparing therapy in a cohort of uveitis and scleritis. Ocul Immunol Inflamm. 2003;11:131–9.
33. Shah SS, Lowder CY, Schmitt MA, et al. Low-dose methotrexate therapy for ocular inflammatory disease. Ophthalmology. 1992;99:1419–23.
34. Samson CM, Waheed N, Baltatzis S, et al. Methotrexate therapy for chronic noninfectious uveitis: analysis of a case series of 160 patients. Ophthalmology. 2001;108:1134–9.
35. Bom S, Zamiri P, Lightman S. Use of methotrexate in the management of sight-threatening uveitis. Ocul Immunol In Flamm. 2001;9:35–40.
36. Malik AR, Pavesio C. The use of low dose methotrexate in children with chronic anterior and intermediate uveitis. Br K Ophthalmol. 2005;89:806–8.
37. Wessels JA, Huizinga TW, Guchelaar HJ. Recent insights in the pharmacological actions of methotrexate in the treatment of rheumatoid arthritis. Rheumatology (Oxford). 2008;47:249–55.
38. Gangaputra S, Newcomb CW, Liesegang TL, et al. Methotrexate for ocular inflammatory diseases. Ophthalmology. 2009;116(11):2188–98.
39. Saw VP, Dart JK. Ocular mucous membrane pemphigoid: diagnosis and management strategies. Ocul Surf. 2008;6:128–42.
40. Van Ede AE, Laan RF, Blom HJ, et al. Methotrexate in rheumatoid arthritis: an update with focus on mechanisms involved in toxicity. Semin Arthritis Rheum. 1998;27:277–97.
41. Walker AM, Funch D, Dreyer NA, et al. Determinants of serious liver disease among patients receiving low-dose methotrexate for rheumatoid arthritis. Arthritis Rheum. 1993;36:329–35.
42. Tolman KG, Clegg DO, Lee RG, et al. Methotrexate and the liver. J Rheumatol Suppl. 1985;12:29–34.
43. Hoekstra M, van Ede AE, Haagsma CJ, et al. Factors associated with toxicity, final dose, and efficacy of methotrexate in patients with rheumatoid arthritis. Ann Rheum Dis. 2003;62:423–6.
44. Lahdenne P, Rapola J, Ylijoki H, et al. Hepatoxicity in patients with juvenile idiopathic arthritis receiving longterm methotrexate therapy. J Rheumatol. 2002;29:2442–5.
45. Suwa A, Hirakata M, Satoh S, et al. Rheumatoid arthritis associated with methotrexate-induced pneumonitis: improvement with i.v. cyclophosphamide therapy. Clin Exp Rheumatol. 1999;17:355–8.
46. Salaffi F, Manganelli P, Carotti M, et al. Methotrexate-induced pneumonitis in patients with rheumatoid arthritis and psoriatic arthritis: report of five cases and review of the literature. Clin Rheumatol. 1997;16:296–304.
47. Cottin V, Tébib J, Massonnet B, et al. Pulmonary function in patients receiving long-term low-dose methotrexate. Chest. 1996;109:933–9.
48. Hilliquin P, Renoux M, Perrot S, et al. Occurrence of pulmonary complications during methotrexate therapy in rheumatoid arthritis. Br J Rheumatol. 1996;35:441–5.
49. Kempen JH, Gangaputra S, Daniel E, et al. Long-term risk of malignancy among patients treated with immunosuppressive agents for ocular inflammation: a critical assessment of the evidence. Am J Ophthalmol. 2008;146:802–12.

50. Miserocchi E, Baltatzis S, Roque MR, et al. The effect of treatment and its related side effects in patients with severe ocular cicatricial pemphigoid. Ophthalmology. 2002;109:111–8.
51. Baker KB, Spurrier NJ, Watkins AS, et al. Retention time for corticosteroid-sparing systemic immunosuppressive agents in patients with inflammatory eye disease. Br J Ophthalmol. 2006;90:1481–5.
52. Bawle EV, Conard JV, Weiss L. Adult and two children with fetal methotrexate syndrome. Teratology. 1998;57:51–5.
53. Lewden B, Vial T, Elefant E, et al. Low dose methotrexate in the first trimester of pregnancy: results of a French collaborative study. J Rheumatol. 2004;31:2360–5.
54. Pasadhika S, Kempen JH, Newcomb CW, et al. Azathioprine for ocular inflammatory diseases. Am J Ophthalmol. 2009;148(4):500–9.
55. Elion GB. The purine path to chemotherapy. Science. 1989;244(4900):41–7.
56. Patel AA, Swerlick RA, McCall CO. Azathioprine in dermatology: the past, the present, and the future. J Am Acad Dermatol. 2006;55(3):369–89.
57. Elion GB, Callahan SW, Hitchings GH, et al. The metabolism of 2-amino-6-(1-methyl-4-nitro-5-imidazolyl) thiopurine (B.W. 57–323) in man. Cancer Chemother Rep 1. 1960;8:47–52.
58. Thiersch JB. Effect of 6-(1'-methyl-4'-nitro-5'-imidazolyl)-mercaptopurine and 2-amino-6-(1'-methyl-4'-nitro-5'-imidazolyl)-mercaptopurine on the rat litter in utero. J Reprod Fertil. 1962;4:297–302.
59. Murray JE, Merrill JP, Harrison JH, et al. Prolonged survival of human-kidney homografts by immunosuppressive drug therapy. New Engl J Med. 1963;268(24):1315–23.
60. Dave VK, Vickers CF. Azathioprine in the treatment of muco-cutaneous pemphigoid. Br J Dermatol. 1974;90:183–6.
61. Ward JR. Role of disease-modifying antirheumatic drugs versus cytotoxic agents in the therapy of rheumatoid arthritis. Am J Med. 1988;85:39–44.
62. Danovitch GM. Choice of immunosuppressive drugs and individualization of immunosuppressive therapy for kidney transplant patients. Transplant Proc. 1999;31:2S–6.
63. Wise M, Callen JP. Azathioprine: a guide for the management of dermatology patients. Dermatol Ther. 2007;20:206–15.
64. Gisbert JP, Niño P, Cara C, et al. Comparative effectiveness of azathioprine in Crohn's disease and ulcerative colitis: prospective, long-term, follow-up study of 394 patients. Aliment Pharmacol Ther. 2008;28:228–38.
65. Lee JC, Gladman DD, Schentag CT, et al. The long-term use of azathioprine in patients with psoriatic arthritis. J Clin Rheumatol. 2001;7:160–5.
66. Goldstein LH, Dolinsky G, Greenberg R, et al. Pregnancy outcome of women exposed to azathioprine during pregnancy. Birth Defects Res A Clin Mol Teratol. 2007;79:696–701.
67. Alstead EM, Ritchie JK, Lennard-Jones JE, et al. Safety of azathioprine in pregnancy in inflammatory bowel disease. Gastroenterology. 1999;99:443–6.
68. Baltatzis S, Tufail F, Yu EN, et al. Mycophenolate mofetil as an immunomodulatory agent in the treatment of chronic ocular inflammatory disorders. Ophthalmology. 2003;110:1061–5.
69. Behrend M. A review of clinical experience with the novel immunosuppressive drug mycophenolate mofetil in renal transplantation. Clin Nephrol. 1996;45:336–41.
70. Zurdel J, Aboalchamat B, Zierhut M, et al. Early clinical experiences with mycophenolate mofetil for immunosuppressive therapy of ocular cicatricial pemphigoid [in German]. Klin Monbl Augenheilkd. 2001;218:222–8.
71. Larkin G, Lightman S. Mycophenolate mofetil: a useful immunosuppressive in inflammatory eye disease. Ophthalmology. 1999;106:370–4.
72. Sollinger HW. Mycophenolate mofetil for the prevention of acute rejection in primary cadaveric renal allograft recipients. Transplantation. 1995;60:225–32.
73. Boumpas DT, Kritikos HD, Daskalakis NG. Perspective on future therapy of vasculitis. Curr Rheumatol Rep. 2000;2:423–9.
74. Adu D, Cross J, Jayne DR. Treatment of systemic lupus erythematosus with mycophenolate mofetil. Lupus. 2001;10:203–8.

75. Meihsler W, Reinisch W, Moser G, et al. Is mycophenolate mofetil an effective alternative in azathioprine-intolerant patients with chronic active Crohn's disease? Am J Gastroenterol. 2001;96:782–7.
76. Schwarz A. New aspects of the treatment of nephrotic syndrome. J Am Soc Nephrol. 2001;12 Suppl 17:S44–7.
77. Chanaud III NP, Vistica BP, Eugui E, et al. Inhibition of experimental autoimmune uveoretinitis by mycophenolate mofetil, an inhibitor of purine metabolism. Exp Eye Res. 1995;61:429–34.
78. Budde K, Glander P, Bauer S, et al. Pharmacodynamic monitoring of mycophenloate mofetil. Clin Chem Lab Med. 2000;38:1213–6.
79. Ahsan N, Johnson C, Gonwa T, et al. Randomized trial of tacrolimus plus mycophenolate mofetil or azathioprine versus cyclosporine oral solution (modified) plus mycophenolate mofetil after cadaveric kidney transplantation: results at 2 years. Transplantation. 2001;72:245–50.
80. Thorne JE, Jabs DA, Qazi FA, et al. Mycophenolate mofetil therapy for inflammatory eye disease. Am Acad Ophthalmology. 2005;112:1472–7.
81. Doycheva D, Deuter C, Blumenstock G, et al. Long-term results of therapy with mycophenolate mofetil in ocular mucous membrane pemphigoid. Ocul Immunol Inflamm. 2011;19:431–8.
82. Nottage JM, Hammersmith KM, Murchison AP, et al. Treatment of mucous membrane pemphigoid with mycophenolate mofetil. Cornea. 2013;32(6):810–5.
83. Daniel E, Thorne JE, Newcomb CW, et al. Mycophenolate mofetil for ocular inflammation. Am J Ophthalmol. 2010;149(3):423–32.
84. Saw VP, Dart JK, Rauz S, et al. Immunosuppressive therapy for ocular mucous membrane pemphigoid strategies and outcomes. Ophthalmology. 2008;115:253–61.
85. Galor A, Jabs DA, Leder HA, et al. Comparison of antimetabolite drugs as corticosteroid-sparing therapy for noninfectious ocular inflammation. Ophthalmology. 2008;115:1826–32.
86. Pleyer U, Ruokonen P, Schmidt N, et al. Mycophenol acid in ocular autoimmune disorders-can we optimize this therapy? [in German]. Klin Monbl Augenheilkd. 2008;225:66–9.
87. Kilmartin DJ, Forrester JV, Dick AD. Rescue therapy with mycophenolate mofetil in refractory uveitis [letter]. Lancet. 1998;352:35–6.
88. Emadi A, Jones RJ, Brodsky RA. Cyclophosphamide and cancer: golden anniversary. Nature Reviews. Clin Oncol. 2009;6(11):638–47.
89. Elder MJ, Jones RJ, Brodsky RA. Role of cyclophosphamide and high dose steroid in ocular cicatricial pemphigoid. Br J Ophthalmology. 1995;79:264–6.
90. Roda PE. Nitrogen mustard therapy of uveitis of unknown etiology. Rev Clin Esp. 1952;44:173–80.
91. Jabs DA, Rosenbaum JT, Foster CS, et al. Guidelines for the use of immunosuppressive drugs in patients with ocular inflammatory disorders: recommendations of an expert panel. Am J Ophthalmol. 2000;130:492–513.
92. Pujari SS, Kempen JH, Newcomb CW, et al. Cyclophosphamide of ocular inflammatory diseases. Ophthalmology. 2010;117(2):356.
93. Hemady R, Tauber J, Foster CS. Immunosuppressive drugs in immune and inflammatory ocular disease. Surv Ophthalmol. 1991;35:369–85.
94. Mondino BJ. Cicatricial pemphigoid and erythema multiforme. Ophthalmology. 1990;97:939–52.
95. Tauber J, Sainz de la Maza M, Foster CS. Systemic chemotherapy for ocular cicatricial pemphigoid. Cornea. 1991;10:185–95.
96. Yesudian PD, Armstrong S, Cawood JI, et al. Mucous membrane pemphigoid: management of advanced ocular disease with intravenous cyclophosphamide and amniotic membrane transplantation. Br J Dermatol. 2005;153:692–4.
97. Pandya AG, Warren KJ, Bergstresser PR. Cicatricial pemphigoid successfully treated with pulse intravenous cyclophosphamide. Arch Dermatol. 1997;133:245–7.
98. Kaçmaz RO, Kempen JH, Newcomb C, et al. Cyclosporine for ocular inflammatory diseases. Ophthalmology. 2010;117(3):576–84.

99. Berkson BM, Lome LG, Shapiro I. Severe cystitis induced by cyclophosphamide, role of surgical management. JAMA. 1973;225:605–6.
100. Park MC, Park YB, Jung SY, et al. Risk of ovarian failure and pregnancy outcome in patients with lupus nephritis treated with intravenous cyclophosphamide pulse therapy. Lupus. 2004;13:569–74.
101. Asten P, Barrett J, Symmons D. Risk of developing certain malignancies is related to duration of immunosuppressive drug exposure in patients with rheumatic disease. J Rheumatol. 1999;26:1705–14.
102. Baltus JA, Boersma JW, Hartman AP, et al. The occurrence of malignancies in patients with rheumatoid arthritis treated with cyclophosphamide: a controlled retrospective follow-up. Ann Rheum Dis. 1983;42:368–73.
103. Baker GL, Kahl LE, Zee BC, et al. Malignancy following treatment of rheumatoid arthritis with cyclophosphamide: long-term case–control follow-up study. Am J Med. 1987;83:1–9.
104. Ostensen M. Treatment with immunosuppressive and disease modifying drugs during pregnancy and lactation. Am J Reprod Immunol. 1992;28:148–52.
105. Rubin B, Palestine AG. Complications of corticosteroid and immunosuppressive drugs. Int Ophthalmol Clin. 1989;29(3):159–71.
106. Kaplan AA. Therapeutic plasma exchange: core curriculum 2008. Am J Kidney Dis. 2008;52(6):1180–96.
107. Siami GA, Siami FS. Membrane plasmapheresis in the United States: a review over the last 20 years. Ther Apher. 2001;5(4):315–20.
108. Szczepiorkowski ZM, Bandarenko N, Kim HC, et al. Guidelines on the use of therapeutic apheresis in clinical practice--evidence-based approach from the Apheresis Applications Committee of the American Society for Apheresis. J Clin Apher. 2010;25(3):83–177.
109. Hashimoto Y, Suga Y, Yoshiike T, et al. A case of antiepiligrin cicatricial pemphigoid successfully treated by plasmapheresis. Dermatology. 2000;201:58–60.
110. Chang B, Tholpady A, Huang R, et al. Clinical and serological responses following plasmapheresis in bullous pemphigoid: two case reports and a review of the literature. Blood Transfus. 2014;12:269–75.
111. Roujeau JC, Revuz J, Touraine R, et al. Cortico-resistant bullous pemphigoid. Favorable results with plasmapheresis [In French]. Nouv Presse Med. 1979;8:3362.
112. Roujeau JC, Guillaume JC, Morel P, et al. Plasma exchange in bullous pemphigoid. Lancet. 1984;2:486–8.
113. Egan CA, Meadows KP, Zone JJ. Plasmapheresis as a steroid saving procedure in bullous pemphigoid. Int J Dermatol. 2000;39(3):230–5.
114. Mazzi G, Raineri A, Zanolli FA, et al. Plasmapheresis therapy in pemphigus vulgaris and bullous pemphigoid. Transfus Apher Sci. 2003;28:13–8.
115. Gurland HJ, Lysaght MJ, Samtleben W, et al. A comparison of centrifugal and membrane-based apheresis formats. Int J Artif Organ. 1984;7(1):35–8.
116. Yamada H, Yaguchi H, Takamori K, et al. Plasmapheresis for the treatment of pemphigus vulgaris and bullous pemphigoid. Therupeutic A. 1997;1(2):178–82.
117. Turner MS, Sutton D, Sauder DN. The use of plasmapheresis and immunosuppression in the treatment of pemphigus vulgaris. J Am Acad Dermatol. 2000;43:1058–64.
118. Bohn J, Jonsson S, Holst R. Successful treatment of recalcitrant cicatricial pemphigoid with a combination of plasma exchange and cyclophosphamide. Br J of Dermatol. 1999;141:536–40.
119. Hashimoto Y, Suga Y, Yoshiike T, et al. A case of antiepiligrin cicatricial successfully treated by plasmapheresis. Dermatology. 2001;201:58–60.
120. Tellier Z. Intravenous immunoglobulin in eye involvement. Clin Rev Allergy Immun. 2005;29:295–306.
121. Ahmed AR, Dahl MV. Consensus statement on the use of intravenous immunoglobulin therapy in the treatment of autoimmune mucocutaneous blistering diseases. Arch Dermatol. 2003;139:1051–9.

122. Kazatchkine MD. Immunomodulation of autoimmune and inflammatory disease with intravenous immune globulin. N Engl J Med. 2001;345:747–55.
123. Tellier Z. Human immunoglobulins in intraocular inflammation. Ann NY Acad Sci. 2007;1110:337–47.
124. Neumann R, Tauber J, Foster CS. Remission and recurrence after withdrawal of therapy for ocular cicatricial pemphigoid. Ophthalmology. 1991;98:858–62.
125. Mondino BJ, Brown SI. Immunosuppressive therapy in ocular cicatricial pemphigoid. Am J Ophthalmol. 1983;96:453–9.
126. Letko E, Miserocchi E, Daoud YJ, et al. A nonradomized comparison of the clinical outcome of ocular involvement in patients with mucous membrane (cicatricial) pemphigoid between conventional immunosuppressive and intravenous immunoglobulin therapies. Clin Immunol. 2004;111:303–10.
127. Foster CS, Ahmed AR. Intravenous immunoglobulin therapy for ocular cicatricial pemphigoid. Am Acad Ophthalmology. 1999;106:2136–43.
128. Sami N, Bhol KC, Razzaque AA, et al. Intravenous immunoglobulin therapy in patients with multiple mucosal involvement in mucous membrane pemphigoid. Clin Immunol. 2002;102:59–67.
129. Foster CS, Chang PY, Ahmed AR. Combination of rituximab and intravenous immunoglobulin for recalcitrant ocular cicatricial pemphigoid. Am Acad Ophthalmology. 2010;117:861–9.
130. Ross AH, Jaycock P, Cook SD, et al. The use of rituximab in refractory mucous membrane pemphigoid with severe ocular involvement. Br J Ophthalmol. 2009;93:421–2, 548.
131. Schumann T, Schmidt E, Booken N, et al. Successful treatment of mucous membrane pemphigoid with the anti-CD-20 antibody rituximab [letter]. Acta Derm Venereol. 2009;89:101–2.
132. Gurcan HM, Keskin DB, Stern JN, et al. A review of the current use of rituximab in autoimmune diseases. Int Immunopharmacol. 2009;9:10–25.
133. El Tal AK, Posner MR, Spigelman Z, et al. Rituximab: a monoclonal antibody to CD20 used in the treatment of pemphigus vulgaris. J Am Acad Dermatol. 2006;55:449–59.

Chapter 6
Mucous Membrane Pemphigoid

Lawrence S. Chan, Young Kwak, and Naveed Sami

Abstract Mucous membrane pemphigoid (MMP) is a term categorizing a group of autoimmune sub-epithelial blistering diseases affecting primarily mucous membrane areas. These diseases mainly affect one or more mucous membranes, and can also affect the skin in a minor fashion. The common features that define this group of diseases are: (1). Mucous membranes are the predominantly affected areas; (2). Pathology of the lesional epithelium demonstrates a sub-epithelial blister; (3). Immunopathology of the peri-lesional epithelium shows linear deposition of immunoglobulin and/or complement component (C3) at the epithelial basement membrane. The therapeutic strategy should be based on both the progressiveness of the disease and the specific mucous membranes affected. Systemic treatments currently available for physicians to employ include dapsone, corticosteroids, immunosuppressives, intravenous immunoglobulin, and, most recently, biologics such as rituximab, an anti-CD20 monoclonal antibody to mature B cells.

Keywords Mucous membrane • Antibody • Antigen • Basement membrane • Immunosuppressives • Corticosteroid • Dapsone • Azathioprine • Mycophenolate mofetil • Rituximab

Nomenclature

Despite a recently published consensus statement on the terminology of this group of diseases [1], several other terms are still being used in the literature. Some authors continue to utilize the term "cicatricial pemphigoid" rather than "mucous membrane pemphigoid" (MMP) [2]. Others employ various terms such as "benign mucous membrane pemphigoid" or "ocular pemphigoid". Thus, some clarification

L.S. Chan, MD (✉)
Department of Dermatology, University of Illinois College of Medicine,
808 S. Wood St., R380, MC624, Chicago, IL 60612, USA
e-mail: larrycha@uic.edu

Y. Kwak, MD, CSM • N. Sami, MD, FAAD
Department of Dermatology, University of Alabama-Birmingham, Birmingham, AL, USA
e-mail: nsami@uabmc.edu; nsderm@gmail.com

N. Sami (ed.), *Autoimmune Bullous Diseases: Approach and Management*,
DOI 10.1007/978-3-319-26728-9_6

still seems necessary in this regard. In a meeting leading to the first international consensus statement on MMP, the rationale of the consenting parties favored the term "MMP" over "cicatricial pemphigoid." This was based on the facts that although cicatricial (scarring) manifestation is a common clinical feature for this group of diseases, it is not a feature present in all affected patients. For example, MMP patients with clinical disease occurring only in the oral mucous membranes usually do not result in a dysfunctional scarring process [1]. Furthermore, the consenting parties agreed to drop the modifying word, "benign," because disease processes involving the ocular, laryngeal, esophageal, or genital mucosae tend to be aggressive in nature, and can lead to significant scar formation. The loss of function in major organs can result in complications such as blindness, or strictures of the larynx, esophagus, or genital orifice. These sequellae, therefore, could not be considered as a benign outcome of the disease [1]. Hence, the modifier does not appear to be appropriate in those circumstances. Moreover, disease processes initially affecting one organ could later impact other organs in the same patient. Therefore, it does not seem appropriate to name a disease in a manner restricted to a single organ. Based on those logics, the consenting parties decided to promote the inclusive term, "MMP," for this group of diseases [1].

Clinical Presentation

Since this group of diseases can affect an individual patient on one or more mucous membrane areas, there is no single typical clinical presentation for MMP. Rather, the disease, if affecting a given mucosal area, can exhibit certain "typical" morphologies. In the following, these morphological presentations are described and displayed to demonstrate the points. Although this group of diseases tends to primarily affect adults in their 50s and 60s, childhood onset has been infrequently reported in the literature [3]. MMP should be distinguished from other forms of autoimmune sub-epidermal blistering skin diseases that can also affect the mucous membranes. These include lichen planus, paraneoplastic pemphigus, Stevens-Johnson syndrome, erythema multiforme, linear IgA bullous dermatosis, epidermolysis bullosa acquisita, bullous pemphigoid, and two other newly characterized bullous dermatoses on a clinical, histological, and immunological basis [1].

Skin Lesions

In addition to the major involvement of mucous membranes, patients afflicted by MMP may or may not have minor skin lesions. When present, these lesions could be blisters, erosions, or a combination of both. While any area of the body can be affected, it is more commonly observed on the upper trunk and head. With treatment, skin lesions tend to respond to medication and resolve more rapidly than those lesions on mucous membranes. Residual scarring tends to be a characteristic feature that can distinguish MMP from other autoimmune blistering diseases such as bullous pemphigoid and pemphigus. The histopathology of a skin lesion would be expected to be similar to that of a mucosal lesion.

Oral Lesions

The oral mucosa is the most commonly affected mucosal surface in MMP [1]. Lesions generally manifest as erythematous patches, erosions, pseudomembrane-covered erosions, and rarely blisters. The common locations of lesions are the palate and attached gingivae, but the mucous membranes of the tongue, buccal area, and labial area can also be involved (Fig. 6.1a–c). Scarring in the oral cavity, however, is rare.

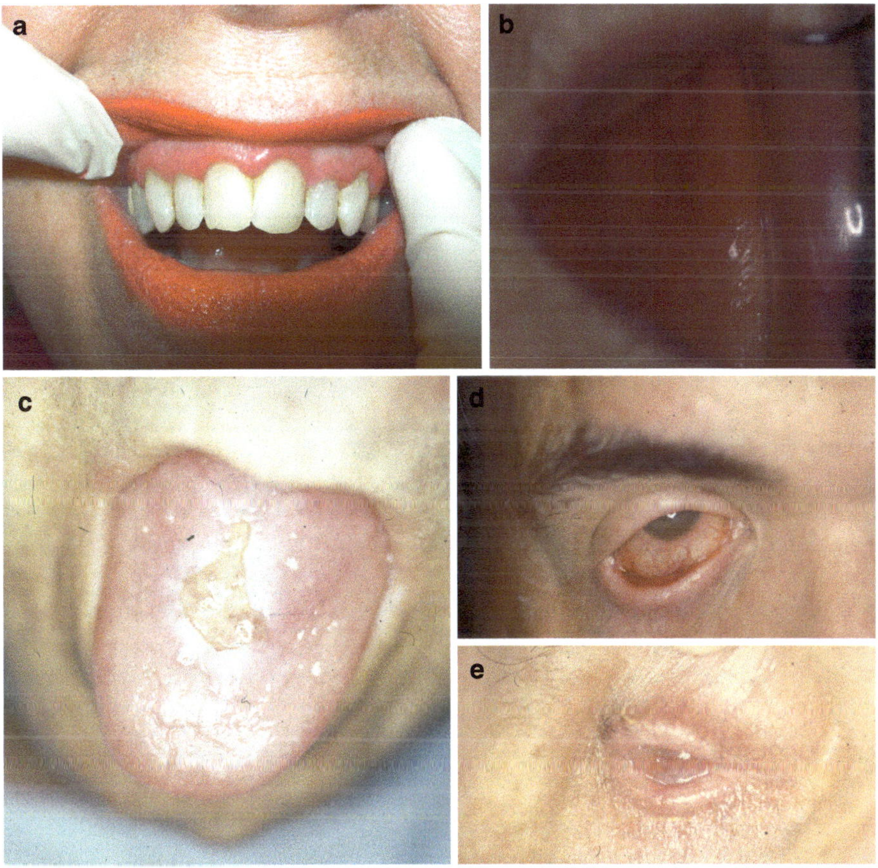

Fig. 6.1 Clinical morphology of MMP. (**a**) Inflammation of attached gingival; (**b**) Involvement of buccal mucosa; (**c**) Erosion of dorsal tongue; (**d**) Ocular inflammation and symblepharon; (**e**) Ocular ankyloblepharon

Ocular Lesions

Ocular involvement represents the second most common mucosal surface involved in MMP [1]. Ocular disease starts with inflammation and erosions on the lower bulbar conjunctiva, and blisters are not commonly observed. As inflammation continues, this process leads to symblepharon formation (Fig. 6.1d, e), and results in shortening of the fornix and in-turning of the eyelashes (entropion). Entropion defects cause irritation to the cornea, leading to corneal neovascularization, corneal opacification (scarring), and eventually blindness. Sometimes, fusion of the medial or lateral corners of the eye can occur, causing ankyloblepharon formation. Ocular involvement and disease staging have been discussed in a separate chapter on the treatment of ocular pemphigoid.

Genital Lesions

Although involvement of MMP on genital mucosae is not commonly observed, it can be very symptomatic in patients. The individual lesional morphology is very similar to that observed in the oral mucosa, and includes inflammation, blisters, erosions, and erythematous patches. However, if not treated at the onset of disease or treated insufficiently, the end result of genital mucosal lesions could involve significant stricturing of the genital orifice, and severe impairment of a patient's normal functions of urination and sexual activities.

Other Mucosal Lesions

Rarely, MMP involves the esophageal, laryngeal, and anal mucosae. Dysphagia, hoarseness, and painful defecation are the symptoms and signs which alert physicians for possible involvement of these sites. To fully identify the lesions, most cases require endoscopic examination. The individual lesional morphology in these areas is not different from those observed in the oral mucosa. As is the case with the genital mucosa, sufficient treatment needs to be provided in a timely manner to prevent dysfunctional scarring from stricture formation.

Diagnostic Methods

Mucous membranes are common areas of involvement in multiple autoimmune blistering diseases that can mimic MMP. For example, the oral mucosa is affected in 70 % of pemphigus vulgaris (PV), and one study reported that more than 50 % of PV presents with the oral cavity as the primary site of involvement [4]. PV can also involve other similar mucosal surfaces as MMP, including the esophagus and genital areas [5, 6]. In addition, paraneoplastic pemphigus, which presents in patients with certain internal malignancies, characteristically manifests as a severe case of mucositis affecting multiple mucous membranes such as the oral, ocular, and genital regions [7]. Thus, utilization of accurate diagnostic methodologies is essential to distinguish MMP from other autoimmune blistering diseases. An algorithm for this purpose is depicted in Fig. 6.2. Starting from blistering diseases affecting mucosal surfaces, the histopathology of a biopsy specimen from lesional epithelial tissue will effectively divide patients into two distinct groups: the pemphigus group with intra-epithelial blisters, and the pemphigoid group with sub-epithelial blisters. Performing direct immunofluorescence (DIF) microscopy on peri-lesional epithelial tissue can allow for

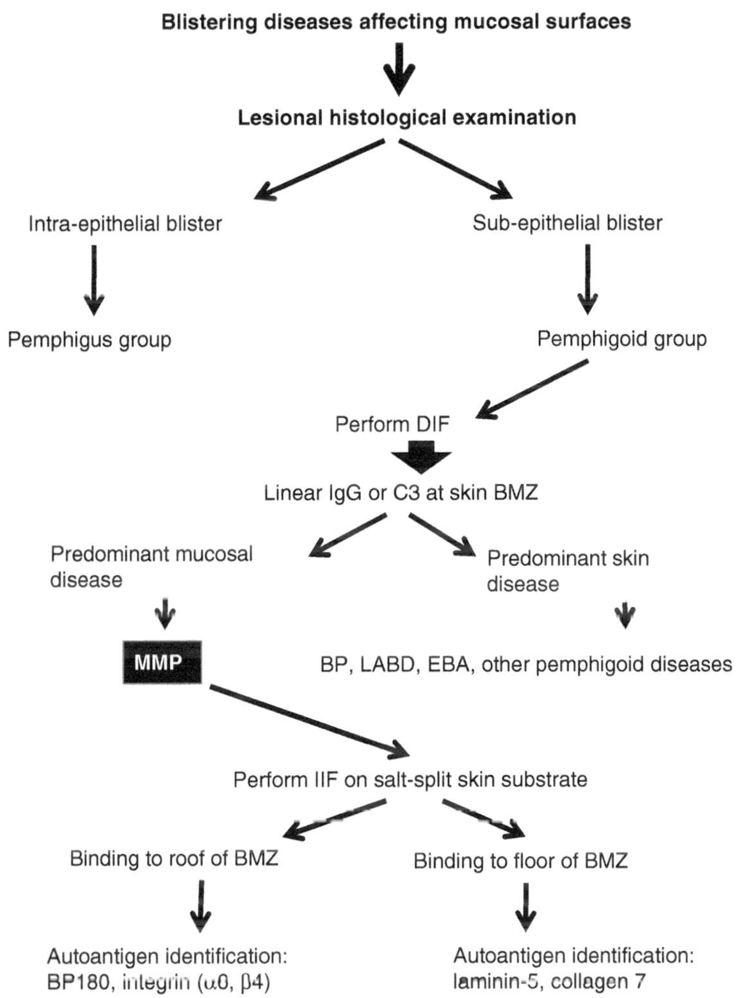

Fig. 6.2 Diagnostic methodology for MMP: an algorithm approach

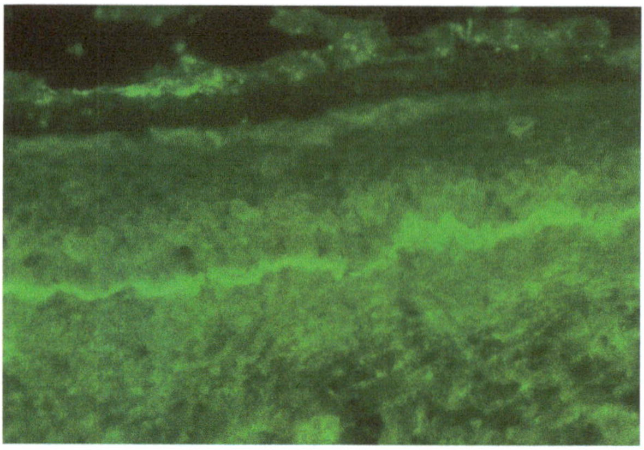

Fig. 6.3 Immunopathology of MMP: direct immunofluorescence microscopic finding of linear IgG deposit in epithelial basement membrane

further examination of the pemphigoid group of patients. This would confirm the diagnosis of "pemphigoid" by the detection of immunoglobulin and/or complement component 3 at the epithelial basement membrane zone [1] (Fig. 6.3). Within this confirmed "pemphigoid" group, patients with predominantly mucosal disease will be classified as "MMP." Based on other clinical and immunological features, patients with disease predominantly involving the skin surface will be categorized into other pemphigoid diseases, including linear IgA bullous dermatosis [8], epidermolysis bullosa acquisita [9], bullous pemphigoid [10], or two other rare pemphigoid diseases [11, 12]. Further sub-classification of MMP can be conducted through indirect immunofluorescence microscopy (IIF) on salt-split skin, and autoantigen identification by immunoblotting or enzyme-linked immunosorbent assay (ELISA) [13–19]. Despite the usefulness of MMP sub-classification, experts in the field consider that the general therapeutic strategy for all subgroups of MMP is essentially independent of this sub-classification result [1].

Treatment

The treatment of MMP can be challenging. This is due to the heterogeneous presentation of the disease along with a variable response to treatment. The current treatment options that are utilized are based on anecdotal case reports and case series. The therapeutic recommendations and algorithms have been made in consensus statements by panels of experts [1, 20]. A summary of the major studies, which were reviewed in a recent consensus statement, are presented in Tables 6.1 and 6.2, and covers the use of topical tacrolimus, laser therapy, and systemic treatments including minocycline, dapsone, azathioprine, mycophenolate mofetil, rituximab, and intravenous immunoglobulin (IVIg) [20–40]. The treatment of ocular pemphigoid was not included since this is reviewed in a separate chapter.

Table 6.1 Mucous membrane pemphigoid treatments

Treatment(s)	Patients	Clinical areas involved	Adjuvant treatment(s)	Results	Time to response	Follow-up	Previous treatments	Notes
Tacrolimus [21] 0.1 % ointment QD	# 1 62 yo F	Genital	**Pred** 40 mg QD × 3 mos until CR, then stopped	CR	3 mos	[a]	Pred 40 mg QD tapered to 10 mg + MMF 2 g QD AZA 150 mg QD	Resolution maintained 3+ mos on tacrolimus oint only
Tacrolimus [22] 0.1 % ointment QD	# 2 67 yo M, 66 yo F	Oral	None	CR	2–3 mos	6–8 mos	Topical & systemic steroids, tetracycline, systemic retinoids, chloroquine[a] Specifics not listed[a]	Applied w dental swabs placed on areas for 15 min BID, mouth rinsed after removal of swabs Ointment Not swallowed Remission maintained during f/u
Tacrolimus [23] 0.1 % ointment TID	# 1 70 yo F	Oral	None	MR	PR – 2 wks MR – 6 wks	14 mos	Triamcinolone 0.1 % paste, intralesional steroid[a], Dex oral rinse (0.5 mg/5 cc) TID – QID	PR = 80 % lesion reduction MR = 95 % lesion reduction
Tacrolimus [24] 0.03 % oral suspension 5 min rinse BID	# 1 84 yo M	Oral	None	CR	2 mos	4 mos	None	Tacrolimus tablets reconstituted in aqueous solution of tacrolimus 0.03 %, carboxymethylene 1 %, methyl parahydroxybenzoate 0.07 %, propylparahydroxybenzoate 0.03 %, water 98.9 %
Minocycline [25] 100 mg BID initially	# 9 Mean 63.5 yo All F	Oral Aerodigestive	5 Pts continued previous compounded **clobetasol** 0.05 % oint & 4 % hydroxyethyl cellulose gel BID	3 × CR 4 × PR 2 × NR	4–16 wks	Mean 4.5 yrs	Compounded clobetasol 0.05 % oint & 4 % hydroxyethyl cellulose gel BID	5 Pts initially with compounded clobetasol 0.05 % oint 5 stopped due to adverse effects (vertigo > GI) High doses (200 mg/day) limited due to frequent adverse effects

(continued)

Table 6.1 (continued)

Treatment(s)	Patients	Clinical areas involved	Adjuvant treatment(s)	Results	Time to response	Follow-up	Previous treatments	Notes
Mycophenolate sodium enteric-coated [26] Initially 360 mg BID, then 720 mg BID	# 2 63 yo M, 68 yo F	Mucosa Cutaneous	**Mpred** initially 1 mg/kg/d IV transitioned to oral 8 mg – 16 mg QD	1 × CR 1 × PR	CR – 3 mos PR – 2 mos	2–4 mos	Systemic corticosteroids[a] CSA[a]	
Cyclophosphamide [27] 2 mg/kg/day	# 13 6 M, 7 F Mean 69 yo (55–86 yo)	Oral Ocular Aerodigestive Genital	10 Pts continued previous **Dap**[a], **Sulfasalazine**[a], topical agents[a]	7 × CR 2 × PR 4 × NR	PR to MR – 4–12 wks CR – 16–52 wks	~12 mos	Dap[a], Sulfasalazine[a], topical agents[a]	3 Pts relapsed after CR (6–18 wks) Lymphopenia most common adverse effect Mean duration of CYCP administration 12 wks (range 2–52 wks)
Multiple regimens [28] **Azathioprine**[a] **Colchicine** 1 mg – 1.5 mg QD (12 Pts) **Cyclophosphamide** 1 g QD (2 Pts) **Dapsone** 100 mg QD (10 Pts)	# 15 F:M = 2.8:1 Mean 63 yo (37–78 yo)	Oral Ocular Aerodigestive Genital	**Pred** 40 mg QD All patients except 1	**Colc** – 5 × CR, 3 × PR **Dap** – 3 × CR **AZA** – 1 × PR **CYCP** – 1 × CR, 1 × PR	[a]	Mean 4 yrs (4 mos – 16 yrs)	[a]	Colc had an overall 67 % response rate Colc 1.5 mg dose did not offer any significant advantage, stopped due to diarrhea

Combination therapy [29] **Dapsone** (initial 50 mg QD) **Mycophenolate mofetil** (initial 1–1.5 g QD) **Prednisolone** (initial 30–80 mg QD)	# 6 4 M, 2 F Mean 64.8 yo (43–86 yo)	Oral Ocular Aerodigestive Genital Cutaneous	**Minocycline** 100 mg then **doxycycline**[a] (1 Pt) Topical corticosteroids[a]	CR	[a]	18 mos	Majority received topical treatment[a] + prednisolone[a] or Dap[a]	MMF (initial dose – 1 g/d × 5 Pts, 1.5 g/d × 1 Pt, adjusted at 18 mos to 0.5–1.5 g QD) Dap (initial dose – 50 mg/d, adjusted to 25–50 mg, 1 Pt stopped) Prednisolone (initial dose – 30 mg/d × 5 Pts, 80 mg/d × 1 Pt, tapered w remission at 18 mos to 5–10 mg QD to QOD)
980 nm diode Laser [30] Low-level laser twice weekly – gallium-aluminum-arsenice diode laser (*Laser settings under Notes*)	# 3 1 M, 2 F Mean 79.4 yo (± 6.71)	Oral	[a]	CR	Mean 9.66 sessions (±4.72)	Mean 13.33 mos (±9.45 mos)	[a]	Laser Settings: diameter 0.6 cm, spot size 0.28 cmq, output power 300 mW, fluence 4 J/cmq @ 2 mm distance, scanning speed 1 cm/s 1 Pt had recurrence during f/u treated successfully with laser

CR complete response, *MR* marked response, *PR* partial response, *NR* no response, *Pt* patient, *Pts* patients, *F* female, *M* male *mos* months, *wks* weeks, *f/u* follow up, *oint* ointment, *soln* solution, *SQ* subcutaneous, *IV* intravenous, *Pred* prednisone, *Mpred* methylprednisolone, *Dex* dexamethasone, *AZA* azathioprene, *MMF* mycophenolate mofetil, *CYCP* cyclophosphamide, *CSA* cyclosporine, *Dap* dapsone, *MTX* methotrexate, *Colc* colchicine, *Yo* year-old, *Wks* weeks

[a]Specifics not listed (i.e. dosage, duration)

Table 6.2 Mucous membrane pemphigoid treatments

Treatment(s)	Patients	Clinical areas involved	Adjuvant treatment(s)	Results	Time to response	Follow-up	Previous treatments	Notes
Etanercept [31] 25 mg SQ twice weekly	# 3 60 yo F, 47 yo F, 49 yo F	Oral Ocular	Pt 1 – **AZA** 100 mg BID + **Dap** 75 mg QD Pt 2 – **IVIg**[a] Pt 3 – nystatin swish + **clobetasol** oint	1 × CR 2 × MR	CR – 1 mo MR – 1 mo	1–2 yrs	Pt 1 – Dap + Pred + AZA; added nystatin swish + clobetasol oint Pt 2 – Dex elixir + topical fluocinonide 0.05 % gel; IVIg + Pred + Dap + nystatin swish + clobetasol oint; IVIg + MMF + nystatin swish + clobetasol oint Pt 3 – nystatin swish + clobetasol oint	Pt 1 – adjuvant dapsone stopped after 1 mo with initial response Pt 2 – marked improvement after 1 mo & IVIg tapered off & Etanercept changed to 50 mg once weekly
Etanercept [32] 25–50 mg SQ once to twice weekly (initial dose 25 mg)	# 1 63 yo F	Oral Ocular Aerodigestive	**AZA** 150–250 mg QD (initial dose 250 mg QD)	MR	PR – 8 wks MR – [a]	2 yrs	CYCP[a], Dap[a], minocycline[a], systemic steroids[a] AZA 250 mg QD	At 8 wks, etanercept changed to 50 mg SQ twice weekly Over 2 yrs, etanercept decreased to 50 mg SQ once weekly, AZA decreased to 150 mg QD
Rituximab [33] 375 mg/m^2 4 doses on 1st & 3rd month	# 1 22 yo M	Oral Ocular Cutaneous	**MMF** 1 g BID + **Pred** 10 mg QD	CR	PR – 4 mos CR – 7 mos	7 mos	Dap, MTX, systemic steroids[a], IVIg × 3 cycles, MMF[a] Specifics not listed[a]	Received 4 additional rituximab maintenance doses over 7 mos
Rituximab [34] 375 mg/m^2 weekly × 4 weeks	# 1 69 yo M	Ocular Perianal Cutaneous	**Dex** 100 mg QD × 3 days pulse dose while tapering **Mpred** Dex pulse dose intervals spaced to 7 wks then stopped 6 mos after rituximab	CR	~6 mos[a]	12 mos	Mpred 0.5 mg/kg + Dap 100 mg QD × 3 wks IV pulse Dex 100 mg QD × 3 days + CYCP 500 mg once at wks 2, 5, 9 + Mpred 20 mg QD between pulses 4 × weekly Dex pulses	Systemic corticosteroids discontinued 6 mos after rituximab infusions

Rituximab [35] 375 mg/m² weekly × 4 weeks 1 cycle or 2 cycles if PR/NR to 1st cycle	# 25 16 F, 9 M Mean 66 yo (17–89 yo)	Ocular Aerodigestive Cutaneous	21 Pts continued prior **Dap** (1 mg/kg/d)/**sulfasalazine** (1–3 g/d)/topical corticosteroids[a] Specifics not listed[a]	17 × CR 6 × PR	CR – median 12 wks (2–32 wks) PR – 4 wks	Median 24 mos (4–72 mos)	Dap[a] and/or Sulfasalazine[a] Pred[a] IVIg[a] CYCP[a], AZA[a], MMF[a], MTX[a]	23 of 25 responded 72 % responded after 1st cycle 92 % responded after 2nd cycle 2 fatal infectious complications
Rituximab [36] 375 mg/m² weekly	# 2 76 yo F, 73 yo F	Oral Ocular Nasal Genital	**Pred** 5–30 mg QD	1 × CR 1 × PR	[a]	4.75–6 mos	Topical corticosteroids[a] Pred 30 mg QD Dap 100 mg QD/MMF 2 g QD/etanercept 50 mg/wk	
IVIg [37] 1.6 g/kg per pulse q 4 weeks × 5 months	# 1 51 yo M	Oral Ocular Aerodigestive	**Pred** 10 mg QD after 5 mos of IVIg	CR	5 mos	7 mos	Pred 60–80 mg QAM + CYCP 100–200 mg QD Pred 60 mg QD + pulse CYCP 1000 mg/month	
IVIg [38] 2 g/kg per cycle monthly over 4 or 5 days	# 4 60 yo F, 65 yo F, 80 yo F, 65 yo[a]	Oral Ocular Genital	2 Pts = none 1 Pt = **Pred + CYCP**[a] 1 Pt = **Pred + CYCP**[a]**/MMF**[a]	1 × CR 2 × PR 1 × NR	CR – 8 mos PR – 3 mos	18–252 mos	Pred + Dap[a]/AZA[a]/CYCP[a] Topical corticosteroids[a], topical tacrolimus	IVIg discontinued in both PR Pts due to adverse effects
IVIg [39] 2 g/kg per cycle q 3–4 weeks	# 1 29 yo F	Oral Laryngeal	**Dap**[a]	CR	6 mos	>5 yrs	Dap 200 mg QD, Pred 60 mg QD	Dapsone slowly tapered and discontinued once response to IVIg was observed Total duration of IVIg ~20 months

(continued)

Table 6.2 (continued)

Treatment(s)	Patients	Clinical areas involved	Adjuvant treatment(s)	Results	Time to response	Follow-up	Previous treatments	Notes
Combination therapy [40] **Cyclophosphamide** 1.5 mg/kg/day × 4 weeks **IVIg** 1 g/kg/day × 2 days **Prednisolone** 2 mg/kg/day	# 1 75 yo F	Oral Ocular Cutaneous	None	Initially MR Eventually NR	1 wk after 1st IVIg dose	2 mos	Prednisolone 1.5 mg/kg/day + Dap 50 mg QD × 3 mos Prednisolone 2 mg/kg/day + IVIg 1 g/kg QD × 2 days for 5 cycles CYCP 1.5 mg/kg/day added to above regimen – stopped after 4 wks for bone marrow suppression	This was a recalcitrant case that responded well to 1st IVIg dose, but gradually lost efficacy with subsequent IVIg doses Patient died

CR complete response, *MR* marked response, *PR* partial response, *NR* no response, *Pt* patient, *Pts* patients, *F* female, *M* male, *mo* month, *mos* months, *wks* weeks, *wkly* weekly, *oint* ointment, *SQ* subcutaneous, *IV* intravenous, *Pred* prednisone, *Mpred* methylprednisolone, *Dex* dexamethasone, *AZA* azathioprene, *MMF* mycophenolate mofetil, *CYCP* cyclophosphamide, *Dap* dapsone, *MTX* methotrexate, *Yo* year-old, *Wks* weeks

[a]Specifics not listed (i.e. dosage, duration)

Therapeutic Strategies

In the first international consensus meeting on MMP, the consenting parties concurred that before appropriate therapies are provided to our patients, it is best to delineate patients into two distinct prognostic groups: (1). Those patients having mucosal disease affecting only the oral cavity are considered to be in the good prognostic group; and (2). Those patients having mucosal disease affecting ocular, laryngeal, esophageal, or genital mucosae are categorized in the poor prognostic group [1]. The rationale for such division is based on the fact that pemphigoid diseases exclusively involving the oral mucosa do not usually lead to a scarring process. For such patients with non-progressive localized oral MMP, topical therapy such as topical tacrolimus (Table 6.1) can be considered and has been discussed in detail in a separate chapter on local therapy. On the contrary, pemphigoid diseases involving ocular, esophageal, laryngeal, or genital mucosae have a greater tendency to form a dysfunctional scarring process, potentially resulting in blindness and organ strictures. Based on this rationale, the consenting parties recommended two distinct paths of therapeutic approaches. A therapeutic algorithm of systemic medications, based in part on the first international consensus and expanded to include updated literature, is depicted in Fig. 6.4 [1]. In addition, topically applied corticosteroids, usually ranging from class I to III potency, could also be added to a systemic regimen (Fig. 6.4).

Treatment for the "Good" Prognostic Group

Since blistering occurring in oral mucosae has little tendency to cause major functional impairment from scarring, patients with lesions restricted to the oral mucosa are considered to be in a "good" prognostic group. However, certain cases may be severe or rapidly progressive. For most cases with mild to moderate severity and without the tendency to progress rapidly, dapsone, usually in a daily dose of 100 mg, could be used as a first line of treatment. A low dose of prednisone, in a daily dose of 10–15 mg, could also be added. The combined regimen of dapsone and prednisone usually has the capacity to control the disease in most cases. For partial responders, additional immunosuppressives, such as azathioprine (usually in a daily dose of 50–100 mg) or mycophenolate mofetil (usually in a daily dose of 500–1,000 mg) could be included in the regimen. A different strategy could be employed for severe and rapidly progressive cases. For example, rather than waiting for a response with a single or double medication regimen, a triple combination of dapsone, prednisone, and an immunosuppressive (azathioprine or mycophenolate mofetil) could be initiated from the outset [1, 29]. In patients where this triple combination does not result in a complete response, the next available course of action would be a different triple combination of dapsone, prednisone, and a stronger immunosuppressive (cyclophosphamide, usually in a daily dose of 100 mg) [1]. Rituximab and IVIg can also be considered as alternatives to cyclophosphamide in recalcitrant disease [33–39, 41–43].

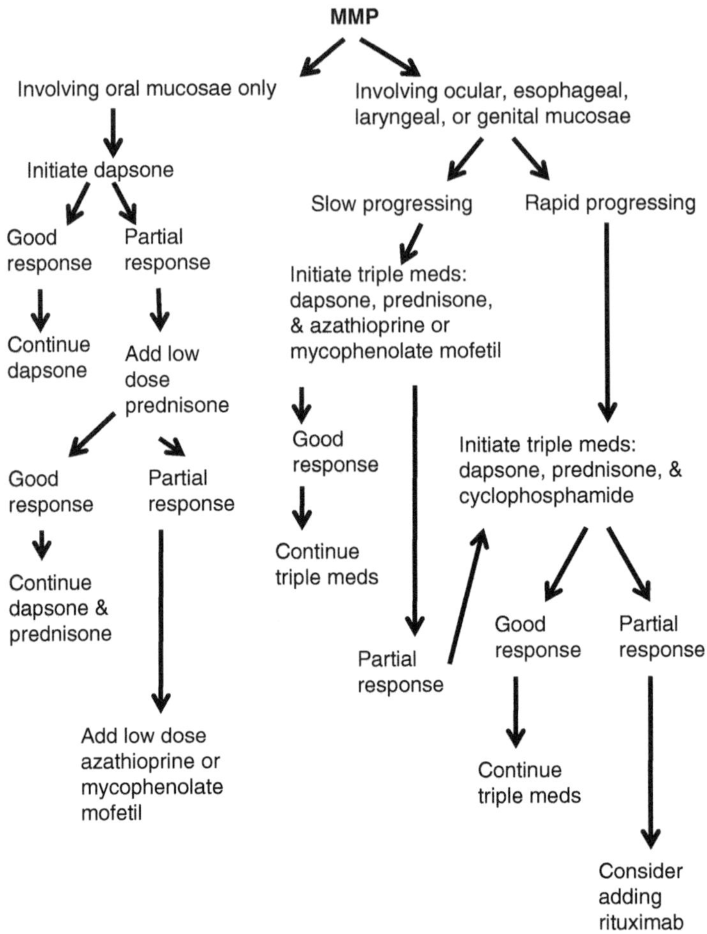

Fig. 6.4 Treatment of MMP: an algorithm of strategy

Treatment for the "Poor" Prognostic Group

The "poor" prognostic group consists of patients with mucous membrane involvement of the ocular, laryngeal, esophageal, or genital region. This is due to the tendency to form scarring from the blistering processes. Scarring in these areas can lead to irreversible functional impairment such as blindness with conjunctival involvement. Even though procedural or surgical interventions are available to relieve scarring and stricture formation, such as dilatation for the esophagus, the outcomes are not optimal. Thus, the best therapeutic strategy is prevention by aggressively controlling the inflammatory process that directly leads to the scarring. Towards that end, a triple combination of dapsone, prednisone, and immunosuppressives should be initiated from the very outset. For rapidly progressing cases, dapsone (usually 100 mg daily), prednisone (usually 50–80 mg daily), and immunosuppressives (daily dose of cyclophosphamide 100 mg) could be initiated [1]. Recent studies suggest that cyclophosphamide can be used to treat severe refractory MMP without systemic corticosteroids [27], and pulsed intravenous cyclophosphamide could be used as an alternative to the oral form [44, 45]. For patients whose disease does not progress rapidly, dapsone (usually 100 mg daily), prednisone (usually 50–80 mg daily), and immunosuppressives (daily dose of azathioprine 100–200 mg or mycophenolate mofetil 2 g) could be alternative options. A recent study also supports the use of mycophenolate mofetil as an initial treatment option for MMP [45]. Additionally, rituximab and IVIg have shown promising results, and may be considered earlier in the treatment algorithm [33–39, 41–43].

Future Directions and Conclusion

Despite continued advances in the treatment of MMP, therapeutic strategies and improved disease understanding are still evolving. Our current understanding and approach is based on the anecdotal experiences of experts spanning over several decades. Randomized clinical trials may not be practical for MMP since the disease is rare and diverse in its presentation, and insufficient therapy can lead to significant functional impairments. However, an attempt to have a standardized disease severity scale for each region of involvement (as currently established for ocular pemphigoid) may facilitate clinical trials examining regional responses to specific treatments.

References

1. Chan LS, Ahmed AR, Anhalt GJ, Bernauer W, Cooper KD, Elder MJ, et al. The first international consensus on mucous membrane pemphigoid. Arch Dermatol. 2002;138(3):370–9.
2. Arafat SN, Suelves AM, Spurr-Michaud S, Chodosh J, Foster CS, Dohlman CH, et al. Neutrophil collagenase, gelatinase, and myeloperoxidase in tears of patients with Stevens-Johnson syndrome and ocular cicatricial pemphigoid. Ophthalmology. 2014;121(1):79–87.
3. Lavallee A, Bourret-Massicotte D, Laughrea PA. Childhood mucous membrane pemphigoid: a case with exclusively ocular involvement. Cornea. 2013;32(10):1399–401.
4. Shamim T, Varghese VI, Shameena PM, Sudha S. Pemphigus vulgaris in oral cavity: clinical analysis of 71 cases. Med Oral Patol Oral Cir Bucal. 2008;13(10):E622–4.
5. Mohan P, Srinivas CR, Leelakrishnan V. A rare initial presentation of esophageal involvement in pemphigus. Dis Esophagus. 2013;26(3):351.
6. Akhyani M, Chams Davatchi C, Naraghi Z, Daneshpazhooh M, Toosi S, Asgari M, et al. Cervicovaginal involvement in pemphigus vulgaris: a clinical study of 77 cases. Br J Dermatol. 2008;158(3):478–82.
7. Anhalt GJ, Kim SC, Stanley JR, Korman NJ, Jabs DA, Kory M, et al. Paraneoplastic pemphigus: an autoimmune mucocutaneous disease associated with neoplasia. N Engl J Med. 1990;323(25):1729–35.
8. Egan CA, Zone JJ. Linear IgA bullous dermatosis. Int J Dermatol. 1999;38(11):818–27.

9. Woodley DT, Briggaman RA, O'Keefe EJ, Inman AO, Queen LL, Gammoan WR. Identification of the skin basement-membrane autoantigen in epidermolysis bullosa acquisita. N Engl J Med. 1984;310(16):1007–13.
10. Diaz LA, Ratrie 3rd H, Saunders WS, Futamara S, Squiquera HL, Anhalt GJ, et al. Isolation of a human epidermal cDNA corresponding to the 180-kD autoantigen recognized by bullous pemphigoid and herpes gestationis sera. Immunolocalization of this protein to the hemidesmosome. J Clin Invest. 1990;86(4):1088–94.
11. Chan LS, Fine JD, Briggaman RA, Woodley DT, Hammerberg C, Drugge RJ, et al. Identification and partial characterization of a novel 105-kDalton lower lamina lucida autoantigen associated with a novel immune-mediated subepidermal blistering disease. J Invest Dermatol. 1993;101(3):262–7.
12. Shimanovich I, Hirako Y, Sitaru C, Hashimoto T, Brocker EB, Butt E, et al. The autoantigen of anti-p200 pemphigoid is an acidic noncollagenous N-linked glycoprotein of the cutaneous basement membrane. J Invest Dermatol. 2003;121(6):1402–8.
13. Zillikens D, Mascaro JM, Rose PA, Liu Z, Ewing SM, Caux F, et al. A highly sensitive enzyme-linked immunosorbent assay for the detection of circulating anti-BP180 autoantibodies in patients with bullous pemphigoid. J Invest Dermatol. 1997;109(5):679–83.
14. Chen M, Chan LS, Cai X, O'Toole EA, Sample JC, Woodley DT. Development of an ELISA for rapid detection of anti-type VII collagen autoantibodies in epidermolysis bullosa acquisita. J Invest Dermatol. 1997;108(1):68–72.
15. Zone JJ, Taylor TB, Kadunce DP, Meyer LJ. Identification of the cutaneous basement membrane zone antigen and isolation of antibody in linear immunoglobulin A bullous dermatosis. J Clin Invest. 1990;85(3):812–20.
16. Chan LS, Majmurdar AA, Tran HH, Meier F, Schumburg-Lever G, Chen M, et al. Laminin-6 and laminin-5 are recognized by autoantibodies in a subset of cicatricial pemphigoid. J Invest Dermatol. 1997;108(6):843–53.
17. Bernard P, Antonicelli F, Bedane C, Joly P, Le Roux-Villet C, Duvert-Lehembre S, et al. Prevalence and clinical significance of anti-laminin 332 autoantibodies detected by a novel enzyme-linked immunosorbent assay in mucous membrane pemphigoid. JAMA Dermatol. 2013;149(5):533–40.
18. Rashid KA, Foster CS, Ahmed AR. Identification of epitopes within integrin b4 for binding of auto-antibodies in ocular cicatricial and mucous membrane pemphigoid: preliminary report. Invest Ophthalmol Vis Sci. 2013;54(12):7707–16.
19. Hayakawa T, Furumura M, Fukano H, Li X, Ishii N, Hamada T, et al. Diagnosis of oral mucous membrane pemphigoid by means of combined serologic testing. Oral Surg Oral Med Oral Pathol Oral Radiol. 2014;117(4):483–96.
20. Taylor J, McMillan R, Shephard M, et al. World Workshop on Oral Medicine VI: a systematic review of the treatment of mucous membrane pemphigoid. Oral Surg Oral Med Oral Pathol Oral Radiol. 2015;120(2):161–71.
21. Günther C, Wozel G, Meurer M, Pfeiffer C. Topical tacrolimus treatment for cicatricial pemphigoid. J Am Acad Dermatol. 2004;50(2):325–6.
22. Assmann T, Becker J, Ruzicka T, Megahed M. Topical tacrolimus for oral cicatricial pemphigoid. Clin Exp Dermatol. 2004;29(6):674–6.
23. Suresh L, Martinez Calixto LE, Radfar L. Successful treatment of mucous membrane pemphigoid with tacrolimus. Spec Care Dentist. 2006;26(2):66–70.
24. Lee HY, Blazek C, Beltraminelli H, Borradori L. Oral mucous membrane pemphigoid: complete response to topical tacrolimus. Acta Derm Venereol. 2011;91(5):604–5.
25. Carrozzo M, Arduino P, Bertolusso G, Cozzani E, Parodi A. Systemic minocycline as a therapeutic option in predominantly oral mucous membrane pemphigoid: a cautionary report. Int J Oral Maxillofac Surg. 2009;38(10):1071–6.
26. Marzano AV, Dassoni F, Caputo R. Treatment of refractory blistering autoimmune diseases with mycophenolic acid. J Dermatolog Treat. 2006;17(6):370–6.

27. Munyangango EM, Le Roux-Villet C, Doan S, et al. Oral cyclophosphamide without corticosteroids to treat mucous membrane pemphigoid. Br J Dermatol. 2013;168(2):381–90.
28. Chaidemenos G, Sidiropoulos T, Katsioula P, Koussidou-Eremondi T. Colchicine in the management of mucous membrane pemphigoid. Dermatol Ther. 2011;24(4):443–5.
29. Staines K, Hampton PJ. Treatment of mucous membrane pemphigoid with the combination of mycophenolate mofetil, dapsone, and prednisolone: a case series. Oral Surg Oral Med Oral Pathol Oral Radiol. 2012;114(1):e49–56.
30. Cafaro A, Broccoletti R, Arduino PG. Low-level laser therapy for oral mucous membrane pemphigoid. Lasers Med Sci. 2012;27(6):124.
31. Canizares MJ, Smith DI, Conners MS, Maverick KJ, Heffernan MP. Successful treatment of mucous membrane pemphigoid with etanercept in 3 patients. Arch Dermatol. 2006;142(11):1457–61.
32. Kennedy JS, Devillez RL, Henning JS. Recalcitrant cicatricial pemphigoid treated with the anti-TNF-alpha agent etanercept. J Drugs Dermatol. 2010;9(1):68–70.
33. Taverna JA, Lerner A, Bhawan J, Demierre M-F. Successful adjuvant treatment of recalcitrant mucous membrane pemphigoid with anti-CD20 antibody rituximab. J Drugs Dermatol. 2007;6(7):731–2.
34. Schumann T, Schmidt E, Booken N, Goerdt S, Goebeler M. Successful treatment of mucous membrane pemphigoid with the anti-CD-20 antibody rituximab. Acta Derm Venereol. 2009;89(1):101–2.
35. Le Roux-Villet C, Prost-Squarcioni C, Alexandre M, et al. Rituximab for patients with refractory mucous membrane pemphigoid. Arch Dermatol. 2011;147(7):843–9.
36. Lourari S, Herve C, Doffoel-Hantz V, et al. Bullous and mucous membrane pemphigoid show a mixed response to rituximab: experience in seven patients. J Eur Acad Dermatol Venereol. 2011;25(10):1238–40.
37. Wozniak K, Waszczykowska E, Hashimoto T, et al. Anti-epiligrin cicatricial pemphigoid initially limited to the upper respiratory tract. Br J Dermatol. 2006;154(4):779–81.
38. Segura S, Iranzo P, Martínez-de Pablo I, et al. High-dose intravenous immunoglobulins for the treatment of autoimmune mucocutaneous blistering diseases: evaluation of its use in 19 cases. J Am Acad Dermatol. 2007;56(6):960–7.
39. Gürcan HM, Ahmed AR. Intravenous immunoglobulin treatment in laryngeal pemphigoid. Clin Exp Dermatol. 2009;34(8):884–6.
40. Yu JT, Chong LY, Lee KC. A recalcitrant case of cicatricial pemphigoid. Hong Kong Med J. 2007;13(2):157–60.
41. Nishmura R, Fujimoto N, Kito K, Uchiyama K, Koga H, Hodohara K, et al. Refractory mucous membrane pemphigoid which developed after allogeneic stem cell transplantation and was successfully treated with rituximab. Eur J Dermatol. 2013;23(4):562–4.
42. Shetty S, Ahmed AR. Critical analysis of the use of rituximab in mucous membrane pemphigoid: a review of the literature. J Am Acad Dermatol. 2013;68(3):499–506.
43. Czemik A, Toosi S, Bystryn JC, Grando SA. Intravenous immunoglobulin in the treatment of autoimmune bullous dermatoses: an update. Autoimmunity. 2012;45(1):111–8.
44. Suelves AM, Arcinue CA, Gonzalez-Martin JM, Kruh JN, Foster CS. Analysis of a novel protocol of pulsed intravenous cyclophosphamide for recalcitrant or severe ocular inflammatory disease. Ophthalmology. 2013;120(6):1201–9.
45. Nottage JM, Hammersmith KM, Murchison AP, Felipe AF, Penne R, Raber I. Treatment of mucous membrane pemphigoid with mycophenolate mofetil. Cornea. 2013;32(6):810–5.

Chapter 7
Linear IgA Bullous Dermatosis

Julia A. Curtis and John J. Zone

Abstract Linear IgA bullous dermatosis (LABD) is a unique autoimmune blistering disease which can present both in children and adults. There are various clinical presentations of the disease which can involve both cutaneous and mucosal tissues. LABD has been reported to be associated with medications, ulcerative colitis, and malignancies. This chapter will discuss the diagnosis, current therapies, and possible treatment algorithms for managing LABD patients.

Keywords Linear IgA bullous disease • Systemic steroids • Dapsone • Azathioprine • Mycophenolate mofetil • Cyclophosphamide • Methotrexate • Rituximab • Intravenous Immunoglobulin

Introduction

Linear IgA bullous dermatosis (LABD) is unique among dermatologic diseases in that it is defined on the basis of a particular immunopathologic finding on direct immunofluorescence – the sharp linear deposition of IgA along the basement membrane zone (BMZ). Some clinicians initially considered it as a variant of pemphigoid (on the basis of the presence of linear basement membrane antibodies) and others considered it a variant of dermatitis herpetiformis (on the basis of identical histopathology); however, it is now generally regarded as its own separate entity [1].

Clinical Findings

The clinical findings associated with this immunopathologic pattern span a wide range of classical immunobullous disorders. These findings include: (1) a papulovesicular variant with erosions on extensor surfaces that resembles classic dermatitis

J.A. Curtis, MD • J.J. Zone, MD (✉)
Department of Dermatology, University of Utah School of Medicine,
30 North 1900 East, 4A330, Salt Lake City, UT 84132, USA
e-mail: john.zone@hsc.utah.edu

N. Sami (ed.), *Autoimmune Bullous Diseases: Approach and Management*,
DOI 10.1007/978-3-319-26728-9_7

herpetiformis; (2) vesicles and bullae of the torso and extremities that resemble bullous pemphigoid or that have a unique annular arrangement of vesicles; (3) annular flexural vesicles and bullae in children (termed chronic bullous disease of childhood); (4) a vesicular erosive disease of the mucous membranes that is clinically identical to mucous membrane pemphigoid with scarring of the conjunctivae, which is identical to ocular cicatricial pemphigoid. Additionally, esophageal and vulvar involvement may occur. Mucous membrane disease can occur alone or in addition to the cutaneous disease [2]. Identification of mucosal disease is critical as it requires aggressive treatment to prevent the potential complications from scarring (Figs. 7.1, 7.2, 7.3, and 7.4).

Diagnosis

The gold standard test for diagnosis is a biopsy of perilesional, clinically normal-appearing skin or mucous membrane immediately adjacent to a lesion that reveals linear IgA deposits along the basement membrane zone on direct immunofluorescence (DIF) testing [3]. The additional presence of linear IgG deposition along the basement membrane has provoked some controversy. Some clinicians have said that IgA alone should be present at the BMZ whereas others have said that IgA and IgG may be present, but IgA must be predominant [4]. A Japanese review of 213 patients with LABD found both antibodies in approximately 20 % of the cases [5]. We

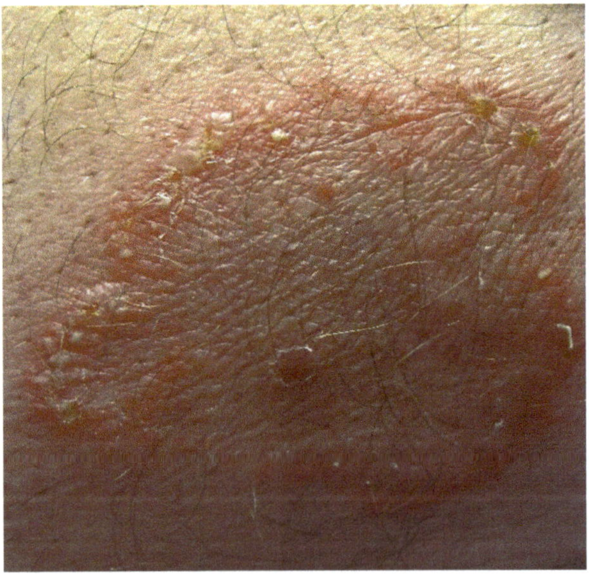

Fig. 7.1 Annular plaque with vesicles at perimeter of lesion

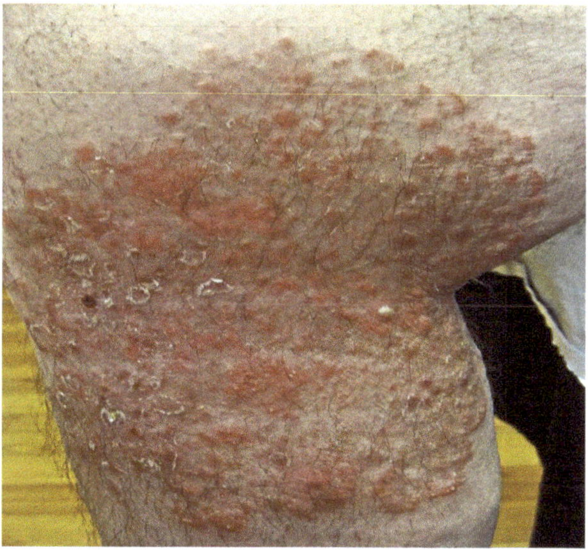

Fig. 7.2 Papulovesicular variant

Fig. 7.3 Involvement of the perineal area

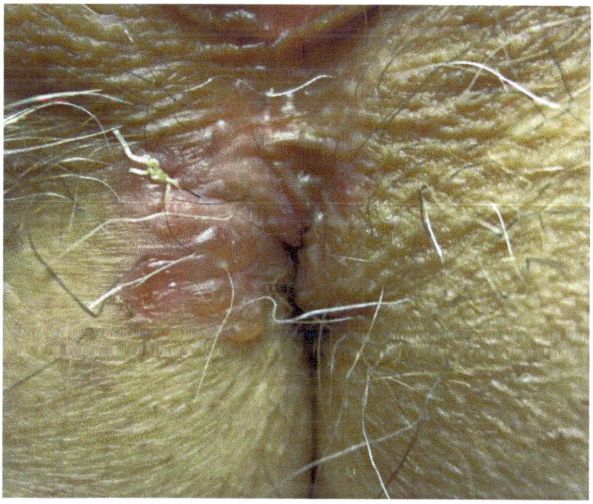

prefer the designation of linear IgA/IgG bullous dermatosis (LAGBD) when both are present [6].

The histopathologic findings with hematoxylin and eosin staining of involved skin are identical to those of dermatitis herpetiformis, showing lymphocytes, occasional eosinophils, and neutrophilic dermal papillary microabscesses [3, 7]. Additionally, another characteristic finding is a subepidermal blister with a diffuse underlying neutrophilic infiltrate in the dermis (Fig. 7.5).

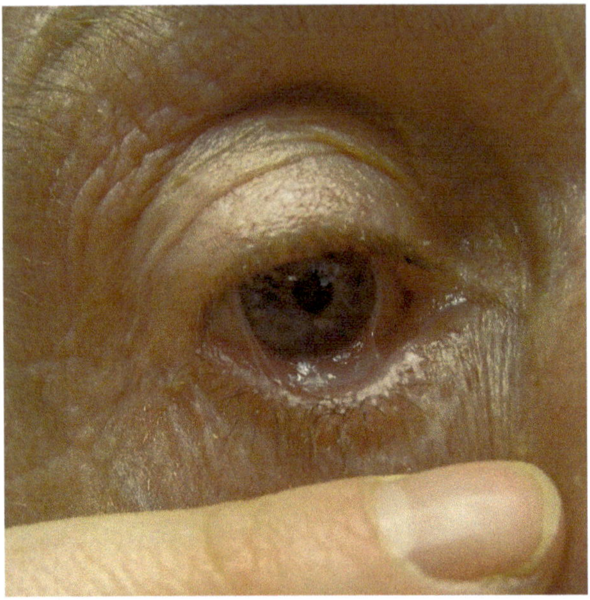

Fig. 7.4 Ocular involvement showing symblepharon and foreshortening of the inferior fornix

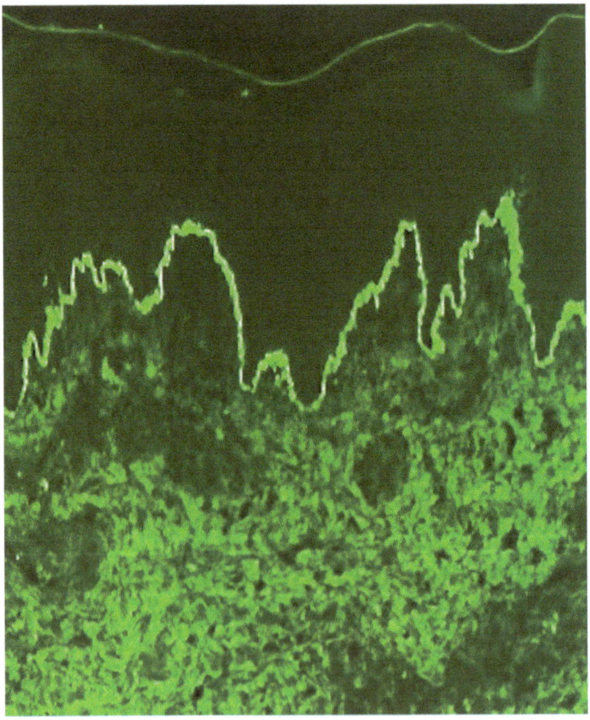

Fig. 7.5 Direct immunofluorescence of IgA in the basement membrane zone

LABD is divided into subtypes based on ultrastructural location of IgA – a sub-lamina densa type and a lamina lucida type. These types can be identified using BMZ salt-split human skin and indirect immunofluorescence. Separation occurs in the lower lamina lucida. Lamina lucida antigens will adhere to the epidermal side of the basement membrane separation, whereas lamina densa and sub-lamina densa antigens will bind to the dermal side. If the patient has positive IgA BMZ antibodies on indirect immunofluorescence with BMZ salt-split skin, the sub-type can be identified (Fig. 7.6). In cases without circulating IgA basement membrane antibodies, immunoelectron microscopy or basement membrane separation of the DIF positive biopsy can identify the type. In most cases this is unnecessary, since treatment for both variants of LABD is the same; however, it is the authors' experience that patients with sub-lamina densa antigens are more resistant to treatment. Furthermore, in both situations antibody titers by indirect immunofluorescence correlate well with response to therapy.

The lamina lucida type predominantly targets a 97-kDa antigen and a 120-kDa antigen that are the proteolytic fragments of the extracellular portion of the bullous pemphigoid antigen 2 (BP180), a key epidermal-dermal adhesion transmembrane protein [8, 9]. Less frequently, LABD is associated with the NC16A epitope of BP180 [10]. The sub-lamina densa type of LABD has been reported to be predominantly Type VII collagen, although a number of other antigens have been proposed [11].

Epidemiology

Reported incidence rates range from less than 0.5–2.3 cases per million individuals yearly. No predilection based on ethnicity or gender for LABD has been established [7]. LABD rarely occurs in neonates [12]. It can develop in children between the ages of 6 months and 10 years. The average age of onset in 25 affected children was

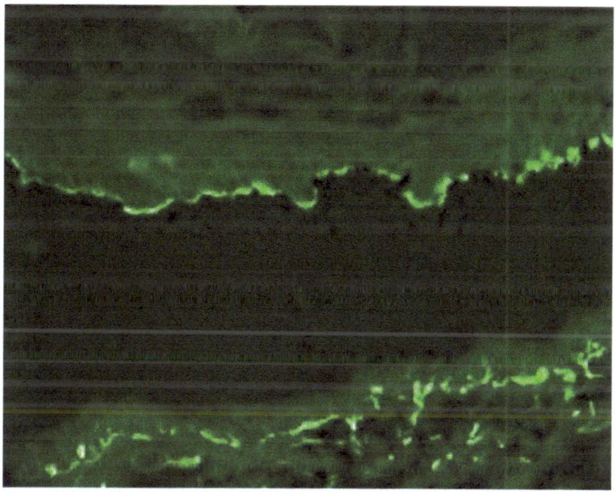

Fig. 7.6 Indirect immunofluorescence of IgA binding to epidermal side in salt-split skin

4.5 years [13]. Childhood cases frequently remit spontaneously in 12–36 months. Adults generally present with LABD later in life, with many cases occurring after age 60. Lastly, drug-induced cases may occur at any age.

The etiology of LABD may be drug-induced or idiopathic. Vancomycin is the most common offending medication; however, over 20 other medications have been incriminated. Beta-lactams and cephalosporins are other inciting antibiotic classes. Non-steroidal anti-inflammatory medications and angiotensin-converting enzyme inhibitors, such as captopril, have been cited in case reports. Some clinicians have said that the idiopathic form of LABD does not differ significantly from the drug-induced form [7]. Both forms of LABD can present exclusively with localized involvement rather than with widespread distribution. They may or may not involve the mucosae. Other clinicians have indicated that the drug-induced form is usually more severe and can even resemble erythema multiforme or toxic epidermal necrolysis [14].

Adults are more frequently afflicted with drug-induced LABD; however, it has also been reported in children [7]. The onset of lesions generally begins within the first month of drug administration and then they resolve gradually over the ensuing several weeks; however, lesions may persist beyond this timeframe in some patients. Furthermore, if the patient is re-exposed to the inciting medication, rapid reappearance of the lesions can occur.

Associations

The most common disorder associated with LABD is ulcerative colitis (UC) [5]. Paige et al. found that of 70 LABD patients, 5 patients (7 %) had UC preceding the diagnosis of LABD by an average of 6 years [15]. A review from Japan of 213 cases of LABD found 4 patients with UC [5]. It is believed that chronic inflammation in the colon exposes BMZ antigens, creates conformational neoantigens, and stimulates the mucosal immune system (IgA) to react to these autoantigens. Some patients have complete resolution of their disease after colectomy, whereas others have persistent disease or recurrences after removal of the colon [16, 17].

Malignant disorders – lymphoproliferative and solid organ type – have also been associated with LABD in multiple case reports [18–23]. Despite these reports and many others, no retrospective analyses have been performed to confirm this association.

Other conditions with reported associations to LABD include systemic lupus erythematosus [5] and psoriasis [24, 25]. Lastly, there are reports of LABD following exposure to ultraviolet light [26].

Prognosis

Idiopathic LABD can persist from months to several years in adults, whereas in children, it typically resolves before puberty [13, 27, 28]. This disease can also prevail for a decade or even longer in some patients. It can also recur after long periods of remission [27]. This circumstance is in contrast to drug-induced LABD, which usually improves within a few days of cessation of the offending drug and resolves within several weeks [29].

The treatment duration for idiopathic LABD is variable. Therapy is generally continued for several weeks after complete resolution of lesions and then gradually tapered off. If at any time lesions recur, the treatment medication must be restarted [27]. Cutaneous lesions typically heal without scarring; however, mucosal lesions may lead to stricture formation or conjunctival and corneal scarring. These sequelae can have a significant impact on patients' oral hygiene and nutritional support.

Treatment

Predisposing Factors

In view of the multiple contributing factors that may be operative in an individual case, several questions must be answered as they will determine the eventual therapeutic approach.

Childhood Disease

Preschool children presenting with idiopathic childhood disease will usually experience remission of symptoms in several months to years. Recommendations are to suppress symptoms, usually with dapsone, as intensive immunosuppression therapy is seldom necessary.

Drug-Induced Disease

Separation of drug-induced LABD from idiopathic disease on the basis of clinical exam alone is virtually impossible. A careful history of medication use must be taken with special attention to medications started within the last month. If a medication is implicated, termination of that medication is very likely to produce complete resolution within weeks using only suppressive therapy with dapsone. In severe or persistent cases prednisone may be used to achieve faster resolution. Therapy should be tapered early in the treatment course, within 4–6 weeks, to ascertain whether the disease is still active, warranting continuation of systemic therapy. A prolonged treatment course is rarely necessary.

Associated Disorders

- **Ulcerative colitis.** Determining the presence of inflammatory bowel disease symptoms such as those associated with ulcerative colitis is essential. Treatment of the underlying inflammatory bowel disease, whether it be with medical or surgical treatment, is likely to improve or clear LABD.

- **Malignancy.** Age-appropriate screening for malignancy is advised with special attention to signs and symptoms of lymphoma, including fevers, chills, night sweats, and weight loss. If identified, treatment of the underlying malignancy is likely to improve or clear the LABD.

Mucosal Disease

- **Ocular disease.** The greatest morbidity in LABD is related to scarring mucosal disease, especially in the eye. Clinicians must examine the conjunctivae for the presence of erythema, symblepharon, and foreshortening of the inferior fornix [13]. If conjunctival disease has manifested, this warrants an ophthalmologic evaluation as well as the initiation of aggressive treatment with immunosuppressants or rituximab or both.
- **Oral and esophageal disease.** Oral and pharyngeal involvement requires evaluation for disease by otolaryngology and gastroenterology. These circumstances may require dilatation of secondary constrictions during and after aggressive systemic treatment.

Additional IgG Antibodies

The additional presence of IgG antibodies is probably associated with resistance to dapsone, and indicates the need for additional systemic treatment with corticosteroids and immunosuppressives.

Systemic Treatment

Dapsone

Dapsone is the first-line medication therapy for LABD [28, 30]. Baseline glucose-6-phosphate dehydrogenase levels must be evaluated to ensure that the oxidative stress of dapsone will not induce a hemolytic crisis. Baseline complete blood count with auto-differential and liver function tests (LFTs) should be also evaluated. Dapsone is started at a low dose: 25–50 mg daily in adults and generally less than 0.5 mg/kg daily in children. This dose is gradually titrated upward over several weeks, depending on tolerance and treatment response. Complete blood counts (CBC) must be monitored every 2–4 weeks for the first 3 months to evaluate for leukopenia or severe hemolysis. Hemolysis to some degree occurs in all patients. Elderly patients or those with cardiac compromise need to be monitored closely as small decreases in the hematocrit or hemoglobin or minimal methemoglobinemia may produce symptoms [31]. Treatment response may occur in 24–48 hours with resolution of lesions within a few days of initiating therapy. If the disease is completely controlled with dapsone, a systematic approach at tapering is recommended. Dapsone should be tapered no more frequently than every 1 to 2 weeks by 12.5–25 mg. Development of an occasional small lesion is not an indication for increasing the dapsone dose as such lesions can be treated topically with potent corticosteroids. Tapering dapsone slowly will eventually allow discontinuation of treatment in cases that undergo spontaneous remission with time. Some patients with more extensive disease, particularly scarring mucosal disease and incomplete response to dapsone therapy may need oral corticosteroids or immediate treatment with rituximab to accelerate improvement of symptoms and effectively suppress the lesions [32, 33].

Sulfapyridine

For patients who are intolerant of dapsone, there are other sulfa-based drugs available: sulfasalazine and sulfapyridine. Although there is no published verification of therapeutic efficacy, patients who are allergic to dapsone or sulfapyridine can be given a trial of the alternate medication at a low dose; and they are generally able to tolerate it. Sulfapyridine is not commercially available in the United States, but can be obtained through compounding pharmacies. Sulfapyridine dosing should be started at 0.5 g 3 times daily and increased up to 6 g daily for control of symptoms. Sulfasalazine is metabolized to sulfapyridine in the intestine; however, the active metabolite level is more predictable when sulfapyridine, itself, is given. Sulfasalazine should be dosed between 1 and 2 g daily [34]. Both medications have the potential adverse effects of agranulocytosis and hypersensitivity reactions, but not hemolysis. Adequate fluid intake and possible alkalinization of the urine with oral bicarbonate is also recommended to reduce the risk of drug-induced nephrolithiasis. As with dapsone, lab monitoring (CBC, LFTs and urinalysis) is recommended periodically.

Oral Corticosteroids

As stated above, those patients with more extensive disease and incomplete response to dapsone may need oral corticosteroids (1 mg/kg daily) for faster resolution of symptoms and effective suppression of the lesions [32, 35, 36]. Corticosteroids may be particularly effective in patients who also have IgG BMZ antibodies on direct immunofluorescence or in the serum. Patients with lone IgA antibodies may not respond to corticosteroids at any dose.

Colchicine

Colchicine can be effective in children with LABD. Some case reports and case series have demonstrated it as a reasonable substitute therapy for dapsone [35, 37–39]. In a series of eight children with systemic glucocorticoid-refractory LABD, the addition of colchicine led to dramatic improvement in 5 patients within 4–6 weeks. Furthermore, these children were able to taper off steroid therapy. The typical dose in children is 0.6 mg twice daily. According to some case reports, adults have also responded to colchicine; however, other authors have not seen such reported results. The adult dosage is 0.6 mg taken 3 to 4 times daily. The dosage is most often limited by gastrointestinal side effects, (especially diarrhea), secondary to the higher dosages of colchicine.

Tetracycline and Niacinamide

This therapeutic combination has been effective for the treatment of bullous pemphigoid and has been applied to LABD. Three adult patients with LABD reported disease resolution within a few weeks of starting therapy [40–42]. The dosing range for tetracycline and nicotinamide are 1000–1500 mg daily and 900–2000 mg daily, respectively. Children under age 9 cannot take tetracycline due to the adverse effect on developing teeth.

Other Antibiotics

Children with LABD may respond to systemic antibiotic therapy. The mechanism for efficacy is not known; whether it is due to anti-inflammatory or antibacterial properties, or another unknown action, remains to be clarified. One case series reported that in 7 children treated with flucloxacillin, all had complete resolution, but only 4 children stayed in remission off therapy [43]. Additional antibiotics reported to effectively treat LABD in children are oxacillin, dicloxacillin, erythromycin and trimethoprim-sulfamethoxazole [36, 44–48].

Immunosuppressive Therapy

When patients with either prolonged disease who require further immunosuppressive therapy or with predominantly mucosal involvement need more aggressive therapy, steroid-sparing agents can be effective. In the authors' estimate, these agents work in refractory disease. The order of preference is dictated by ease of use and severity of side effects [49–61].

- **Mycophenolate mofetil:** This antimetabolite immunosuppressant is a prodrug of mycophenolic acid and is FDA-approved as an organ transplant rejection medication. It reversibly inhibits inosine-monophosphate-dehydrogenase, an enzyme in lymphocytes responsible for *de novo* guanosine nucleoside synthesis. Its use in dermatologic diseases, for which none are FDA-approved, has been increasing since its effective use in psoriasis. There are a few case reports of its successful use in cutaneous and oral LABD in children and adults [49, 50, 55, 56, 58].
- **Azathioprine:** This corticosteroid-sparing immunosuppressant is a prodrug of 6-mercaptopurine, whose active metabolite is 6-thioguanine monophosphate. Its use in immunobullous disease is also not FDA-approved; however, its efficacy

has been widely proven with numerous reviews on its use in this class of dermatologic diseases [62–64].

- **Cyclophosphamide:** This alkylating agent is a nitrogen mustard derivative that directly damages DNA by cross-linking it, thereby inducing cell apoptosis. It is FDA-approved for mycosis fungoides; however, it is not approved for any immunobullous disease. This agent has shown particular efficacy when there is ocular involvement [65].

Intravenous Immunoglobulin (IVIg)

This non-immunosuppressive agent is pooled purified plasma from blood donors that contains supraphysiologic quantities of IgG and trace other immunoglobulins [66]. Its immunomodulatory effects are still not fully elucidated; however a few of its mechanisms of action include: suppression of the complement activation pathway through inhibiton of the membrane attack complex formation and the enzymes C3 and C5 convertase, neutralization of circulating autoantibodies, and blockade of the Fc receptors on macrophages and Fas ligand receptors on keratinocytes [67]. IgA levels must be checked before use of this medication as it can precipitate anaphylaxis in patients with IgA deficiency. IVIg has been successfully used alone and in combination with corticosteroids in patients with chronic renal failure and LABD, treatment-refractory LABD, and in those with chronic ocular involvement [52–54].

Rituximab

In resistant cases of immunobullous disease and scarring mucosal disease, particularly in the eyes, rituximab has been frequently used with great success. There is a single report in the literature of this being successful in ocular cicatricial pemphigoid [68]. The author (JZ) has treated 2 unreported cases. The first had no circulating antibodies and improved slowly over a number of years; however, it was difficult to ascertain whether the rituximab produced the remission. In the second case the patient improved significantly 2–3 months after receiving rituximab. A subsequent course of it induced further improvement, as well as maintenance of remission with the addition of low-dose dapsone. The treatment course used for these cases was 2 doses of 1000 mg intravenous infusions on day 0 and day 14. The efficacy of rituximab in LABD needs further investigation with controlled trials or case reports.

Future Directions for Treatment

The treatments for childhood disease reported here are largely empirical. Dapsone effectively treats IgA dermatoses, therefore it is not surprising that children with LABD improve. Colchicine delivers this same effect. Additionally, tetracycline antibiotics and niacinamide improve this condition for unknown reasons. In the case of childhood disease this type of empirical treatment is generally adequate since spontaneous remission usually occurs.

Alternatively, adult LABD can be very resistant to treatment. Rituximab and its ability to eliminate short-term memory B cells has been effective in several immunobullous diseases and therefore, by extension, is very likely efficacious in LABD. The future of immunobullous disease will likely become more focused with treatments that specifically target antigen-specific B cells that in turn will be useful in LABD. Complicating this possibility is that there are many different antigens in the various types of LABD. Instead we believe it would be most effective to target progenitor B cells of IgA-producing plasma cells, a small subset of B cells with an alpha chain on their surface, as this will likely not interfere with the IgG and IgM antibodies that are predecessors in the progressive class-switching process. Targeting IgA-producing B cells may well provoke a relative IgA deficiency; however, a spontaneously occurring IgA-deficiency state is not associated with severe disease, and elimination of IgA-producing cells may well be very effective for patients afflicted with severe IgA dermatoses.

Algorithms

Algorithm 1 (Fig. 7.7)

After the diagnosis of LABD is made by direct immunofluorescence, the possibility of drug-induced disease or disease with an associated underlying malignancy or bowel disease needs to be evaluated. If this is the case, then stopping the medication or treating the underlying disease may produce a remission. If remission is not produced or if there is no evidence of an associated medication or disease, treatment with dapsone is initiated. If there is no ocular disease present, proceed to algorithm #2. If ocular disease is present and dapsone does not halt its progression, immediate treatment with rituximab is indicated. If response of ocular disease to rituximab is inadequate, treatment with cyclophosphamide or other immunosuppressants should be undertaken.

Algorithm 2 (Fig. 7.8)

Many cases of LABD respond effectively to dapsone and the medication is well-tolerated. In this situation suppressive therapy should be maintained while awaiting a remission. If the patient is intolerant of dapsone or if there is an inadequate response, sequential treatment with sulfapyridine, colchicine, tetracycline and niacinamide, mycophenolate, azathioprine, or rituximab is undertaken. When a good response is obtained maintenance of suppressive therapy is once again undertaken while awaiting a remission. This may involve combinations of the above agents.

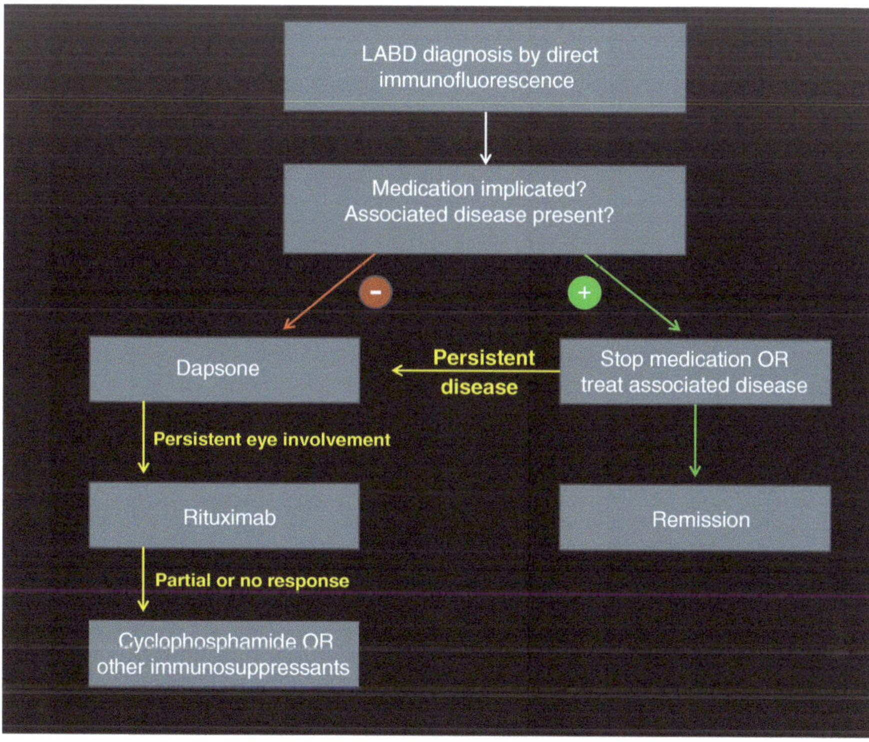

Fig. 7.7 Algorithm 1

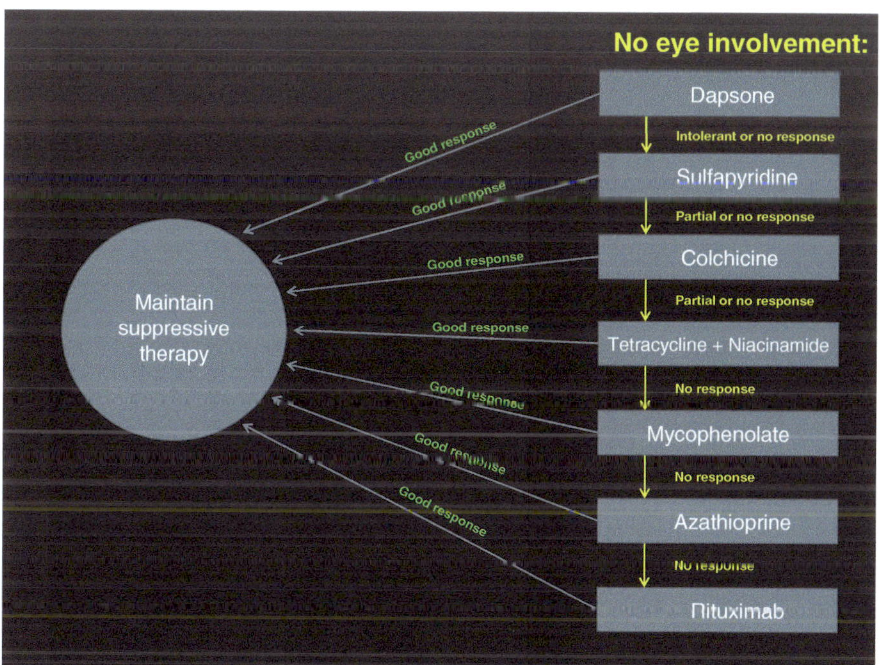

Fig. 7.8 Algorithm 2

References

1. Chorzelski T, Jablonska S. Evolving concept of IgA linear dermatosis. Semin Dermatol. 1988;7(3):225–32.
2. Egan CA, Zone JJ. Linear IgA bullous dermatosis. Int J Dermatol. 1999;38(11):818–27.
3. Guide SV, Marinkovich MP. Linear IgA bullous dermatosis. Clin Dermatol. 2001;19(6):719–27.
4. Antiga E, Caproni M, Fabbri P. Linear immunoglobulin a bullous dermatosis: need for an agreement on diagnostic criteria. Dermatology. 2013;226(4):329–32.
5. Horiguchi Y, Ikoma A, Sakai R, Masatsugu A, Ohta M, Hashimoto T. Linear IgA dermatosis: report of an infantile case and analysis of 213 cases in Japan. J Dermatol. 2008;35(11):737–43.
6. Sakaguchi M, Bito T, Oda Y, et al. Three cases of linear IgA/IgG bullous dermatosis showing IgA and IgG reactivity with multiple antigens, particularly laminin-332. JAMA Dermatol. 2013;149(11):1308–13.
7. Fortuna G, Salas-Alanis JC, Guidetti E, Marinkovich MP. A critical reappraisal of the current data on drug-induced linear immunoglobulin A bullous dermatosis: a real and separate nosological entity? J Am Acad Dermatol. 2012;66(6):988–94.
8. Marinkovich MP, Taylor TB, Keene DR, Burgeson RE, Zone JJ. LAD-1, the linear IgA bullous dermatosis autoantigen, is a novel 120-kDa anchoring filament protein synthesized by epidermal cells. J Invest Dermatol. 1996;106(4):734–8.
9. Zone JJ, Taylor TB, Kadunce DP, Meyer LJ. Identification of the cutaneous basement membrane zone antigen and isolation of antibody in linear immunoglobulin A bullous dermatosis. J Clin Invest. 1990;85(3):812–20.
10. Ishii N, Ohyama B, Yamaguchi Z, Hashimoto T. IgA autoantibodies against the NC16a domain of BP180 but not 120-kDa LAD-1 detected in a patient with linear IgA disease. Br J Dermatol. 2008;158(5):1151–3.
11. Tsuchisaka A, Ohara K, Ishii N, Nguyen NT, Marinkovich MP, Hashimoto T. Type VII collagen is the major autoantigen for sublamina densa-type linear IgA bullous dermatosis. J Invest Dermatol. 2015;135:626–9.
12. Gluth MB, Witman PM, Thompson DM. Upper aerodigestive tract complications in a neonate with linear IgA bullous dermatosis. Int J Pediatr Otorhinolaryngol. 2004;68(7):965–70.
13. Kelly SE, Frith PA, Millard PR, Wojnarowska F, Black MM. A clinicopathological study of mucosal involvement in linear IgA disease. Br J Dermatol. 1988;119(2):161–70.
14. Chanal J, Ingen-Housz-Oro S, Ortonne N, et al. Linear IgA bullous dermatosis: comparison between the drug-induced and spontaneous forms. Br J Dermatol. 2013;169(5):1041–8.
15. Paige DG, Leonard JN, Wojnarowska F, Fry L. Linear IgA disease and ulcerative colitis. Br J Dermatol. 1997;136(5):779–82.
16. Caldarola G, Annese V, Bossa F, Pellicano R. Linear IgA bullous dermatosis and ulcerative colitis treated by proctocolectomy. Eur J Dermatol EJD. 2009;19(6):651.
17. Walker SL, Banerjee P, Harland CC, Black MM. Remission of linear IgA disease associated with ulcerative colitis following panproclocolectomy. Br J Dermatol. 2000;143(6):1341–2.
18. Dippel E, Orfanos CE, Zouboulis C. Linear IgA dermatosis presenting with erythema annulare centrifugum lesions: report of three cases in adults. J Eur Acad Dermatol Venereol JEADV. 2001;15(2):167–70.
19. Adamic M, Potocnik M, Pavlovic MD. Linear IgA bullous dermatosis in a patient with advanced pancreatic carcinoma. Clin Exp Dermatol. 2008;33(4):503–5.
20. Gantzer A, Bouaziz JD, Valeyrie-Allanore L, Ingen-Housz-Oro S, Ortonne N, Bagot M. Acute linear IgA bullous dermatosis with circulating IgA monoclonal antibody associated with Hodgkin's disease. Ann Dermatol Venereol. 2010;137(12):819–20.
21. Hollo P, Preisz K, Nemes L, Biro J, Karpati S, Horvath A. Linear IgA dermatosis associated with chronic clonal myeloproliferative disease. Int J Dermatol. 2003;42(2):143–6.

22. Nassar D, Gabillot-Carre M, Ortonne N, et al. Atypical linear IgA dermatosis revealing angio-immunoblastic T-cell lymphoma. Arch Dermatol. 2009;145(3):342–3.
23. Usmani N, Baxter KF, Child JA, Sheehan-Dare R. Linear IgA disease in association with chronic lymphocytic leukaemia. Br J Dermatol. 2004;151(3):710–1.
24. Cooke N, Jenkinson H, Wojnarowska F, McKenna K, Alderdice J. Coexistence of psoriasis and linear IgA disease in a patient with recent herpes zoster infection. Clin Exp Dermatol. 2005;30(6):643–5.
25. Takagi Y, Sawada S, Yamauchi M, Amagai M, Niimura M. Coexistence of psoriasis and linear IgA bullous dermatosis. Br J Dermatol. 2000;142(3):513–6.
26. Salmhofer W, Soyer HP, Wolf P, Fodinger D, Hodl S, Kerl H. UV light-induced linear IgA dermatosis. J Am Acad Dermatol. 2004;50(1):109–15.
27. Chorzelski TP, Jablonska S, Maciejowska E. Linear IgA bullous dermatosis of adults. Clin Dermatol. 1991;9(3):383–92.
28. Mintz EM, Morel KD. Clinical features, diagnosis, and pathogenesis of chronic bullous disease of childhood. Dermatol Clin. 2011;29(3):459–62. ix.
29. Navi D, Michael DJ, Fazel N. Drug-induced linear IgA bullous dermatosis. Dermatol Online J. 2006;12(5):12.
30. Ng SY, Venning VV. Management of linear IgA disease. Dermatol Clin. 2011;29(4):629–30.
31. Wojnarowska F, Kirtschig G, Khumalo N. Treatment of subepidermal immunobullous diseases. Clin Dermatol. 2001;19(6):768–77.
32. Venning VA. Linear IgA disease: clinical presentation, diagnosis, and pathogenesis. Dermatol Clin. 2011;29(3):453–8. ix.
33. Ang P, Goh BK, Giam YC. Case reports of linear IgA bullous dermatosis of childhood. Ann Acad Med Singapore. 1999;28(6):849–54.
34. Willsteed E, Lee M, Wong LC, Cooper A. Sulfasalazine and dermatitis herpetiformis. Australas J Dermatol. 2005;46(2):101–3.
35. Ang P, Tay YK. Treatment of linear IgA bullous dermatosis of childhood with colchicine. Pediatr Dermatol. 1999;16(1):50–2.
36. Kenani N, Mebazaa A, Denguezli M, et al. Childhood linear IgA bullous dermatosis in Tunisia. Pediatr Dermatol. 2009;26(1):28–33.
37. Banodkar DD, al-Suwaid AR. Colchicine as a novel therapeutic agent in chronic bullous dermatosis of childhood. Int J Dermatol. 1997;36(3):213–6.
38. Tay YK, Ang P. Treatment of linear IgA bullous dermatosis of childhood with colchicine: in reply. Pediatr Dermatol. 2000;17(2):157.
39. Zeharia A, Hodak E, Mukamel M, Danziger Y, Mimouni M. Successful treatment of chronic bullous dermatosis of childhood with colchicine. J Am Acad Dermatol. 1994;30(4):660–1.
40. Chaffins ML, Collison D, Fivenson DP. Treatment of pemphigus and linear IgA dermatosis with nicotinamide and tetracycline: a review of 13 cases. J Am Acad Dermatol. 1993;28(6):998–1000.
41. Peoples D, Fivenson DP. Linear IgA bullous dermatosis: successful treatment with tetracycline and nicotinamide. J Am Acad Dermatol. 1992;26(3 Pt 2):498–9.
42. Yomada M, Komai A, Hashimato T. Sublamina densa-type linear IgA bullous dermatosis successfully treated with oral tetracycline and niacianamide. Br J Dermatol. 1999;141(3):608–9.
43. Alajlan A, Al-Khawajah M, Al-Sheikh O, et al. Treatment of linear IgA bullous dermatosis of childhood with flucloxacillin. J Am Acad Dermatol. 2006;54(4):652–6.
44. Farrant P, Darley C, Carmichael A. Is erythromycin an effective treatment for chronic bullous disease of childhood? a national survey of members of the British Society for Paediatric Dermatology. Pediatr Dermatol. 2008;25(4):479–82.
45. Mervic L, Dragos V, Pavlovic MD. Linear IgA bullous dermatosis of childhood: successful treatment with miocamycin and topical corticosteroid. Clin Exp Dermatol. 2009;34(7):e391–2.
46. Monia K, Aida K, Amel K, Ines Z, Becima F, Ridha KM. Linear IgA bullous dermatosis in tunisian children: 31 cases. Indian J Dermatol. 2011;56(2):153–9.

47. Siegfried EC, Sirawan S. Chronic bullous disease of childhood: successful treatment with dicloxacillin. J Am Acad Dermatol. 1998;39(5 Pt 1):797–800.
48. Cooper SM, Powell J, Wojnarowska F. Linear IgA disease: successful treatment with erythromycin. Clin Exp Dermatol. 2002;27(8):677–9.
49. Farley-Li J, Mancini AJ. Treatment of linear IgA bullous dermatosis of childhood with mycophenolate mofetil. Arch Dermatol. 2003;139(9):1121–4.
50. Glaser R, Sticherlin M. Successful treatment of linear IgA bullous dermatosis with mycophenolate mofetil. Acta Derm Venereol. 2002;82(4):308–9.
51. Goebeler M, Seitz C, Rose C, et al. Successful treatment of linear IgA disease with salazosulphapyridine and intravenous immunoglobulins. Br J Dermatol. 2003;149(4):912–4.
52. Khan IU, Bhol KC, Ahmed AR. Linear IgA bullous dermatosis in a patient with chronic renal failure: response to intravenous immunoglobulin therapy. J Am Acad Dermatol. 1999;40(3):485–8.
53. Kroiss MM, Vogt T, Landthaler M, Stolz W. High-dose intravenous immune globulin is also effective in linear IgA disease. Br J Dermatol. 2000;142(3):582.
54. Letko E, Bhol K, Foster CS, Ahmed AR. Linear IgA bullous disease limited to the eye: a diagnostic dilemma: response to intravenous immunoglobulin therapy. Ophthalmology. 2000;107(8):1524–8.
55. Lewis MA, Yaqoob NA, Emanuel C, Potts AJ. Successful treatment of oral linear IgA disease using mycophenolate. Oral Surg Oral Med Oral Pathol Oral Radiol Endod. 2007;103(4):483–6.
56. Marzano AV, Ramoni S, Spinelli D, Alessi E, Berti E. Refractory linear IgA bullous dermatosis successfully treated with mycophenolate sodium. J Dermatolog Treat. 2008;19(6):364–7.
57. Segura S, Iranzo P, Martinez-de Pablo I, et al. High-dose intravenous immunoglobulins for the treatment of autoimmune mucocutaneous blistering diseases: evaluation of its use in 19 cases. J Am Acad Dermatol. 2007;56(6):960–7.
58. Talhari C, Mahnke N, Ruzicka T, Megahed M. Successful treatment of linear IgA disease with mycophenolate mofetil as a corticosteroid sparing agent. Clin Exp Dermatol. 2005;30(3):297–8.
59. Wetter DA, Davis MD, Yiannias JA, et al. Effectiveness of intravenous immunoglobulin therapy for skin disease other than toxic epidermal necrolysis: a retrospective review of Mayo Clinic experience. Mayo Clin Proc. 2005;80(1):41–7.
60. Young HS, Coulson IH. Linear IgA disease: successful treatment with cyclosporin. Br J Dermatol. 2000;143(1):204–5.
61. Cauza K, Hinterhuber G, Sterniczky B, et al. Unusual clinical manifestation of linear IgA dermatosis: a report of two cases. J Am Acad Dermatol. 2004;51(2 Suppl):S112–7.
62. Anstey AV, Wakelin S, Reynolds NJ; British Association of Dermatologists Therapy; Guidelines and Audit Subcommittee. Guidelines for prescribing azathioprine in dermatology. Br J Dermatol. 2004;151(6):1123–32.
63. Belgi G, Friedmann PS. Traditional therapies: glucocorticoids, azathioprine, methotrexate, hydroxyurea. Clin Exp Dermatol. 2002;27(7):546–54.
64. Snow JL, Gibson LE. A pharmacogenetic basis for the safe and effective use of azathioprine and other thiopurine drugs in dermatologic patients. J Am Acad Dermatol. 1995;32(1):114–6.
65. Smith JR, Kupa A, Coster DJ. Linear IgA disease. Aust N Z J Ophthalmol. 1999;27(6):443–6.
66. Wolverton SE. Comprehensive dermatologic drug therapy. Philadelphia: Saunders; 2001.
67. Mouthon L, Kaveri SV, Spalter SH, et al. Mechanisms of action of intravenous immune globulin in immune-mediated diseases. Clin Exp Immunol. 1996;104 Suppl 1:3–9.
68. Lozinski A, Baum S, Sagi L, Volkov A, Trau H, Barzilai A. Rituximab (Mabthera) for treatment of rare autoimmune bullous skin disorders. Harefuah. 2012;151(10):562–5. 606.

Chapter 8
Epidermolysis Bullosa Acquisita

Olivia Y. Lai, Michael Kasperkiewicz, Brittney K. DeClerck, Mei Chen, and David T. Woodley

Abstract Epidermolysis bullosa acquisita (EBA) is a blistering skin disease that is caused by an autoantibody to type VII collagen (C7). C7 is the main component of large structures called anchoring fibrils localized at the dermal-epidermal junction (DEJ) of skin and critical for epidermal – dermal adherence. Classically, EBA presents as a mechanobullous disease with skin fragility and scarring reminiscent of hereditary dystrophic epidermolysis bullosa (DEB) or porphyria cutanea tarda. Nevertheless, if the disease is defined as autoimmunity to type VII collagen, EBA can have clinical presentations that are reminiscent of inflammatory bullous pemphigoid (BP), mucous membrane pemphigoid (MMP), and Brunsting-Perry pemphigoid. Very rarely, EBA involving IgA autoantibodies to C7 presents clinically similar to linear IgA bullous dermatosis (LABD) with small pruritic symmetrical papulovesicles. Anecdotal reports have linked EBA to several underlying systemic diseases with the most common being inflammatory bowel disease (IBD) and systemic bullous erythematosus (SLE). Interestingly, in the gastrointestinal track there is an anchoring fibril equivalent composed of C7, and patients with Crohn's Disease and other IBDs have anti-C7 antibodies in their plasma. EBA is diagnosed using salt-split skin indirect and direct immunofluorescence (IIF and DIF), ELISA or Western blot analysis to detect anti-C7 antibodies in the blood, and, at research centers, by immuno-electron microscopy. EBA is notoriously difficult to treat. Systemic steroids and immunosuppressant agents (azathiaprine, mycophenolate mofetil, cyclophosphamide, and methotrexate) are inconsistently effective. Colchicine and

O.Y. Lai, BS
Department of Dermatology, USC Keck School of Medicine, Los Angeles, CA, USA

M. Kasperkiewicz, MD
Department of Dermatology, University of Lübeck, Lübeck, Germany

B.K. DeClerck, MD
Department of Pathology and Dermatology, Keck School of Medicine of the University of Southern California, Los Angeles, CA, USA

M. Chen, PhD
Department of Dermatology, University of Southern California, Los Angeles, CA, USA

D.T. Woodley, MD (✉)
Department of Dermatology, Keck School of Medicine, University of Southern California, 1441 Eastlake Avenue, Topping Tower, Suite 3405, Los Angeles, CA 90033, USA
e-mail: David.Woodley@med.usc.edu; dwoodley@med.usc.edu

N. Sami (ed.), *Autoimmune Bullous Diseases: Approach and Management*,
DOI 10.1007/978-3-319-26728-9_8

cyclosporine may be helpful, but the former cannot be used in patients who have concomitant IBD and the latter requires very high doses. Other treatments with varying success include dapsone, photophoresis, IVIG and plasmapheresis. Recently, rituximab, an anti-CD20 monoclonal antibody, has shown promise in EBA.

Keywords Epidermolysis bullosa • Type VII collagen • Anchoring fibrils

Abbreviations

BMZ	Basement membrane zone
BP	Bullous pemphigoid
C7	Collagen VII
CBDC	Chronic bullous disease of childhood
CP	Cicatricial pemphigoid
CsA	Cyclosporin A
DEB	Dystrophic epidermolysis bullosa
DIF	Direct immunofluorescence
EB	Epidermolysis bullosa
EBA	Epidermolysis bullosa acquisita
ECP	Extracorporeal photochemotherapy
ELISA	Enzyme-linked immunosorbent assay
EM	Electron microscopy
GI	Gastrointestinal
HLA	Human leukocyte antigen
IBD	Inflammatory bowel disease
IEM	Immunoelectron microscopy
IgG	Immunoglobulin G
IIF	Indirect immunofluorescence
IVIG	Intravenous immunoglobulin
LABD	Linear IgA bullous dermatosis
mg/m^2	Milligrams per square meter
PCT	Porphyria cutanea tarda
SLE	Systemic lupus erythematosus
SSS	Salt-split skin
TNF-α	Anti–tumor necrosis factor-α
TPMT	Thiopurine methyltransferase

Introduction

In 1895, Elliott described two cases of an acquired, adult-onset blistering disease that clinically resembled hereditary dystrophic epidermolysis bullosa (DEB) [1]. Clinically, these patients had skin fragility, bullae and erosions over trauma prone areas of the skin such as the extensor surfaces, prominent scarring, nail loss and milia, within their scars. Over the years other similar cases were reported, but infrequently. It was clear that this acquired form of EB, so-called epidermolysis bullosa acquisita (EBA), was a very rare bullous disorder. In 1971, Roenigk et al. [2] reported three new cases of epidermolysis bullosa acquisita (EBA), reviewed the EBA world literature and recommended the first diagnostic criteria for EBA, namely:

A. A negative personal and family history for blistering disorders,
B. An adult onset of the eruption,
C. Trauma-induced or spontaneous blisters that resemble those of DEB, and
D. The exclusion of all other bullous diseases.

This paper was prior to the advent of indirect immunofluorescence (IIF) and direct immunofluorescence (DIF), which were not included in the first diagnostic criteria for EBA. Nevertheless, soon afterward, it became clear that patients with EBA had linear IgG (and often other classes of immunoglobulins and complement) deposits at their dermal-epidermal junctions (DEJ) detected by DIF and also circulating serum antibodies that labeled the epidermal basement membrane zone (BMZ) of human skin or monkey esophagus frozen sections by IIF [3–6]. Therefore, a positive DIF for IgG deposits at the DEJ was added to the diagnostic criteria. Moreover, by immuno-electron microscopy (IEM) it was shown that the IgG immune deposits in EBA were localized in the DEJ in a different place than those of bullous pemphigoid (BP), another autoimmune bullous disease that is more inflammatory than EBA and usually does not scar [6]. In BP, the immune deposits were within the hemidesmosomes and lamina lucida of the DEJ, while in EBA the immune deposits were below the lamina densa of the DEJ [3–7]. Later, it was shown that these IgG autoantibodies in the blood and skin of EBA patients targeted a 290 kDa protein in the skin that turned out to be type VII (anchoring fibril) collagen [8, 9].

Pathogenesis

The etiology of EBA is unknown. For some un-explained reason, patients with EBA begin to express IgG autoantibodies that target their own C7 within their anchoring fibrils. Therefore, EBA has been classified as an autoimmune bullous disease. As mentioned above, anchoring fibrils are critical for epidermal dermal adherence. When these EBA IgG autoantibodies bind to the patient's anchoring fibrils, the function of the anchoring fibrils is perturbed and the patient experiences a sub-epidermal bulla. Anchoring fibrils emanate perpendicularly down from the lamina densa area of the DEJ into the papillary dermis. This location is exactly where the EBA IgG immune deposits are seen by immuno-electron microscopy (IEM). It is known that C7 has specific binding sub-domains with affinity to other DEJ components such as laminin 332 and type IV collagen as well as to other components of the papillary dermis such as type I collagen and fibronectin [10, 11]. Most likely, the

EBA IgG autoantibodies disrupt these C7 connections to other extracellular matrix components allowing the epidermis to separate from the dermis. EBA patients have immunoglobulin G (IgG) deposits at the dermal- epidermal junction. It has been shown clearly that like patients with hereditary DEB, patients with EBA have a paucity of anchoring fibrils [12].

Genetic factors may also predispose patients to developing EBA. Gammon et al. [13] reported that the human leukocyte antigen (HLA)-DR2 phenotype was significantly increased in both black and white EBA patients [13]. This study found that the risk of developing EBA was 13.1 times more frequent in HLA-DR2+ Caucasians and 4.81 times more frequent in HLA-DR2+ African-Americans. Although the study results also suggested that DR2 is merely a genetic marker for the unknown gene that may predispose patients to EBA, the association between DR2+ and EBA indicates that immunogenetic factors may predispose certain patients to developing EBA [13].

Clinical Presentations

As previously mentioned, all patients with EBA possess autoimmunity to type VII (anchoring fibril) collagen [7, 8, 14]. EBA, however, has several distinct clinical presentations and occasionally these can overlap. Using autoimmunity to C7 as the diagnostic hallmark for EBA, there are five recognized EBA presentations.

1. A mechano-bullous hereditary DEB-like classical presentation [2, 7, 8, 14]
2. An inflammatory bullous BP-like eruption presentation [15–18],
3. A mucosal-centered presentation reminiscent of MMP/CP [18, 19],
4. A Brunsting-Perry pemphigoid-like presentation with scarring lesions localized to the head and neck region [20, 21],
5. A linear IgA bullous dermatosis (LABD)/chronic bullous disease of childhood (CBDC)-like presentation [22–27].

Classic Presentation

EBA classically presents as a non-inflammatory mechanobullous disease. These patients may experience skin fragility in an acral distribution, erosions, tense blisters (which can be hemorrhagic and/or present with crusts, erosions, or scales), scarring and milia cysts that occur primarily over trauma-prone areas (e.g. the knuckles, toes, elbows, knees, dorsum of the hands, and sacral area). The disease can be mild, with a clinical presentation similar to that of porphyria cutanea tarda (PCT). In these milder cases, clinical features such as nail dystrophy and possible cicatricial alopecia may be seen. These patients, however, lack other features of PCT such as elevated urinary porphyrins, hirsutism, scleroderma-like alterations, or photodistribution of the lesions. In more severe cases, EBA can resemble the hereditary form of recessive dystrophic EB, although the disease is not typically as severe. EBA patients with the classical presentation of the disease can also experience the same sequelae as patients with hereditary forms of recessive dystrophic EB. These sequelae include esophageal stenosis, hand and finger fibrosis, scarring, and hair loss [2, 7, 8, 14, 15, 18].

Bullous Pemphigoid–Like Presentation

About 25–30 % of EBA patients have a clinical presentation that appears less like a mechanobullous disorder and more like BP. Patients with the BP-like presentation of EBA present with inflammatory, widespread, pruritic disease. Vesicles and tense bullae that involve the extremities, the trunk and central body, and the skin folds and flexural areas are also present [15–18]. Inflamed, erythematous, urticarial skin may be seen surrounding skin blisters, but large swathes of inflamed skin may be found even when these blisters are not present. Fragile skin, scarring, and milia formation are not present.

Cicatricial Pemphigoid/Mucous Membrane Pemphigoid-Like Presentation

Although both the BP-like and classic presentations of EBA can involve the mucosa, a cicatricial pemphigoid (CP)/mucous membrane pemphigoid (MMP) – like presentation of EBA with predominant mucous membrane involvement also exists [19]. Less than 10 % of patients with EBA have a clinical presentation that resembles pure CP. The CP-like form of the disease can present with erosions, blisters, and scarring in the ocular, vaginal, and oral mucous membranes. Lesions on the glabrous skin may also occur occasionally.

Brunsting-Perry Pemphigoid-Like Presentation

Brunsting-Perry pemphigoid is an autoimmune, chronic, vesiculobullous condition that is mostly confined to the head and neck region. The disease is characterized by IgG deposits at the dermal-epidermal junction, little to no mucosal involvement, subepidermal bullae, and significant scarring. When this disorder was first described, many of the laboratory methods used today were not available and no antigenic target in the skin was described for the IgG autoantibodies. Kurzhals et al. [20] described a patient with the typical clinical features of Brunsting-Perry pemphigoid. Direct immunelectron microscopy of a subepidermal blister from this patient revealed IgG and C3 deposits below the lamina densa that were directed against anchoring fibrils suggesting EBA. Tanaka and colleagues have reported another similar case that responded well to oral colchicine [21]. We have seen two similar patients and tested their circulating anti-BMZ antibodies using salt-split indirect immunofluorescence, Western blot analysis against purified type VII collagen and an ELISA against purified type VII collagen. These studies showed that their IgG autoantibodies bound to the dermal floor of salt-split human skin and were directed against type VII (anchoring fibril) collagen.

Linear Immunoglobulin A Bullous Dermatosis-Like Presentation

Linear IgA bullous dermatosis (LABD) is a well-described entity in which the patients have IgA autoantibodies directed against the more carboxyl end to the bullous pemphigoid 180 kDa antigen (a.k.a type XVII collagen). An LABD- like presentation of EBA also exists, albeit extremely rarely [22–26]. There is the question of whether this should be called "EBA with IgA autoantibodies" or "LABD with autoantibodies to type VII collagen" [28]. When EBA has IgA autoantibodies against C7, it appears clinically similar to LABD, chronic bullous disease of childhood (CBDC) or dermatitis herpetiformis (DH) with small symmetrical, pruritic papulovesicles. The patients have IgA and often IgG linear deposits at the DEJ observed by DIF. The sub-epidermal blisters often show a neutrophil rich dermal infiltrated on histology. Mucous membrane involvement and circularly arranged, tense vesicles reminiscent of CBDC may also be seen. This form of EBA has a number of clinical manifestations and can appear similar to DH, CBDC, or LABD [22–24].

Childhood EBA

Childhood EBA, which is a rare disease with considerable clinical variation, frequently presents with severe mucosal involvement. Out of 14 pediatric patients described in the medical literature, four presented with classic EBA, five presented with the BP-like form, and five presented with the LABD-like form. In general, the prognosis for childhood EBA is better than adult-onset EBA [27].

Associated Clinical Issues

Patients with EBA may also experience a number of associated clinical issues that negatively affect their quality of life. These clinical conditions, all of which may also be seen in hereditary dystrophic EB, may include scarring, nail loss, esophageal stenosis [15], oral lesions and milia cyst formation (small white, pearl-like lesions studded within scarred areas). This constellation of findings is sequelae from the classical mechanobullous type of EBA and is not seen in the BP-like form of EBA, which is generally non-scarring. Nevertheless, occasionally EBA patient can present with a blend of the classical form and the BP-like form. It is important to know that EBA can present clinically, histologically, and immunologically like BP and CP/MMP.

Associated Systemic Diseases

Anecdotal case reports have linked EBA to other systemic autoimmune and inflammatory diseases. These include rheumatoid arthritis, systemic lupus erythematosus (SLE), thyroiditis, amyloidosis, chronic lymphocytic leukemia, pulmonary fibrosis, multiple endocrinopathy syndrome, diabetes, inflammatory bowel disease, and thymoma [2, 28–31].

Diagnosis

As mentioned above, the diagnostic criteria for EBA outlined by Roengik and coworkers [2] was modified when it was found that EBA patients had IgG autoantibodies at their DEJ as detected by DIF and IEM [3–6]. Today the diagnostic criteria for EBA include the following:

1. A sub-epidermal bullous disorder
2. No family history of a bullous disorder
3. Deposition of IgG at the DEJ viewed by DIF of perilesional skin
4. IgG deposits localized to the lower lamina densa and sublamina densa
5. An auto-antibodies to C7 detected by ELISA or Western blot analysis

Histopathology

The histopathology of EBA lesions reveals a sub-epidermal blister. Classical EBA blisters are characterized by a paucity of inflammatory cells in the dermis and significant scarring. The BP-like presentation of EBA often reveals a mixed inflammatory infiltrate of neutrophils, macrophages, eosinophils and lymphocytes. In those rare LABD like presentation of EBA, a dermal infiltrate rich in neutrophils has been described [22, 26].

Direct Immunofluorescence (DIF)

Patients with EBA have immune deposits (predominantly IgG) at their DEJ that are detected by a positive DIF of perilesional skin [3–6]. The appearance of the immunoglobulin deposits may provide clues as to whether the patient has EBA versus BP or other immunobullous diseases [32].

Serology

Many but not all EBA patients have anti-C7 antibodies circulating in their blood that can be detected by IIF. The anti-BMZ antibodies detected by IIF against monkey esophagus substrate, guinea pig esophagus substrate or normal human skin substrate are often low titer between 1:20 and 1:40. DIF and IIF using salt-split skin test can be used to demonstrate autoantibody binding to the dermal floor (anchoring fibrils) in EBA [33–35]. However, the dermal binding can also be seen in diseases including antiepiligrin (or anti laminin 332) CP [36], protein 200 pemphigoid [37], Chan's Disease (a BP-like disease with antibodies to a 105 kDa DEJ protein) [38] and the autoimmune bullous disease of Goodpasture's Syndrome [39, 40].

Western immunoblotting and ELISA demonstrating anti-C7 antibodies are more sensitive and specific in confirming the diagnosis of EBA [7, 41]. An ELISA for autoantibodies to C7 is commercially available [11, 42, 43].

Treatment of EBA

EBA can be refractory to multiple therapies and is notoriously difficult to treat. If the patient has the classical mechanobullous type of EBA some common sense and supportive measures are useful such as avoiding trauma, avoiding harsh soaps, cleaning the skin in a very gentle manner, immediately treating skin infections and good consistent wound care with non-adhesive dressings. No clear-cut treatment algorithm has been widely agreed upon for EBA [44], but an EBA consensus group is currently developing guidelines. A summary of these treatments is outlined in Fig. 8.1.

Colchicine

Colchicine therapy is used to treat gout and has a relatively benign side effect profile. It has been used as an initial treatment for EBA with reasonable success [45]. Colchicine is a microtubule inhibitor that has the additional therapeutic benefit of down-regulating autoimmunity and inhibiting antigen presentation to T-cells [46]. Colchicine causes dose-dependent diarrhea. Therefore, it is started at 0.6 mg/day and increased as tolerated. In practice, we give 0.6 mg per day for 1 week and then increase it to 0.6 mg twice a day for a week. If there are no gastrointestinal problems, we then increase it to 0.6 mg three times a day for another week. The dosage of the prednisone is increased in this fashion each week until the patient experiences diarrhea, and then subsequently decreased by one colchicines tablet per day to the previously tolerated maximum dosage for the patient. In general, for colchicine to be effective, a dose greater than 1.8 mgs per day must be reached. About a quarter of patients with EBA have associated inflammatory bowel disease (IBD). Given the gastrointestinal side effects of colchicine, we do not use colchicine in EBA patients who have associated IBD.

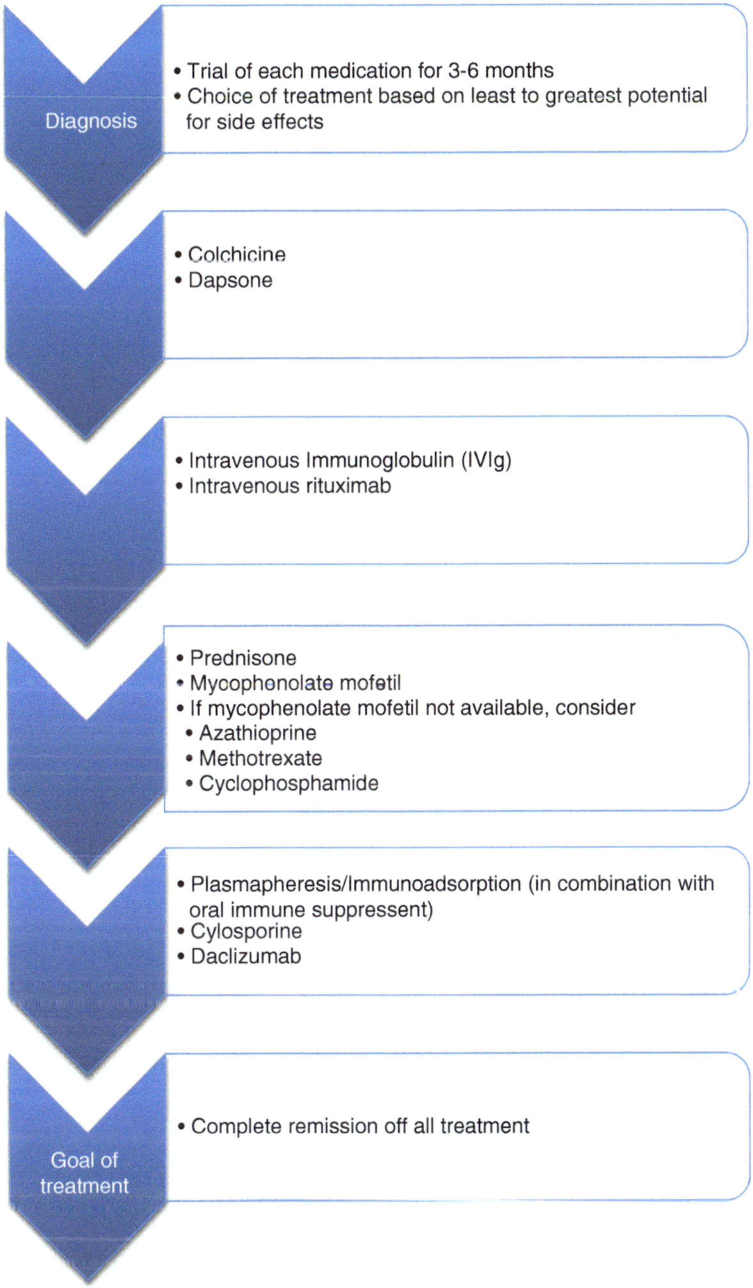

Fig. 8.1 Outline of treatments for EBA

Prednisone and Non-steroidal Immunosuppressive Agents

Other autoimmune bullous diseases such as BP and pemphigus are often well controlled with immunosuppressive agents such as systemic corticosteroids in combination with other potent immunosuppressive agents (methotrexate, azathioprine, cyclophosphamide, cyclosporine A, and mycophenolate mofetil). Unfortunately, EBA's response to these measures in less predictable than other autoimmune immunobullous diseases, particularly with the non-inflammatory classical mechanobullous presentation of EBA. If these agents are tried, prednisone 1–2 mg/kg is given once a day after the patient has had breakfast alone or in conjunction with non-steroidal immunosuppressive agents. Prednisone may be used in conjunction with oral methotrexate (10–50 mg per week), oral mycophenolate mofetil (1000–3000 mg daily), oral azathioprine (50–250 mg per day based on TPMT levels), or oral cyclophosphamide (50–250 mg per day). Mycophenolate mofetil is our first non-steroidal immunosuppressive agent of choice because it appears, relative to other immunosuppressive agents, to have a lower incidence of side effects. These measures may be useful to some degree at controlling the inflammatory BP-like presentation of EBA.

Another non-steroidal immunosuppressive agent, cyclosporine A, has shown promise in EBA [47, 48]. The problem with cyclosporine A is that high doses (6 or more mgs/kg) are needed to control EBA and the drug's nephrotoxicity, which is time and dose dependent, limits its long-term use.

Dapsone

Dapsone is an antibiotic that has the secondary property of inhibiting the migration of inflammatory cells in the skin, particularly neutrophils. A small subset of EBA patients has a neutrophil rich inflammatory infiltrate and some EBA patients have responded positively to treatment with dapsone [50]. Dapsone is given orally starting with 50 mg per day and going up as high as 300 mg per day if needed to control the disease. All patients on dapsone will get a methemoglobinemia and a concomitant drop of 1–2 g in their hemoglobin is not uncommon. For that reason, the doses of dapsone are increased slowly such that the patient can adjust and tolerate the iatrogenic anemia. Prior to starting dapsone, the patient should be evaluated for a deficiency in glucose-6-phosphate dehydrogenase (G6PD), which is a genetic disorder in which the patient has a predisposition toward hemolytic anemia. Dapsone is contraindicated in G6PD deficient patients. A simple blood test for plasma G6PD levels should be done on all patients prior to starting dapsone. Rare side effects of dapsone include bone marrow suppression, a chemical hepatitis, and drug reaction with eosinophilia and systemic symptoms (DRESS). Although these side effects may occur anytime during the patient's course on dapsone, usually they occur early in treatment. For that reason, it is important to obtain frequent complete blood counts and comprehensive metabolic panels on patients who are on dapsone.

Rituximab

Although the number of cases of EBA treated so far is small, it appears that rituximab, a monoclonal anti-CD20 antibody, can control some patients with recalcitrant EBA refractory to other therapies [51–56]. In these reports, rituximab was often given in conjunction with other immunosuppressive agents, which were then tapered when the patient's EBA came under control. McKinley and co-workers [49] treated a pediatric patient with EBA and achieved a sustained clinical response even after rituximab was discontinued. In general, it appears that EBA has a better prognosis in children than in adults. Rituximab is given intravenously at a dose of 375 mg/m^2 of the patient's body surface at weekly intervals for a total of 4 weeks, the same regimen as that given for a B cell lymphoma. For connective tissue diseases, rheumatologists administer rituximab intravenously at a dose of 1000 mg given 1 week and repeated 2 weeks later. This regimen has also been used for autoimmune bullous diseases with success, but so far it has not been used in EBA patients. Although rituximab may be beneficial for controlling EBA, one problem with the reported cases to date is that the EBA patients had been given prior immunosuppressive agents and were usually continued on immunosuppressive agents in addition to rituximab when control of their EBA occurred. It is not clear if monotherapy with rituximab would be beneficial for EBA.

Photopheresis and Plasmapheresis

Extracorporeal photochemotherapy (ECP), or photopheresis, has reportedly been successful in treating a number of autoimmune bullous conditions. Gordon and colleagues (58) studied three patients with recalcitrant EBA who were treated with ECP. The patients were given 1.5 mg/kg of oral crystalline 8-methoxypsoralen 90 min prior to the photopheresis treatments with a Therakos UVAR machine. Treatments were given on two consecutive days every month for a total of 6 or 7 months and then followed for 6 months post treatment. In these patients, ECP led to an improvement in clinical symptoms, an increase in dermal epidermal adherence as measured by suction blister times, and a decrease in the level of circulating anti-BMZ antibodies [57]. There is another case report of a patient with life-threatening EBA who responded favorably and was put into remission with ECP [58]. In another report, plasmapheresis alone resulted in lower circulating anti-C7 antibodies in the blood of an EBA patient and concomitant remission of the disease [59].

Intravenous Immunoglobulin

Intravenous immunoglobulin (IVIG) has also shown efficacy in treating EBA patients [60–67]. The usual total dose of IVIG was 2 g/kg of body weight administered intravenously in divided doses over 3–5 days each month for 9–24 months. In many of these reports, the IVIG was concomitantly administered with other systemic immunosuppressives. Often conventional immunosuppression was given first and with lack of a satisfactory response, the IVIG was added and appeared to make a significant difference in controlling the patient [67]. No serious side effects have been reported in any of the EBA patients treated with IVIG.

Conclusion

EBA is an autoimmune blistering skin disease due to auto-immunity to C7, the collagen in anchoring fibrils. These autoantibodies perturb the function of anchoring fibrils leading to epidermal-dermal separation. EBA can present in a number of different ways and can be diagnosed by clinical findings, histopathology, DIF, IIF, IEM, ELISA, and Western blotting. EBA is associated with IBD and has significant clinical complications such as exuberant scarring and nail loss. EBA is notoriously difficult to treat, and there is a lack of large controlled studies, so most of the data are anecdotal case reports and small case series.

References

1. Elliott G. Two cases of epidermolysis bullosa. J Cutan Genitourin Dis. 1895;13:10–8.
2. Roenigk Jr HH, Ryan JG, Bergfeld WF. Epidermolysis bullosa acquisita. Report of three cases and review of all published cases. Arch Dermatol. 1971;103(1):1–10.
3. Gibbs RB, Minus HR. Epidermolysis bullosa acquisita with electron microscopical studies. Arch Dermatol. 1975;111(2):215–20.
4. Kushniruk W. The immunopathology of epidermolysis bullosa acquisita. Can Med Assoc J. 1973;108(9):1143–6.
5. Nieboer C, Boorsma DM, Woerdeman MJ, Kalsbeek GL. Epidermolysis bullosa acquisita. Immunofluorescence, electron microscopic and immunoelectron microscopic studies in four patients. Br J Dermatol. 1980;102(4):383–92.
6. Yaoita H, Briggaman RA, Lawley TJ, Provost TT, Katz SI. Epidermolysis bullosa acquisita: ultrastructural and immunological studies. J Invest Dermatol. 1981;76(4):288–92.
7. Woodley DT, Briggaman RA, O'Keefe EJ, Inman AO, Queen LL, Gammon WR. Identification of the skin basement-membrane autoantigen in epidermolysis bullosa acquisita. N Engl J Med. 1984;310(16):1007–13.
8. Woodley DT, Burgeson RE, Lunstrum G, Bruckner-Tuderman L, Reese MJ, Briggaman RA. Epidermolysis bullosa acquisita antigen is the globular carboxyl terminus of type VII procollagen. J Clin Invest. 1988;81(3):683–7.
9. Woodley DT, O'Keefe EJ, McDonald JA, Reese MJ, Briggaman RA, Gammon WR. Specific affinity between fibronectin and the epidermolysis bullosa acquisita antigen. J Clin Invest. 1987;79(6):1826–30.
10. Lapiere JC, Chen JD, Iwasaki T, Hu L, Uitto J, Woodley DT. Type VII collagen specifically binds fibronectin via a unique subdomain within the collagenous triple helix. J Invest Dermatol. 1994;103(5):637–41.
11. Chen M, Marinkovich MP, Veis A, Cai X, Rao CN, O'Toole EA, et al. Interactions of the amino-terminal noncollagenous (NC1) domain of type VII collagen with extracellular matrix components. A potential role in epidermal-dermal adherence in human skin. J Biol Chem. 1997;272(23):14516–22.

12. Ray TL, Levine JB, Weiss W, Ward PA. Epidermolysis bullosa acquisita and inflammatory bowel disease. J Am Acad Dermatol. 1982;6(2):242–52.
13. Gammon WR, Heise ER, Burke WA, Fine JD, Woodley DT, Briggaman RA. Increased frequency of HLA-DR2 in patients with autoantibodies to epidermolysis bullosa acquisita antigen: evidence that the expression of autoimmunity to type VII collagen is HLA class II allele associated. J Invest Dermatol. 1988;91(3):228–32.
14. Woodley D. Epidermolysis bullosa acquisita. Prog Dermatol. 1988;22:1–13.
15. Stewart MI, Woodley DT, Briggaman RA. Epidermolysis bullosa acquisita and associated symptomatic esophageal webs. Arch Dermatol. 1991;127(3):373–7.
16. Gammon WR, Briggaman RA, Woodley DT, Heald PW, Wheeler Jr CE. Epidermolysis bullosa acquisita--a pemphigoid-like disease. J Am Acad Dermatol. 1984;11:820–32.
17. Provost TT, Maize JC, Ahmed AR, Strauss JS, Dobson RL. Unusual subepidermal bullous diseases with immunologic features of bullous pemphigoid. Arch Dermatol. 1979;115(2):156–60.
18. Richter BJ, McNutt NS. The spectrum of epidermolysis bullosa acquisita. Arch Dermatol. 1979;115(11):1325–8.
19. Dahl MG. Epidermolysis bullosa acquisita--a sign of cicatricial pemphigoid? Br J Dermatol. 1979;101(4):475–84.
20. Kurzhals G, Stolz W, Meurer M, Kunze J, Braun-Falco O, Krieg T. Acquired epidermolysis bullosa with the clinical feature of Brunsting-Perry cicatricial bullous pemphigoid. Arch Dermatol. 1991;127(3):391–5.
21. Tanaka N, Dainichi T, Ohyama B, et al. A case of epidermolysis bullosa acquisita with clinical features of Brunsting-Perry pemphigoid showing an excellent response to colchicine. J Am Acad Dermatol. 2009;61:715–9.
22. Hashimoto T, Ishiko A, Shimizu H, et al. A case of linear IgA bullous dermatosis withIgA anti-type VII collagen autoantibodies. Br J Dermatol. 1996;134:336–9.
23. Bauer JW, Schaeppi H, Metze D, Muss W, Pohla-Gubo G, Hametner R, et al. Ocular involvement in IgA-epidermolysis bullosa acquisita. Br J Dermatol. 1999;141(5):887–92.
24. Park SB, Cho KH, Youn JL, Hwang DH, Kim SC, Chung JH. Epidermolysis bullosa acquisita in childhood--a case mimicking chronic bullous dermatosis of childhood. Clin Exp Dermatol. 1997;22(5):220–2.
25. Callot-Mellot C, Bodemer C, Caux F, Bourgault-Villada I, Fraitag S, Goudie G, et al. Epidermolysis bullosa acquisita in childhood. Arch Dermatol. 1997;133(9):1122–6.
26. Lee CW. Serum IgA autoantibodies in patients with epidermolysis bullosa acquisita: a high frequency of detection. Dermatology. 2000;200:83–4.
27. Edwards S, Wakelin SH, Wojnarowska F, Marsden RA, Kirtschig G, Bhogal B, et al. Bullous pemphigoid and epidermolysis bullosa acquisita: presentation, prognosis, and immunopathology in 11 children. Pediatr Dermatol. 1998;15(3):184–90.
28. Burke WA, Briggaman RA, Gammon WR. Epidermolysis bullosa acquisita in a patient with multiple endocrinopathies syndrome. Arch Dermatol. 1986;122(2):187–9.
29. Chan L, Woodley D. Pemphigoid: bullous and cicatricial. In: Lichenstein L, Fauci AS, editors. Rheumatology. 5th ed. St. Louis: Mosby; 1996. p. 93.
30. Chen M, O'Toole EA, Sanghavi J, Mahmud N, Weir D, Kelleher D, Fairley JA, Woodley DT. The EBA antigen is present in human colon and patients with Crohn's disease have autoantibodies to type VII collagen. J Invest Dermatol. 2002;118:1059–64.
31. Ishii N, Recke A, Mihai S, Hirose M, Hashimoto T, Zillikens D, et al. Autoantibody-induced intestinal inflammation and weight loss in experimental epidermolysis bullosa acquisita. J Pathol. 2011;224(2):234–44.
32. Vodegel RM, Jonkman MR, Pas HH, de Jong MC. U-serrated immunodeposition pattern differentiates type VII collagne targeting bullous diseases from other subjepidermal bullous autoimmune diseases. Br J Dermatol. 2004;151:112–8.
33. Woodley D, Sauder D, Talley MJ, Silver M, Grotendorst G, Qwarnstrom E. Localization of basement membrane components after dermal-epidermal junction separation. J Invest Dermatol. 1983;81(2):149–53.

34. Gammon WR, Briggaman RA, Inman 3rd AO, Queen LL, Wheeler CE. Differentiating anti-lamina lucida and anti-sublamina densa anti-BMZ antibodies by indirect immunofluorescence on 1.0 M sodium chloride-separated skin. J Invest Dermatol. 1984;82(2):139–44.
35. Gammon WR, Kowalewski C, Chorzelski TP, Kumar V, Briggaman RA, Beutner EH. Direct immunofluorescence studies of sodium chloride-separated skin in the differential diagnosis of bullous pemphigoid and epidermolysis bullosa acquisita. J Am Acad Dermatol. 1990;22(4):664–70.
36. Domloge-Hultsch N, Anhalt GJ, Gammon WR, Lazarova Z, Briggaman R, Welch M, et al. Antiepiligrin cicatricial pemphigoid. A subepithelial bullous disorder. Arch Dermatol. 1994;130(12):1521–9.
37. Goletz S, Hashimoto T, Zillikens D, Schmidt E. Anti-p200 pemphigoid. J Am Acad Dermatol. 2014;71(1):185–91.
38. Chan LS, Wang XS, Lapiere JC, Marinkovich MP, Jones JC, Woodley DT. A newly identified 105-kD lower lamina lucida autoantigen is an acidic protein distinct from the 105-kD gamma 2 chain of laminin-5. J Invest Dermatol. 1995;105(1):75–9.
39. Ghohestani RF, Hudson BG, Claudy A, Uitto J. The alpha 5 chain of type IV collagen is the target of IgG autoantibodies in a novel autoimmune disease with subepidermal blisters and renal insufficiency. J Biol Chem. 2000;275(21):16002–6.
40. Ghohestani RF, Rotunda SL, Hudson B, Gaughan WJ, Farber JL, Webster G, et al. Crescentic glomerulonephritis and subepidermal blisters with autoantibodies to α5 and α6 chains of type IV collagen. Lab Invest. 2003;83:605–11.
41. Gammon WR, Woodley DT, Dole KC, Briggaman RA. Evidence that anti-basement membrane zone antibodies in bullous eruption of systemic lupus erythematosus recognize epidermolysis bullosa acquisita autoantigen. J Invest Dermatol. 1985;84(6):472–6.
42. Chen M, Chan LS, Cai X, O'Toole EA, Sample JC, Woodley DT. Development of an ELISA for rapid detection of anti-type VII collagen autoantibodies in epidermolysis bullosa acquisita. J Invest Dermatol. 1997;108(1):68–72.
43. Woodley DT, O'Keefe EJ, Reese MJ, Mechanic GL, Briggaman RA, Gammon WR. Epidermolysis bullosa acquisita antigen, a new major component of cutaneous basement membrane, is a glycoprotein with collagenous domains. J Invest Dermatol. 1986;86(6):668–72.
44. Kirtschig G, Murrell D, Wojnarowska F, Khumalo N. Interventions for mucous membrane pemphigoid and epidermolysis bullosa acquisita. Cochrane Database Syst Rev. 2003;(1):CD004056.
45. Cunningham BB, Kirchmann TT, Woodley D. Colchicine for epidermolysis bullosa acquisita. J Am Acad Dermatol. 1996;34:781–4.
46. Mekori YA, Chowers Y, Ducker I, Klajman A. Inhibition of delayed hypersensitivity reactions by colchicine. II. Colchicine inhibits interferon-gamma induced expression of HLA-DR on gut epithelial cell line. Clin Exp Immunol. 1989;78(2):230–2.
47. Connolly SM, Sander HM. Treatment of epidermolysis bullosa acquisita with cyclosporine. J Am Acad Dermatol. 1987;16(4):890.
48. Crow LL, Finkle JP, Gammon WR, Woodley DT. Clearing of epidermolysis bullosa acquisita with cyclosporine. J Am Acad Dermatol. 1988;19:937–42.
49. McKinley SK, Huang JT, Tan J, Kroshinsky D, Gellis S. A case of recalcitrant epidermolysis bullosa acquisita responsive to rituximab therapy. Pediatr Dermatol. 2014;31(2):241–4.
50. Hughes AP, Callen JP. Epidermolysis bullosa acquisita responsive to dapsone therapy. J Cutan Med Surg. 2001;5:397–9.
51. Saha M, Cutler T, Bhogal B, Black MM, Groves RW. Refractory epidermolysis bullosa acquisita: successful treatment with rituximab. Clin Exp Dermatol. 2009;34:e979–80.
52. Li Y, Foshee JB, Sontheimer RD. Sustained clinical response to rituximab in a case of life-threatening overlap subepidermal autoimmune blistering disease. J Am Acad Dermatol. 2011;64(4):773–8.
53. Sadler E, Schafleitner B, Lanschuetzer C, Laimer M, Pohla-Gubo G, Hametner R, et al. Treatment-resistant classical epidermolysis bullosa acquisita responding to rituximab. Br J Dermatol. 2007;157:417–9.

54. Crichlow SM, Mortimer NJ, Harman KE. A successful therapeutic trial of rituximab in the treatment of a patient with recalcitrant, high-titre epidermolysis bullosa acquisita. Br J Dermatol. 2007;156:194–6.
55. Schmidt E, Benoit S, Brocker EB, Zillikens D, Goebeler M. Successful adjuvant treatment of recalcitrant epidermolysis bullosa acquisita with anti-CD20 antibody rituximab. Arch Dermatol. 2006;142(2):147–50.
56. Niedermeier A, Eming R, Pfutze M, Neumann CR, Happel C, Reich K, et al. Clinical response of severe mechanobullous epidermolysis bullosa acquisita to combined treatment with immunoadsorption and rituximab (anti-CD20 monoclonal antibodies). Arch Dermatol. 2007;143(2):192–8.
57. Gordon KB, Chan LS, Woodley DT. Treatment of refractory epidermolysis bullosa acquisita with extracorporeal photochemotherapy. Br J Dermatol. 1997;136(3):415–20.
58. Miller JL, Stricklin GP, Fine JD, King LE, Arzubiaga MC, Ellis DL. Remission of severe epidermolysis bullosa acquisita induced by extracorporeal photochemotherapy. Br J Dermatol. 1995;133(3):467–71.
59. Furue M, Iwata M, Yoon HI, Kubota Y, Ohto H, Kawashima M, et al. Epidermolysis bullosa acquisita: clinical response to plasma exchange therapy and circulating anti-basement membrane zone antibody titer. J Am Acad Dermatol. 1986;14:873–8.
60. Sami N, Ahmed AR. Results of intravenous immunoglobulin therapy in ocular involvement in epidermolysis bullosa acquisita. Invest Ophthalmol Vis Sci. 2003;44:1388.
61. Kim JH, Kim YH, Kim SC. Epidermolysis bullosa acquisita: a retrospective clinical analysis of 30 cases. Acta Derm Venereol. 2011;91:307–12.
62. Harman KE, Black MM. High-dose intravenous immune globulin for the treatment of autoimmune blistering diseases: an evaluation of its use in 14 cases. Br J Dermatol. 1999;140:864–74.
63. Caldwell JB, Yancey KB, Engler RJ, et al. Epidermolysis bullosa acquisita: efficacy of high-dose intravenous immunoglobulins. J Am Acad Dermatol. 1994;31:827–8.
64. Gourgiotou K, Exadaktylou D, Aroni K, Rallis E, Nicolaidou E, Paraskevakou H, Katsambas AD. Epidermolysis bullosa acquisita: treatment with intravenous immunoglobulins. J Eur Acad Dermatol Venereol. 2002;16:77–88.
65. Osada S-I, Yoshida R, Kikuchi I, Tsuruta D, Ansai S-I, Hashimoto T, Kawana S. Successful treatment of intravenous immunoglobulins in a patient with intractable epidermolysis bullosa acquisita with autoantibodies to type VII collagen and laminin alpha-3. J Clin Exp Dermatol Res. 2013;4:1–3.
66. Meier F, Sonnichsen K, Schaumburg-Lever G, Dopfer R, Rassner G. Epidermolysis bullosa acquisita: efficacy of high-dose intravenous immunoglobulins. J Am Acad Dermatol. 1993;29:334–7.
67. Ahmed AR, Gurcan HM. Treatment of epidermolysis bullosa acquisita with intravenous immunoglobulin in patients non-responsive to conventional therapy: clinical outcome and post-treatment long-term follow-up. J Eur Acad Dermatol Venereol. 2012;26:1074–83.

Chapter 9
Pemphigoid Gestationis

Elizabeth M. Moore and Victoria P. Werth

Abstract Pemphigoid gestationis (PG) is an autoimmune blistering disease that occurs during pregnancy or soon after delivery. It is possibly caused by cross-reactivity between placental antigens and collagen XVII in the skin. Patients typically present with an intensely pruritic, vesiculobullous rash that starts periumbilically and spreads outwards across the trunk and extremities. Treatment is with immunosuppressive agents; however, given that PG is very rare—estimated to occur in 1 in 50,000 pregnancies—there is a paucity of evidence around specific treatments. Treatment of PG is also complicated by the need to consider the health of the fetus. Often, evidence for the use of immunosuppressant medications in pregnant women for other diseases can be extrapolated to PG. We review the literature and present an algorithm for treatment in the pre- and post-partum periods for women with PG based on the evidence available. We also list areas of focus for the future.

Keywords Pemphigoid Gestationis • PG • Autoimmune • Blistering • Pregnancy • BP180

Abbreviations

ABSIS	Autoimmune Bullous Skin Disorder Intensity Score
BP	Bullous pemphigoid
DIF	Direct immunofluorescence
ELISA	Enzyme-linked immunosorbent assay
IA	Immunoadsorption
IIF	Indirect immunofluorescence
LBW	Low birth weight

E.M. Moore, BA
Department of Dermatology, University of Pennsylvania, Philadelphia, PA, USA

V.P. Werth, MD (✉)
Department of Dermatology, Corporal Michael J. Crescenz Veterans Affairs Medical Center, University of Pennsylvania, Philadelphia, PA, USA

Department of Dermatology, Perelman Center for Advanced Medicine, Suite 1-330A, 3400 Civic Center Boulevard, Philadelphia, PA 19104, USA
e-mail: werth@mail.med.upenn.edu

N. Sami (ed.), *Autoimmune Bullous Diseases: Approach and Management*,
DOI 10.1007/978-3-319-26728-9_9

LHRH	Luteinizing hormone releasing hormone
PDAI	Pemphigus Disease Area Index
PG	Pemphigoid gestationis
TSH	Thyroid stimulating hormone

Introduction

Pemphigoid gestationis (PG) is an autoimmune blistering disease that occurs either during pregnancy or immediately after delivery. It is rare, with an incidence estimated around 1 in 50,000 pregnancies [1]. Typically erupting in a woman's first or second trimester, PG presents with erythematous papules and plaques and is associated with a high degree of pruritus. Lesions tend to first appear periumbilically and spread centrifugally [2]. In the later stages of the eruption, vesicles and bullae predominate and affect the trunk and extremities, while sparing the palms, soles of feet, face, and mucous membranes [3] (see Fig. 9.1). While not associated with systemic maternal health risks, the pruritus can be incapacitating [3].

There appears to be a hormonal component to disease activity, with many patients experiencing improvements in late pregnancy, but flares after delivery [5]. Flares can also occur during menstruation and with oral contraceptive use [6]. PG can present initially in the postpartum period in a reported 25 % of cases, sometimes within hours of delivery [3]. It can recur with subsequent pregnancies, sometimes earlier in the gestation and more severe in quality [3].

Pathogenesis

The histologic and immunologic features of PG are similar to those of bullous pemphigoid (BP) [7]. Like BP, PG is associated with antibodies to two hemidesmosomal proteins: BP180 (collagen XVII, a transdermal hemidesmosomal protein) and, to a lesser degree, BP230. Both antibodies are members of the IgG1 subclass [8]. The purported mechanism of PG is initiated in the placenta, where MHCII molecules are thought to be aberrantly expressed and expose the maternal immune system to the BP180 antigen. Normally, the fetal trophoblastic cells do not express these MHC molecules, so the maternal immune system is tolerant to the fetoplacental unit [9]. Because the BP180 antigen is present in both the skin and the placenta, cross-reactivity can occur, resulting in an autoimmune reaction targeting the basement membrane of the epidermis [10]. Destruction of hemidesmosomal proteins leads to vesicles and bullae. The involved autoantibodies are also capable of activating complement and precipitating infiltration of neutrophils and eosinophils [6].

Certain individuals can be predisposed to developing PG during pregnancy. There is an association between PG and HLA-DR3 in up to 80 % of patients and with HLA-DR4 in up to 53 % of patients; both are expressed in up to 50 % patients with PG, but in only 3 % of the general population [10].

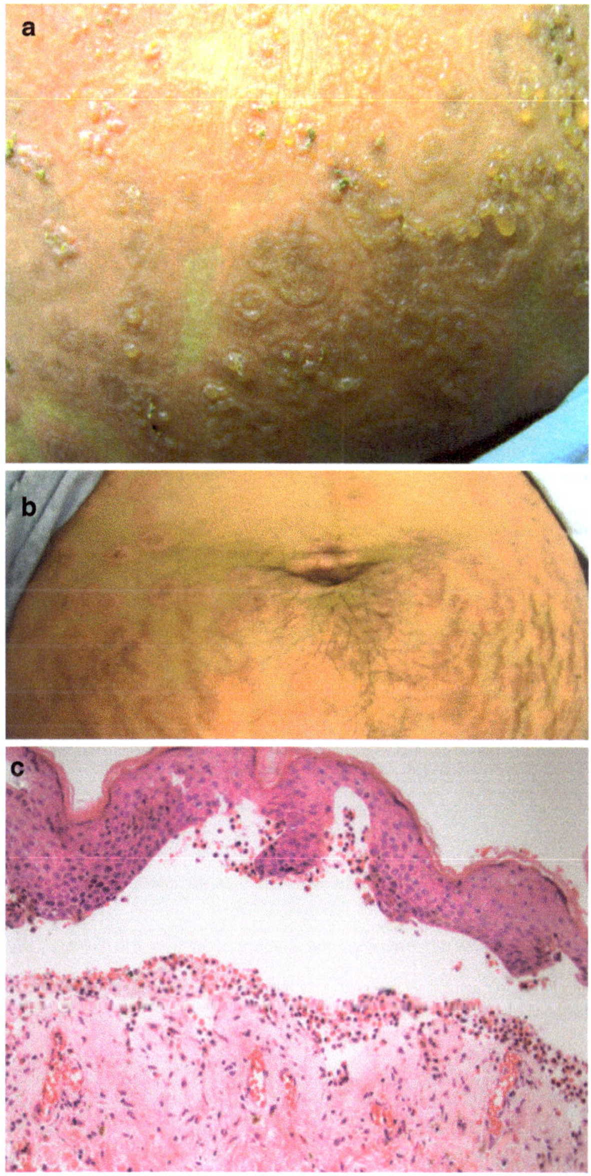

Fig. 9.1 (**a**) vesicles and erythematous plaques on the chest, (**b**) targetoid plaques on the abdomen, (**c**) punch biopsy of vesicle with H&E staining (From Morganroth and McHargue [4]. Reprinted with permission from American Medical Association)

Diagnosis

Diagnosis of PG can be confirmed based on clinical, histologic, and direct immunofluorescence (DIF) findings. On histology, urticarial lesions demonstrate a perivascular lymphocytic and eosinophilic infiltrate. In their plaque form, lesions demonstrate dermal edema and spongiosis as well as basal cell necrosis on dermal papillae tips. Vesiculobullous lesions demonstrate subepidermal blistering and bullae can contain eosinophils [6] (see Fig. 9.1). On DIF, lesions demonstrate linear C3 deposition at the basement membrane zone. IgG can also be present along the basement membrane [11]. DIF is the gold standard of diagnosis when combined with the appropriate clinical picture.

Indirect immunofluorescence (IIF), additionally, can detect IgG antibodies at the basement membrane in around 20 % of patients [11]. ELISA testing can also be helpful for diagnosis through detection of BP180 antibodies. In 2004, a commercially available BP180-NC16a domain enzyme-linked immunoassay became available. ELISA was shown in 2008 to have a higher sensitivity for BP and PG than IIF (93 % compared to 74 %) with a similar specificity [12].

Treatment

Remission of PG can occur without intervention within weeks of delivery [3]. In general, the pruritus associated with PG in not tolerable to patients and treatment should be started upon presentation. Immunosuppression with steroids is the mainstay of therapy, with steroid-sparing agents generally started after delivery to avoid fetal exposure to these agents.

Topical Agents/Antihistamines

Topical steroids can be started during the early stages of PG before the presence of blistering. Typically, a potent corticosteroid such as clobetasol propionate 0.05 % or betamethasone 0.05 % dipropionate can be applied twice a day [13]. They can be used along with emollients and oral antihistamines to alleviate pruritus and prevent eruption of blisters. FDA category B antihistamines are generally considered safer to use after the first trimester.

Oral Corticosteroids

Once a patient has blistering, systemic corticosteroids are typically added to the treatment plan. Oral prednisone and prednisolone are mainstays of therapy that are used during pregnancy as well as postpartum. There is some evidence for a more liberal approach to starting oral corticosteroids; a retrospective analysis of 13 patients in Iran found that those in whom oral corticosteroids were implemented sooner had faster improvement [14].

The accepted dosage for severe PG during the post-partum period is 0.5–1.0 mg/kg/day of prednisone that can be tapered when tolerated [6]. It is important to monitor patients for appropriate response and make changes as necessary. In general, a patient should respond to an appropriate dose after 3 days of treatment (as defined below); if the patient does not respond, a 2 mg/kg/day dose is given. Once the patient responds, the steroids can be tapered and maintained at the lowest effective dose [10].

The use of oral corticosteroids during pregnancy is important for the treatment of many autoimmune diseases. Along with topical agents, systemic corticosteroids are the only mainstay of therapy for PG that is used during pregnancy. Transplacental passage of steroids differs by type, with non-fluorinated corticosteroids such as prednisone largely deactivated before passage to the fetus [15]. The fluorinated compounds, meanwhile, such as betamethasone, do pass to the fetus. Prednisone is therefore the preferred corticosteroid during pregnancy.

Some studies have shown that prednisone can lead to intrauterine growth retardation, premature rupture of membranes, and preterm delivery [15]. There have also been reports of corticosteroids causing cleft palate in animals [16], with small studies replicating this finding in humans when steroids are given between 4 weeks prior to conception to 12 weeks after [17]. Larger human studies have not replicated these findings [18].

In 2013, a cohort study of over 1700 children compared survival and neurodevelopmental disability between those whose mothers were treated with one *vs* multiple courses of systemic corticosteroids; the study found no significant difference between the groups [19]. However, follow-up ended when children were 5 years old, leaving open the possibility of differences between groups in late-presenting neurobehavioral functioning. Chi et al., additionally, found an association with blistering diseases of pregnancy and fetuses that were born small for gestational age, but concluded that the use of oral corticosteroids was not a risk factor [20].

Once steroids are discontinued, the patient and the fetus should be examined for adrenal insufficiency, depending on the duration of use [21]. Some recommend a maximum dose of 7.5 mg/day of prednisone when use is prolonged in a pregnant patient; doses greater than 20 mg daily should be avoided [18].

Alternatives to corticosteroids can be considered in steroid-refractory cases during pregnancy, as well as postpartum to avoid the side effect profile of long-term corticosteroid use. Steroid-sparing therapies also have the potential to cause serious side effects and their risks and benefits should be considered.

Azathioprine

While there are no prospective controlled trials of azathioprine, there are several case studies showing varying degrees of benefit of this drug. It is typically given at doses of 50–150 mg/day [13]. Kreuter et al. described a patient whose disease continued to progress on 150 mg/day prednisone after 10 days of therapy. Azathioprine 100 mg/day was implemented, which improved the patient clinically and enabled prednisone to be lowered to 50 mg/day, though not below this point [22]. Cianchini et al. documented a woman with severe PG who was started on daily doses of prednisone 100 mg, azathioprine 150 mg, and dapsone 125 mg with partial response [23].

Azathioprine is a category D drug; it is therefore generally used in the postpartum period only in cases of PG [13]. However, there is data supporting its safety during pregnancy, much of which is from studies on azathioprine use for organ transplants as well as other autoimmune diseases such as systemic lupus erythematosus [18]. No associations with congenital malformations have been noted, although there may be a slightly increased risk of atrial or ventricular septal defects [24]. There have been reports of cytopenias in neonates born to women taking azathioprine, however since initiating a protocol to halve azathioprine doses at 32 weeks gestation, there have not been reports of cytopenias [25].

Dapsone

Dapsone can also be used as an adjuvant therapy for PG, typically given at 50–150 mg/day. Amato et al. reported on a patient on prednisone, azathioprine, dapsone, and plasmapheresis who had a limited response [26]. The Cianchini case described above also used both azathioprine and dapsone as adjuvant agents with limited response.

Dapsone is pregnancy category C. Prior to starting dapsone, G6PD levels should be checked to avoid hemolysis in vulnerable patients. Fetal risks include hyperbilirubinemia and hemolytic anemia; when patients use dapsone while breastfeeding, infants should be monitored for hemolysis.

Cyclophosphamide

Cyclophophamide is also category D in pregnancy and only used postpartum in severe, steroid-refractory cases of PG. One case report published in 1996 described a patient with severe persistent PG who also had anti-phospholipid syndrome. This patient achieved complete remission on cyclophosphamide 0.75 g/m^2, given in monthly doses by intravenous infusion over the course of 8 weeks, and another dose 5 months later. This patient's illness was severe enough that she was delivered by emergency c-section at 32 weeks when prednisone 120 mg/day did not control symptoms. High dose prednisone and azathioprine were unable to control the disease postpartum as well [13, 27].

Intravenous Immunoglobulin (IVIg)

Unlike most therapies for PG, IVIg is not immunosuppressive, and has a less concerning side effect profile; as such, its use has expanded in recent years [7]. Its use in pregnancy has not been shown to harm the fetus during human gestation (category C). Typically it is added to therapy when systemic corticosteroids plus adjuvant dapsone or azathioprine are unable to control blistering. As with other PG therapies, only a handful of case reports are available as evidence for the effectiveness of IVIg, all reporting a favorable response to IVIg. The dose in all was 1–2 g/kg in monthly cycles; complete remission was achieved in 3–4 months with no reported side effects [7]. As mentioned above, Kreuter et al. described a patient whose disease worsened on azathioprine and prednisone when the prednisone was tapered; upon addition of IVIg, the patient's lesions completely resolved [22]. Rodrigues et al. reported a very similar case [28].

The use of IVIg is better established in pemphigus than PG or BP, with over 100 publications favoring the use of IVIg in pemphigus. Most of the reports utilized IVIg at a dose of 2 g/kg/cycle given over 2–5 days and showed a positive clinical outcome, decrease in pathologic autoantibodies, and a steroid-sparing effect [13].

Plasmapheresis

Plasmapheresis works by removing autoantibodies from the serum. There are a small number of case reports documenting the use of plasmapheresis in PG, both during pregnancy and after delivery. Amato et al. demonstrated a partial response when plasmapheresis was added to prednisone, azathioprine, and dapsone [26]. Van de Wiel et al. reported a patient who acquired PG in the 20th week of her pregnancy. She received plasmapheresis at 26 weeks, at delivery, and postpartum, with complete resolution of disease [29].

Immunoadsorbtion (IA)

Like plasmapheresis, IA removes autoantibodies from circulation, but can specifically remove IgG and does not require plasma product replacement. Recommendations for treatment of autoimmune blistering diseases with IA have even been published by German, Austrian, and Swiss experts [30]. Unfortunately, again, the evidence for IA in PG is provided by only case reports. Westerman et al. reported on a postpartum woman whose lesions progressed despite treatment with topical and oral corticosteroids. Because she was breastfeeding, the patient's prednisolone dose was not increased beyond 60 mg/day, and the decision was made to perform 10 immunoadsorptions over 4 weeks. During this period her clinical status improved dramatically, enabling prednisolone to be reduced. More recently, a case report was published of a woman who received 15 AI treatments, nearly all during the prepartum period, and responded well [31].

Other Treatments

There are additionally case reports of successful adjuvant therapy with rituximab [23] and goserelin [13, 23]. The Cianchini et al. case described above documented a woman on daily doses of prednisone 100 mg, azathioprine 150 mg, and dapsone 125 mg; IVIg enabled temporary benefit, but complete response was not achieved until the addition of rituximab 375 mg/m^2 weekly for 4 consecutive weeks. Goserelin is an LHRH agonist that effectively oophorectimizes the patient. The hormonal component of PG has been established, given the observations that symptoms often recur during menstruation and can flare with use of oral contraceptive pills [32]. A study in 2002 found that goserelin helped cleared symptoms of PG [33].

Approach to a Patient with PG

The approach to the PG patient can be difficult given the lack of systematic evidence and lack of established clinical guidelines for such a rare disease. In general, treatment choices for a patient with PG is determined first by whether the patient is prepartum or postpartum, and next based on the severity of the condition. Important to the discussion of how to treat PG patients are criteria for evaluating the disease as mild, moderate, or severe.

Evaluation of Condition Severity and Failure of Treatment

While there are no established criteria for determining whether PG is mild, moderate, or severe, clinicians can borrow from the criteria of other autoimmune blistering diseases. Using such scoring systems for initial assessment and monitoring of cutaneous involvement of disease has proven useful. Three scoring systems have already been validated for similar diseases. These are the Autoimmune Bullous Skin Disorder Intensity Score (ABSIS), the Pemphigus Disease Area Index (PDAI) and the BP Disease Area Index (BPDAI) [34].

ABSIS was created to monitor patients with pemphigus, and has also been used in epidermolysis bullosa acquisita and BP [35]. This system comprises body surface area involved along with a weighting factor (i.e., a factor of 1.5 is assigned to exudative and erosive lesions, 1.0 to dry erosive lesions, and 0.5 to lesions that have re-epithelialized.) The body surface area (BSA) measurement uses the established system of measuring burns (i.e., the head and each arm are 9 % total BSA, abdomen and back are each 18 %, and legs are each 18 %).

The PDAI was developed by the International Pemphigus Definitions Committee. This score system comprises scores for the skin, scalp, and mucous membranes [34]. The skin component, in turn, comprises scores for both activity and damage.

"Activity" is the extent of erosions, blisters, or new erythema, while "damage" depends on whether there is postinflammatory hyperpigmentation or erythema from a resolving lesion. The scalp score assesses the number of quadrants of the scalp affected by disease, and the mucous membranes score is similar to the skin activity score with presence of any lesions counted for each mucous membrane area.

In 2011, the International Pemphigoid Committee proposed the BP Disease Area Index (BPDAI) [34]. The BPDAI is similar to the PDAI, but allows more emphasis for lesions on the extremities than the scalp and mucosa. This scoring system measures bullous lesions as well as urticarial and eczematous lesions [34]. A study in 2012 found that ABSIS and BPDAI scores correlated with BP180 titers [36].

The BPDAI is likely the best fit to use for assessing and monitoring patients with PG given that PG tends to spare the scalp and mucous membranes, areas that are given more value in the PDAI. It also includes points for urticarial lesions, which play a role in PG prior to blistering. Using a score for PG that was developed for BP is also appropriate given the similarities of the conditions. Both result from BP180 autoantibodies, and there are several cases in the literature of long-term PG that is thought to have perhaps converted to BP.

Control and Failure of Treatment

It is also important to define whether a treatment is controlling the disease or failing. Again, guidelines have not been developed specifically for PG, but clinicians and researchers can borrow from those developed for other conditions. Disease control consensus statement guidelines were released in 2008 for pemphigus and in 2012 for bullous pemphigoid [37, 38]. These definitions were proposed:

1. Control: The time at which new lesions cease to form and established lesions begin to heal
2. Complete remission: The absence of new or established lesions, either on systemic therapy or off, for at least 2 months
3. Partial remission off therapy: Presence of transient new lesions that heal within 1 week without treatment and while the patient is off all systemic therapy for at least 2 months
4. Partial remission on therapy: The presence of transient new lesions that heal within 1 week while the patient is receiving minimal therapy, including topical steroids
5. Relapse/flare: Appearance of at least three new lesions per month that do not heal spontaneously within 1 week, or the extension of established lesions, in a patient who has achieved disease control
6. Failure on conventional therapy: Continued new blister formation, extension of existing vesicles, or lack of healing while on prednisone 1.5 mg/kg for 1 weeks

These definitions may be applicable to PG and can be helpful in making treatment choices.

Summary: Prepartum Treatment

Options for prepartum treatment are limited to topical agents, systemic corticosteroids, and, in severe cases, azathioprine, IVIg, IA, and plasmapheresis. In general, we recommend starting with topical agents for mild PG without blistering. Once PG progresses to the blistering stage, oral corticosteroids can be added with the goal of keeping doses within the limits described above. Clinicians should keep in mind that long-term steroid use is associated with hypertension, gestational diabetes, osteopenia and Cushing's syndrome; appropriate monitoring should be implemented for at-risk patients [13].

There are additionally reports of success in treating PG with azathioprine, plasmapheresis, IVIg, and immunoadsorption during pregnancy. These therapies should be used in severe cases that are not responsive to steroids (as defined above). There is not enough evidence to recommend one of these adjuvant therapies over the others.

Summary: Postpartum Treatment

There are more options for postpartum treatment. In general, postpartum treatment is initially identical to prepartum treatment, with topical agents used first and then systemic corticosteroids. Steroid-sparing therapies should be added and steroids tapered when control has been achieved in order to reduce steroid-related side effects. Case reports and small series have demonstrated the effectiveness of azathioprine, dapsone, cyclosporine, and cyclophosphamide. We recommend starting with azathioprine, dapsone, or cyclosporine before cyclophosphamide given the toxicity of the latter – notably, permanent infertility in young women.

If disease activity persists (as defined above) on two or more of these agents, IVIg, plasmapheresis, or immunoadsorption should be considered as an addition. Again, the literature is not adequate to recommend one treatment over the others.

If treatment again fails after using corticosteroids in addition to several steroid-sparing agents and either IVIg, plasmapheresis, or immunoadsorption, there is minimal evidence for attempting treatment with goserelin (which is not safe for use during pregnancy) or rituximab (which is pregnancy Category C). There are also reports of benefit from tetracycline antibiotics [39, 40]. Notably, however, pre-partum use of these antibiotics is contraindicated given their association with permanent discoloration of teeth and hypoplasia of enamel in fetuses.

Dosages sited in the PG literature of these steroid-sparing agents are the following [13] (see Fig. 9.2).

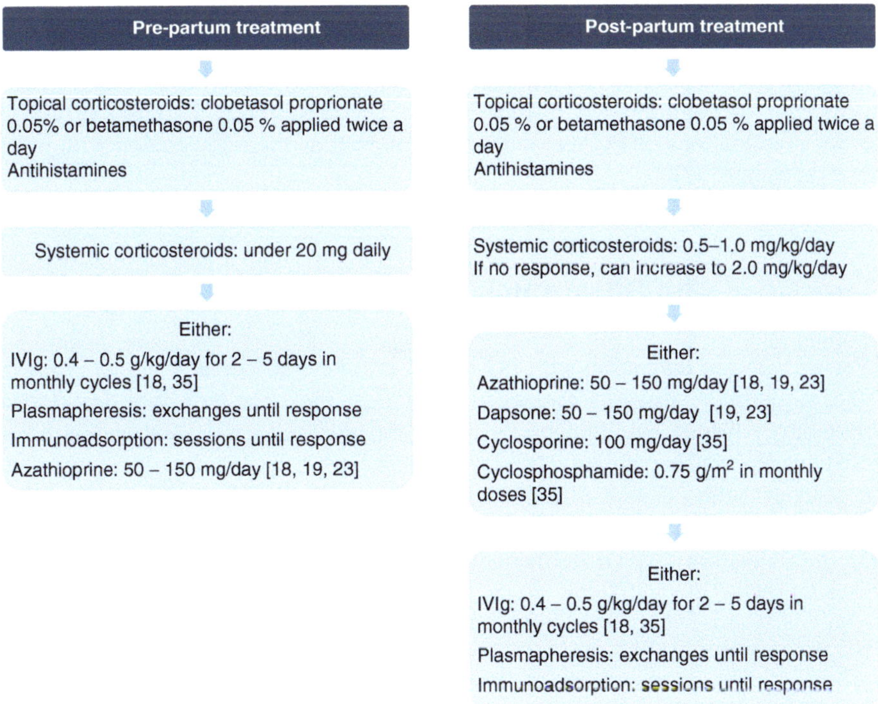

Fig. 9.2 Treatment algorithm for PG with dosages cited in the literature

Fetal Outcomes

Given that PG almost exclusively (with the rare exception of a hydatidiform mole) occurs around the time of a pregnancy, it is important to consider the health of the fetus. Chi et al. found that PG was associated with neonates who were small for gestational age and born prematurely; fortunately, the study did not find an association with fetal mortality. This replicated findings of earlier studies [41]. This report concluded that early onset of PG, in particular in the 2nd and 3rd trimesters, was associated with LBW children. It also concluded that treatment with oral corticosteroids did not impact pregnancy outcomes, and that its benefits significantly outweighed its risks [20].

There are rare reports of neonates of mothers with PG born with blistering. The mechanism is thought to be passage of IgG antibodies across the placenta from mother to fetus [42]. Affected newborns demonstrate transient blistering that resolves untreated in days to weeks; wound care can be implemented as necessary [9].

One case study reports a patient who experienced intrauterine fetal demise at 25 weeks and subsequently underwent a C-section. The patient returned to the hospital 2 days later with pruritic bilateral palmar dyshidrosis and one blister on the abdomen; PG was confirmed on histopathology. This case raises the possibility that minor presentations of PG may be missed, as well as their association with poor fetal outcomes [43].

Association with Other Autoimmune Diseases

Women who are diagnosed with PG should also be considered at higher risk for other autoimmune diseases. Graves' disease is the most common, and Hashimoto thyroiditis, vitiligo, autoimmune thrombocytopenia, and pernicious anemia have also been reported in patients with a history of PG [6]. A case study in 2014 reported on a patient with PG as well as autoantibodies to type VII collagen, which is the antigenic target in EBA; the authors implicated epitope spreading in this case as a rare mechanism by which PG patients may present with additional autoimmune diseases [11].

Areas for Future Study

Given the rarity of PG, it is unsurprising that there are deficiencies in the literature. Evidence regarding treatment is largely in the form of case studies; ideally, randomized controlled trials would eventually be used to determine the most effective treatment for PG. However, a prospective trial is unlikely given the scarcity of patients. The creation of a global database was suggested by Semkova et al. [44]. We agree that a database that includes disease characteristics, treatments, and outcomes would be the most feasible way to collect sufficient information on PG to draw more powerful conclusions on comparative effectiveness of treatments.

Additionally, researchers and clinicians would benefit from a validated measurement tool for PG. The BPDAI has been found to correlate with BP180 antibody titers in bullous pemphigoid; by studying antibody titers in PG, the BPDAI could be either validated or discarded.

Finally, it is unclear whether there are benefits to screening women with a history of PG for other autoimmune diseases—e.g., monitoring TSH—and whether there is a place for monitoring their antibody levels during subsequent pregnancies. Screening for concurrent autoimmune diseases may enable early treatment; however, it could potentially encourage overtreatment of asymptomatic patients. Monitoring antibody levels in women with a history of PG during subsequent pregnancies could potentially allow for the use of prophylactic corticosteroids before skin symptoms occur. However, it could also lead to unnecessary fetal exposure to steroids.

Acknowledgements This material is supported by the Veterans Health Administration, Office of Research and Development, Biomedical Laboratory Research and Development.

Funding Sources None

References

1. Yancey KB. Herpes gestationis. Dermatol Clin. 1990;8(4):727–35.
2. Shornick JK, et al. Herpes gestationis: clinical and histologic features of twenty-eight cases. J Am Acad Dermatol. 1983;8(2):214–24.
3. Lehrhoff S, Pomeranz MK. Specific dermatoses of pregnancy and their treatment. Dermatol Ther. 2013;26(4):274–84.
4. Morganroth PA, McHargue CA. Vesicles and targetoid lesions in a postpartum woman. JAMA Dermatol. 2014;150(4):445–6.
5. Shornick JK. Dermatoses of pregnancy. Semin Cutan Med Surg. 1998;17(3):172–81.
6. Lipozencic J, Ljubojevic S, Bukvic-Mokos Z. Pemphigoid gestationis. Clin Dermatol. 2012;30(1):51–5.
7. Czernik A, et al. Intravenous immunoglobulin in the treatment of autoimmune bullous dermatoses: an update. Autoimmunity. 2012;45(1):111–8.
8. Chimanovitch I, et al. IgG1 and IgG3 are the major immunoglobulin subclasses targeting epitopes within the NC16A domain of BP180 in pemphigoid gestationis. J Invest Dermatol. 1999;113(1):140–2.
9. Intong LR, Murrell DF. Pemphigoid gestationis: pathogenesis and clinical features. Dermatol Clin. 2011;29(3):447–52, ix.
10. Roth MM. Pregnancy dermatoses: diagnosis, management, and controversies. Am J Clin Dermatol. 2011;12(1):25–41.
11. Yang B, et al. A case of pemphigoid gestationis with concurrent IgG antibodies to BP180, BP230 and type VII collagen. Australas J Dermatol. 2014;55(1):e15–8.
12. Barnadas MA, et al. Enzyme-linked immunosorbent assay (ELISA) and indirect immunofluorescence testing in a bullous pemphigoid and pemphigoid gestationis. Int J Dermatol. 2008;47(12):1245–9.
13. Intong LR, Murrell DF. Pemphigoid gestationis: current management. Dermatol Clin. 2011;29(4):621–8.
14. Rassai S, et al. Pemphigoid gestationis: a retrospective study in southwest Iran. Acta Med Iran. 2013;51(6):408–10.
15. Makol A, Wright K, Amin S. Rheumatoid arthritis and pregnancy: safety considerations in pharmacological management. Drugs. 2011;71(15):1973–87.
16. Pradat P, et al. First trimester exposure to corticosteroids and oral clefts. Birth Defects Res A Clin Mol Teratol. 2003;67(12):968–70.
17. Carmichael SL, et al. Maternal corticosteroid use and orofacial clefts. Am J Obstet Gynecol. 2007;197(6):585.e1–7; discussion 683–4, e1–7.
18. Braunstein I, Werth V. Treatment of dermatologic connective tissue disease and autoimmune blistering disorders in pregnancy. Dermatol Ther. 2013;26(4):354–63.
19. Asztalos EV, et al. Multiple courses of antenatal corticosteroids for preterm birth study: outcomes in children at 5 years of age (MACS-5). JAMA Pediatr. 2013;167(12):1102–10.
20. Chi CC, et al. Pemphigoid gestationis: early onset and blister formation are associated with adverse pregnancy outcomes. Br J Dermatol. 2009;160(6):1222–8.
21. Cobo MF, et al. Pemphigoid gestationis: clinical and laboratory evaluation. Clinics (Sao Paulo). 2009;64(11):1043–7.
22. Kreuter A, et al. Intravenous immune globulin in the treatment of persistent pemphigoid gestationis. J Am Acad Dermatol. 2004;51(6):1027–8.

23. Cianchini G, et al. Severe persistent pemphigoid gestationis: long-term remission with rituximab. Br J Dermatol. 2007;157(2):388–9.
24. Gisbert JP. Safety of immunomodulators and biologics for the treatment of inflammatory bowel disease during pregnancy and breast-feeding. Inflamm Bowel Dis. 2010;16(5):881–95.
25. Davison JM, Dellagrammatikas H, Parkin JM. Maternal azathioprine therapy and depressed haemopoiesis in the babies of renal allograft patients. Br J Obstet Gynaecol. 1985;92(3):233–9.
26. Amato L, et al. A case of chronic herpes gestationis: persistent disease or conversion to bullous pemphigoid? J Am Acad Dermatol. 2003;49(2):302–7.
27. Castle SP, et al. Chronic herpes gestationis and antiphospholipid antibody syndrome successfully treated with cyclophosphamide. J Am Acad Dermatol. 1996;34(2 Pt 2):333–6.
28. Rodrigues Cdos S, et al. Persistent herpes gestationis treated with high-dose intravenous immunoglobulin. Acta Derm Venereol. 2007;87(2):184–6.
29. Van de Wiel A, et al. Plasma exchange in herpes gestationis. Br Med J. 1980;281(6247):1041–2.
30. Westermann L, et al. Glucocorticosteroid-resistant pemphigoid gestationis: successful treatment with adjuvant immunoadsorption. J Dermatol. 2012;39(2):168–71.
31. Marker M, et al. Successful immunoapheresis of bullous autoimmune diseases: pemphigus vulgaris and pemphigoid gestationis. J Dtsch Dermatol Ges. 2011;9(1):27–31.
32. Thomas S, et al. Postpartum pemphigoid gestationis. Indian J Dermatol. 2012;57(2):146–8.
33. Garvey MP, Handfield-Jones SE, Black MM. Pemphigoid gestationis – response to chemical oophorectomy with goserelin. Clin Exp Dermatol. 1992;17(6):443–5.
34. Daniel BS, et al. Severity score indexes for blistering diseases. Clin Dermatol. 2012;30(1):108–13.
35. Pfutze M, et al. Introducing a novel Autoimmune Bullous Skin Disorder Intensity Score (ABSIS) in pemphigus. Eur J Dermatol. 2007;17(1):4–11.
36. Patsatsi A, et al. Association of autoantibodies to BP180 with disease activity in Greek patients with bullous pemphigoid. Clin Dev Immunol. 2012;2012:854795.
37. Murrell DF, et al. Consensus statement on definitions of disease, end points, and therapeutic response for pemphigus. J Am Acad Dermatol. 2008;58(6):1043–6.
38. Murrell DF, et al. Definitions and outcome measures for bullous pemphigoid: recommendations by an international panel of experts. J Am Acad Dermatol. 2012;66(3):479–85.
39. Loo WJ, Dean D, Wojnarowska F. A severe persistent case of recurrent pemphigoid gestationis successfully treated with minocycline and nicotinamide. Clin Exp Dermatol. 2001;26(8):726–7.
40. Amato L, et al. Successful treatment with doxycycline and nicotinamide of two cases of persistent pemphigoid gestationis. J Dermatolog Treat. 2002;13(3):143–6.
41. Shornick JK, Black MM. Fetal risks in herpes gestationis. J Am Acad Dermatol. 1992;26(1):63–8.
42. Tunzi M, Gray GR. Common skin conditions during pregnancy. Am Fam Physician. 2007;75(2):211–8.
43. Perez J, et al. Dyshidrosiform presentation (pompholyx-like) of pemphigoid gestationis with intrauterine fetal death. Int J Dermatol. 2013;53(11):1383–5.
44. Semkova K, Black M. Pemphigoid gestationis: current insights into pathogenesis and treatment. Eur J Obstet Gynecol Reprod Biol. 2009;145(2):138–44.

Chapter 10
Dermatitis Herpetiformis

Timothy Patton and Neil J. Korman

Abstract Dermatitis herpetiformis is an immunobullous skin disease that is closely related to gluten sensitive enteropathy. Classic clinical characteristics of intensely pruritic vesiculopapules on the elbows, knees, and scalp are well defined, although some clinical variation exists. In most cases the diagnosis is firmly established by the presence of granular IgA in the dermal papillae on direct immunofluorescent studies. Sulfonamide compounds were first described as effective therapy several decades ago and remain the mainstay of medical therapy, while a strict gluten free diet will keep patients free of cutaneous manifestations in the majority of cases. Our understanding of dermatitis herpetiformis continues to grow, as does our understanding of the relationship between the gut and the skin.

Keywords Immunobullous • Immunofluorescence • Dapsone • Gluten sensitive enteropathy • Autoimmune

Abbreviations

DH	Dermatitis herpetiformis
DIF	Direct immunofluorescence
GSE	Gluten sensitive enteropathy
H&E	Hematoxylin and eosin
IgA	Immunoglobulin A

T. Patton, DO (✉)
Department of Dermatology, University of Pittsburgh,
580 South Aiken Ave., Suite 200, Pittsburgh, PA 15232, USA
e-mail: pattontj@upmc.edu

N.J. Korman, MD, PhD
Department of Dermatology, University Hospitals Case Medical Center, Cleveland, OH, USA
e-mail: njk2@case.edu

N. Sami (ed.), *Autoimmune Bullous Diseases: Approach and Management*,
DOI 10.1007/978-3-319-26728-9_10

History

The term "dermatitis herpetiformis" (DH) was first used as the title of an article by Louis Duhring published in the Journal of the Medical Association in 1884, describing a pruritic skin disease that he felt did not fit into previously well-established dermatologic conditions [1]. In Duhring's original description and for several decades after, the disease was described as being notoriously difficult to treat [2]. The effectiveness of sulfonamide compounds in DH was described in 1947 [3], and its association with GSE was first described by Marks in 1966 [4]. Improvement in the skin disease following a gluten free diet was described soon after [5].

Epidemiology

Earlier reports in Northern European populations found that the prevalence of DH varied from about 10–39 per 100,000 [6–8]. A more recent population based study performed in the United Kingdom from 1990 to 2011 demonstrated a comparable prevalence of DH of about 1 out of 3300 people, with a 4 % decrease per year in the incidence of DH over the same time period [9], while a recent study from Finland found a much higher prevalence of DH of 75 per 100,000 [10]. The prevalence of DH in African American and Asian populations is much lower [11, 12]. Earlier studies demonstrated a male to female ratio of almost 2:1 [13]; however, the male to female ratio in the two most recent epidemiologic studies was 0.95:1 and 1.1:1, respectively [9, 10].

Relationship to Gluten Sensitive Enteropathy

Since the initial report of Marks et al. describing the small bowel changes that were present in patients with DH, the evidence linking DH and celiac disease was reinforced over the next several decades. Histologic abnormalities of the small bowel consistent with changes of gluten sensitive enteropathy can be detected in a high percentage of DH patients [13, 14], and genetic studies have detected higher rates of certain HLA types in patients with both gluten sensitive enteropathy and DH, particularly HLA-B8, HLADQ2, and HLADQ8 [15, 16]. Despite the presence of histologic changes that are consistent with GSE in the vast majority of DH patients, symptomatic gastrointestinal disease is uncommon, present in only about 10–15 % of patients [17, 18]. Even in the absence of gastrointestinal symptoms, following a strict gluten free diet will improve the skin lesions in almost all patients diagnosed with DH [19].

Pathophysiology of the Skin Disease

The human transglutaminases are a family of proteins that are expressed in different human tissues that act by performing posttranslational remodeling through calcium dependent crosslinking of proteins [20, 21]. There are eight transglutaminases that have been identified in the human genome, each with differing functions and distributions in tissue (Table 10.1).

In the gut, tissue transglutaminase deamidates the insoluble wheat protein, gliadin, altering its solubility as well as its immunogenicity. In patients with celiac disease, antibodies are generated against both gliadin as well as the tissue transglutaminase protein [22]. These IgA antibodies can be detected in the serum in a high percentage of celiac disease patients [95–98 %] and a slightly lower percentage of patients with DH [75 %] [23]. In patients with DH, perhaps through a process of epitope spreading, antibodies against epidermal transglutaminase are also present and can be detected in the granular deposits of IgA in the dermal papillae [24]. These anti-epidermal antibodies can be measured in the serum of 95 % of DH patients not on a gluten free diet [25]. Antigen-antibody complexes deposit in the dermal papillae of the skin, which leads to neutrophil recruitment, activation, and subsequent destruction of structural proteins present at the dermoepidermal junction which leads to sub-epidermal cleft formation [26].

Clinical Presentation

The classic clinical presentation of patients with DH is that of a papulovesicular eruption that is present on the extensor surfaces of the extremities, sacrum, and scalp (Fig. 10.1). Pruritus is significant, often dramatically affecting quality of

Table 10.1 Human transglutaminase proteins

Protein	Synonyms	Location	Function
Factor XIIIa	Fibrin stabilizing factor	Platelets, chondrocytes, other cells	Blood Coagulation
TG1	Keratinocyte TG	Keratinocytes, brain	Keratinocyte differentiation
TG2	Tissue TG	Ubiquitous	Multiple functions
TG3	Epidermal TG	Squamous epithelium, brain	Hair follicle differentiation
TG4	Prostate TG	Prostate	Decreased immunogenicity of sperm
TG5	TGx	Ubiquitous	Cellular differentiation
TG6	TGy	Unknown	Unknown
TG7	TGz	Ubiquitous	Unknown

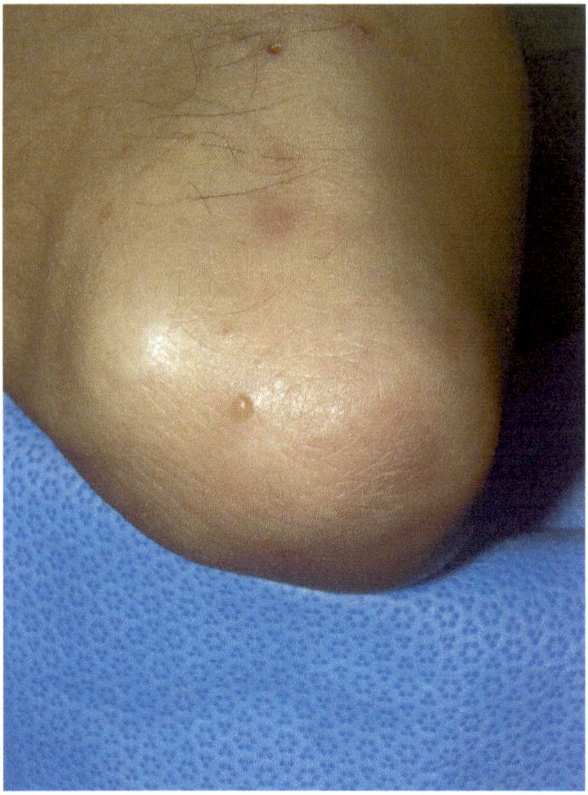

Fig. 10.1 Excoriations, postinflammatory erythema, and a vesicle on the right elbow

life, and can be confined to the specific skin lesions or generalized. Due to the degree of pruritus that is present, the classic skin lesions of papulovesicles are often difficult to find as secondary changes of scratching such as excoriations or dermatographism may be the predominant clinic findings (Fig. 10.2). With more advanced cutaneous disease, the papulovesicles can coalesce, forming large, scaling patches or plaques with serous crusts and vesicles present at the periphery of the lesions. If the presence of the vesicles is not appreciated in these larger lesions, the location and appearance of the plaques can mimic psoriasis (Fig. 10.3). Other presentations can include urticarial plaques, bullous lesions, and larger erosions (Fig. 10.4). Occasionally, the presentation can be nonspecific, with only faint erythema and minimal scaling present on clinical examination (Fig. 10.5).

An unusual presentation of DH is that of isolated digital or palmar petechiae, purpura, and microvesicles. This is a more common presentation in children [27], but adult cases have been described as well [28]. As the digital lesions can be the only manifestation of disease in these patients, a high degree of clinical suspicion is required.

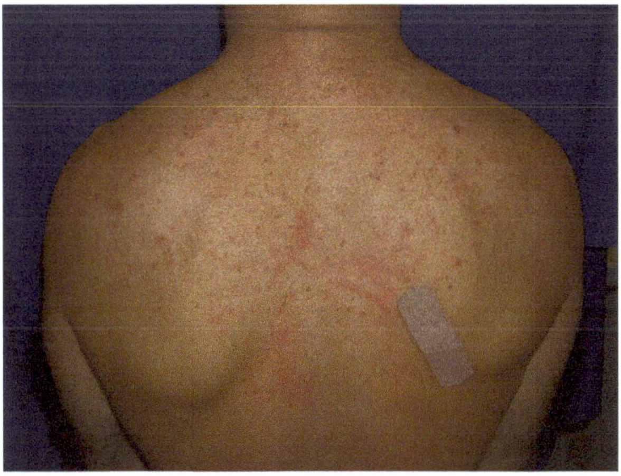

Fig. 10.2 Widespread excoriations with dermatographism on the upper back

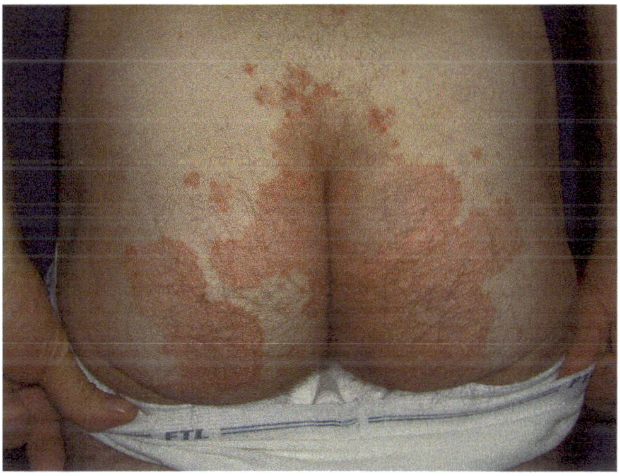

Fig. 10.3 Erythematous scaling patches with peripheral microvesicles, excoriations, and erosions

Diagnosis

There are several diagnostic procedures that can be considered in making a diagnosis of DH, starting with a skin biopsy. Tissue can be taken from a vesicle or excoriated papule and sent for standard H&E analysis, with an additional biopsy from normal peri-lesional skin to be sent for immunofluorescence studies. Classic H&E findings in DH include a subepidermal bullae with sterile microabscesses present within one or more dermal papillae [29], although nonspecific histologic findings may be present in up to 22–37 % of cases [18, 30]. A much more sensitive test is that of direct immunofluorescence [DIF] of perilesional normal skin,

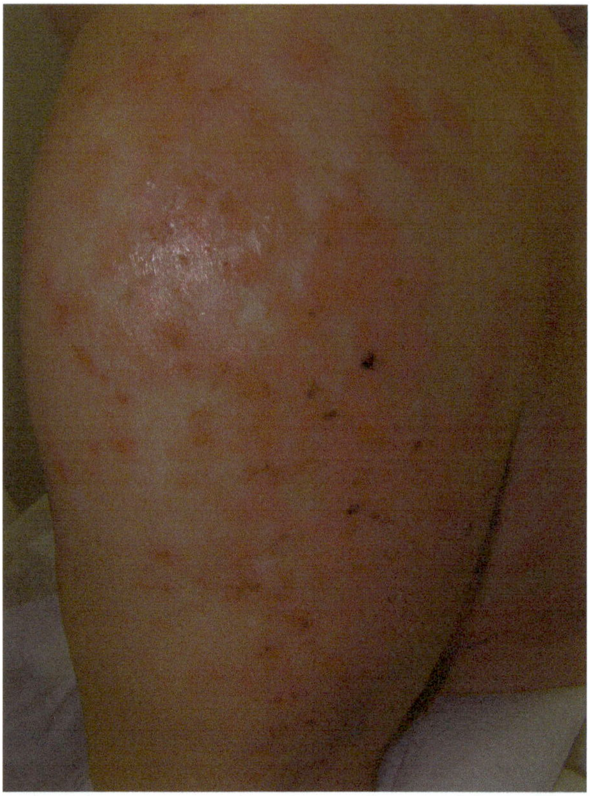

Fig. 10.4 Larger erosions, hemorrhagic crusting, postinflammatory erythema, and one larger bulla on the lateral upper arm

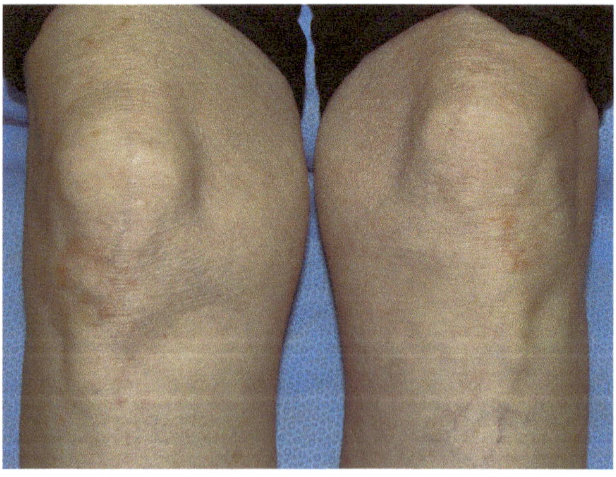

Fig. 10.5 Faint erythema with minimal scaling on bilateral knees

which will demonstrate granular deposition of IgA in the dermal papillae in 97 % of cases [18]. Rare cases have been reported in the literature in which both the histology and DIF studies of patients with DH were negative [31]. In cases without classic H&E and immunofluorescence findings, the presence of circulating IgA anti-tissue transglutaminase antibodies and/or IgG/IgA anti-gliadin antibodies, in association with a pruritic eruption of erythematous papules and plaques, may raise the possibility of an atypical form of DH, and patients may respond to DH therapy. Serum testing for gliadin or transglutaminase antibodies is not completely sensitive, and the widely available IgA anti-tissue transglutaminase test will be positive in approximately 70 % of patients [18, 25]. Tests which can measure IgA anti-epidermal transglutaminase are more sensitive [95 %] [25], but are not widely commercially available.

Therapy

Medical Therapy

Dapsone is the only FDA approved medication for the treatment of DH. Initial doses are usually 50–100 mg a day, with adjustments as needed based on patient tolerance and response to therapy. Up to 300 mg a day may be required in some cases. Improvement in pruritus is noted almost immediately, while the resolution of the skin lesions may take several more days. Despite resolution of the skin lesions, immunoreactants are still present in patients taking dapsone who continue to consume a normal, gluten-containing diet [32], and the intestinal abnormalities that can be present are not influenced by dapsone therapy. In general, dapsone is tolerated well, although patients must be monitored on a regular basis. A glucose 6-phosphate dehydrogenase level should be checked prior to initiation of systemic dapsone therapy, and weekly CBC should be performed for the first month due to the possibility of agranulocytosis. A slight hemolytic anemia and methemoglobinemia, usually not significant enough to cause any symptoms, is expected in most patients. A hypersensitivity reaction can be seen rarely, and can occur up to 8 weeks following initiation of therapy. Long term side effects are also rare but include a peripheral neuropathy, most frequently a small muscle motor neuropathy, although sensory neuropathy has also been reported [33]. The mechanism of action of dapsone in the treatment of DH is largely unknown.

In patients that cannot tolerate dapsone, sulfasalazine has been reported as an effective therapy for DH [34], but the response in patients overall is less consistent when compared with dapsone. Isolated case reports describe the effectiveness of colchicine [35], and tetracycline and nicotinamide [36]. These options could be considered in patients who have documented allergies to sulfonamide medications.

Dietary Therapy

A strict gluten free diet will allow most patients to discontinue any medical therapy needed to control the skin lesions [19, 37]. Fry demonstrated that 80 % of DH patients that adhered to a gluten free diet were able to decrease the dose of dapsone required to control their skin disease, with some patients being able to discontinue the dapsone dose completely [37]. No patient was able to reduce the dapsone dose prior to 5 months on the gluten-free diet, and the time that it took to discontinue dapsone varied from 8 to 48 months [37]. Hence it is important to counsel patients that the response to the gluten-free diet is not immediate. Because of the severity of the pruritus and the time that it takes to respond to a gluten free diet, almost all DH patients are initially started on dapsone therapy, with initiation of the gluten free diet in order to decrease or discontinue the dapsone altogether. Iodine, either in dietary form or as a component of contrast agents, can cause a flare of skin lesions.

Additional Workup

Because of the presence of intestinal abnormalities present in DH patients – even those that are asymptomatic – malabsorption and nutritional deficiencies may occur [38, 39], although screening all DH patients for nutritional deficiencies is not indicated. A comparison between patients with DH and celiac disease demonstrated similar values for levels of Vitamin D, folate, iron, and Vitamin B_{12} [40] although in neither group were levels outside of the reference range. Another study of 86 DH patients did not find significant nutritional abnormalities when compared to controls, although hematologic abnormalities from drug therapy were common [41].

Patients with celiac disease, as well as their first degree relatives, are at higher risk of having another autoimmune disease, including autoimmune thyroid disease and insulin dependent diabetes mellitus when compared to the background population [42]. Higher rates of thyroid disease and diabetes have been demonstrated in patients with DH as well [40, 43]. Other autoimmune diseases, including lupus, Sjogren's, vitiligo, and alopecia areata also occur more commonly in patients with DH when compared to controls [40, 43].

Increased rates of malignancy have been reported in patients with dermatitis herpetiformis [44, 45], with increased rates of lymphoma occurring at particularly higher frequency when compared to the background population. A large retrospective study of dermatitis herpetiformis patients suggested that a gluten free diet may play a protective role in the development of lymphoma [46].

Long Term Prognosis

Remission has been reported in patients with DH [47, 48]. In one study, 10 of 86 DH patients did not require medical therapy to control their skin disease despite not complying with a gluten free diet for a period of 2 years [48]. It seems reasonable to occasionally address the need for both medical therapy as well as a gluten free diet in patients with a diagnosis of DH, with the realization that most DH patients that are controlled on a gluten free diet will have a flare of their skin disease upon reintroduction of gluten. Discontinuing a gluten free diet should be addressed in the setting of the fact that gut pathology, even if it is asymptomatic, may develop in DH patients not adhering to a gluten free diet.

Future Directions and Conclusion

Future therapies directed at the treatment of celiac disease may play a role in the treatment of DH as well. These experimental therapies include enzymes that digest gluten; substances which bind to gluten, thereby decreasing absorption; medications which decrease intestinal permeability; tissue transglutaminase inhibitors; and multiple other therapies directed against the immune response involved in gluten sensitivity [49].

Dermatitis herpetiformis is a pruritic vesiculobullous skin disease that occurs in the setting of GSE. Correlation with other autoimmune conditions is well established. While older therapies such as dapsone and a gluten free diet are mainstays of therapy for DH to this day, our understanding of DH and the broader relationship of skin and the gastrointestinal system continues to grow.

References

1. Duhring LA. Dermatitis herpetiformis. JAMA. 1884;3(9):212–6.
2. Kalis JB, Malkinson FD. Landmark perspective: dermatitis herpetiformis. A commentary. JAMA [United States]. 1983;250(2):217–21.
3. COSTELLO MJ. Dermatitis herpetiformis (papular type) successfully treated with sulfapyridine. Arch Derm Syphilol. 1947;55(5):725. Not Available.
4. Marks J, Shuster S, Watson AJ. Small-bowel changes in dermatitis herpetiformis. Lancet [England]. 1966;2(7476):1280–2.
5. Fry L, McMinn RM, Cowan JD, Hoffbrand AV. Effect of gluten-free diet on dermatological, intestinal, and haematological manifestations of dermatitis herpetiformis. Lancet [England]. 1968;1(7542):557–61.
6. Reunala T, Lokki J. Dermatitis herpetiformis in Finland. Acta Derm Venereol [Sweden]. 1978;58(6):505–10.
7. Mobacken H, Kastrup W, Nilsson LA. Incidence and prevalence of dermatitis herpetiformis in western Sweden. Acta Derm Venereol [Sweden]. 1984;64(5):400–4.
8. Moi H. Incidence and prevalence of dermatitis herpetiformis in a country in central Sweden, with comments on the course of the disease and IgA deposits as diagnostic criterion. Acta Derm Venereol [Sweden]. 1984;64(2):144–50.
9. West J, Fleming KM, Tata LJ, Card TR, Crooks CJ. Incidence and prevalence of celiac disease and dermatitis herpetiformis in the UK over two decades: population-based study. Am J Gastroenterol [United States]. 2014;109(5):757–68.
10. Salmi TT, Hervonen K, Kautiainen H, Collin P, Reunala T. Prevalence and incidence of dermatitis herpetiformis: a 40-year prospective study from Finland. Br J Dermatol [Internet]. 2011;165(2):354–9. [cited 2014 Dec 14].
11. Hall RP, Clark RE, Ward FE. Dermatitis herpetiformis in two American blacks: HLA type and clinical characteristics. J Am Acad Dermatol [United States]. 1990;22(3):436–9.

12. Ohata C, Ishii N, Hamada T, Shimomura Y, Niizeki H, Dainichi T, et al. Distinct characteristics in Japanese dermatitis herpetiformis: a review of all 91 Japanese patients over the last 35 years. Clin Dev Immunol [Internet]. 2012;2012:562168. [cited 2014 Dec 14].
13. Gawkrodger DJ, Blackwell JN, Gilmour HM, Rifkind EA, Heading RC, Barnetson RS. Dermatitis herpetiformis: diagnosis, diet and demography. Gut [England]. 1984;25(2):151–7.
14. Salmi TT, Hervonen K, Laurila K, Collin P, Mäki M, Koskinen O, et al. Small bowel transglutaminase 2-specific IgA deposits in dermatitis herpetiformis. Acta Derm Venereol [Internet]. 2014;94(4):393–7. [cited 2014 Dec 14].
15. Katz SI, Falchuk ZM, Dahl MV, Rogentine GN, Strober W, Service D, et al. HL-A8: a genetic link between dermatitis herpetiformis and gluten-sensitive enteropathy. J Clin Invest. 1972;51(11):2977–80.
16. Spurkland A, Ingvarsson G, Falk ES, Knutsen I, Sollid LM, Thorsby E. Dermatitis herpetiformis and celiac disease are both primarily associated with the HLA-DQ (alpha 1*0501, beta 1*02) or the HLA-DQ (alpha 1*03, beta 1*0302) heterodimers. Tissue Antigens [Denmark]. 1997;49(1):29–34.
17. Reunala T, Kosnai I, Karpati S, Kuitunen P, Torok E, Savilahti E. Dermatitis herpetiformis: jejunal findings and skin response to gluten free diet. Arch Dis Child [Internet]. 1984;59(6):517–22.
18. Alonso-llamazares J, Gibson LE, Rogers III RS. Clinical, pathologic, and immunopathologic features of dermatitis herpetiformis: review of the Mayo Clinic experience. Int J Dermatol. 2007;46:910–9.
19. Garioch JJ, Lewis HM, Sargent SA, Leonard JN, Fry L. 25 years' experience of a gluten-free diet in the treatment of dermatitis herpetiformis. Br J Dermatol [England]. 1994;131(4):541–5.
20. Lorand L, Graham RM. Transglutaminases: crosslinking enzymes with pleiotropic functions. Nat Rev Mol Cell Biol [Internet]. 2003;4(2):140–56. [cited 2014 Dec 8]. Available from
21. Martin A, De Vivo G, Gentile V. Possible role of the transglutaminases in the pathogenesis of Alzheimer's disease and other neurodegenerative diseases. Int J Alzheimers Dis [Internet]. 2011;2011(Cd):865432. [cited 2014 Dec 7].
22. Alaedini A, Green PHR. Narrative review: celiac disease: understanding a complex autoimmune disorder. Ann Intern Med [United States]. 2005;142(4):289–98.
23. Porter WM, Unsworth DJ, Lock RJ, Hardman CM, Baker BS, Fry L. Tissue transglutaminase antibodies in dermatitis herpetiformis Gastroenterology. 1999;117(3):749–50.
24. Sardy M, Karpati S, Merkl B, Paulsson M, Smyth N. Epidermal transglutaminase (TGase 3) is the autoantigen of dermatitis herpetiformis. J Exp Med [United States]. 2002;195(6):747–57.
25. Rose C, Armbruster FP, Ruppert J, Igl BW, Zillikens D, Shimanovich I. Autoantibodies against epidermal transglutaminase are a sensitive diagnostic marker in patients with dermatitis herpetiformis on a normal or gluten-free diet. J Am Acad Dermatol [Internet]. 2009;61(1):39–43. Elsevier Inc. [cited 2014 Dec 14].
26. Zone JJ, Egan CA, Taylor TB, Meyer LJ. Iga autoimmune disorders: development of a passive transfer mouse model. J Investig Dermatology Symp Proc. 2004;9(1):47–51.
27. Heinlin J, Knoppke B, Kohl E, Landthaler M, Karrer S. Dermatitis herpetiformis presenting as digital petechiae. Pediatr Dermatol [Internet]. 2012;29(2):209–12. [cited 2014 Dec 14].
28. Flann S, Degiovanni C, Derrick EK, Munn SE. Two cases of palmar petechiae as a presentation of dermatitis herpetiformis. Clin Exp Dermatol [Internet]. 2010;35(2):206–8. [cited 2014 Dec 14].
29. Blenkinsopp WK, Haffenden GP, Fry L, Leonard JN. Histology of linear IgA disease, dermatitis herpetiformis, and bullous pemphigoid. Am J Dermatopathol [United States]. 1983;5(6):547–54.
30. Warren SJP, Cockerell CJ. Characterization of a subgroup of patients with dermatitis herpetiformis with nonclassical histologic features. Am J Dermatopathol. 2002;24(4):305–8.
31. Huber C, Trueb RM, French LE, Hafner J. Negative direct immunofluorescence and nonspecific histology do not exclude the diagnosis of dermatitis herpetiformis Duhring. Int J Dermatol [England]. 2013;52:248–9.
32. Katz SI, Hertz KC, Crawford PS, Gazze LA, Frank MM, Lawley TJ. Effect of sulfones on complement deposition in dermatitis herpetiformis and on complement-mediated guinea-pig reactions. J Invest Dermatol [United States]. 1976;67(6):688–90.

33. Mery L, Dega H, Prost C, Dubertret L. [Dapsone-induced sensory peripheral neuropathy]. Ann Dermatol Venereol [France]. 2003;130(4):447–9.
34. Willsteed E, Lee M, Wong LC, Cooper A. Sulfasalazine and dermatitis herpetiformis. Australas J Dermatol [Internet]. 2005;46(2):101–3.
35. Silvers DN, Juhlin EA, Berczeller PH, McSorley J. Treatment of dermatitis herpetiformis with colchicine. Arch Dermatol [United States]. 1980;116(12):1373–84.
36. Zemtsov A, Neldner KH. Successful treatment of dermatitis herpetiformis with tetracycline and nicotinamide in a patient unable to tolerate dapsone. J Am Acad Dermatol [United States]. 1993;28(3):505–6.
37. Fry L, Seah PP, Riches DJ, Hoffbrand AV. Clearance of skin lesions in dermatitis herpetiformis after gluten withdrawal. Lancet [England]. 1973;1(7798):288–91.
38. Kastrup W, Mobacken H, Stockbrugger R, Swolin B, Westin J. Malabsorption of vitamin B12 in dermatitis herpetiformis and its association with pernicious anaemia. Acta Med Scand [Sweden]. 1986;220(3):261–8.
39. Denman SL, Freeman NJ. Asymptomatic anemia in three men with dermatitis herpetiformis. Hosp Pract [United States]. 1992;27(4):187, 189–90.
40. Krishnareddy S, Lewis SK, Green PH. Dermatitis herpetiformis: clinical presentations are independent of manifestations of celiac disease. Am J Clin Dermatol [Internet]. 2014;15(1):51–6. [cited 2014 Dec 14].
41. Gawkrodger DJ, Ferguson A, Barnetson RS. Nutritional status in patients with dermatitis herpetiformis. Am J Clin Nutr [United States]. 1988;48(2):355–60.
42. Neuhausen SL, Steele L, Ryan S, Mousavi M, Pinto M, Osann KE, et al. Co-occurrence of celiac disease and other autoimmune diseases in celiacs and their first-degree relatives. J Autoimmun [England]. 2008;31(2):160–5.
43. Reunala T, Collin P. Diseases associated with dermatitis herpetiformis. Br J Dermatol [England]. 1997;136(3):315–8.
44. Leonard JN, Tucker WF, Fry JS, Coulter CA, Boylston AW, McMinn RM, et al. Increased incidence of malignancy in dermatitis herpetiformis. Br Med J (Clin Res Ed) [England]. 1983;286(6358):16–8.
45. Sigurgeirsson B, Agnarsson BA, Lindelof B. Risk of lymphoma in patients with dermatitis herpetiformis. BMJ Clin Res. 1994;308:13–5.
46. Lewis HM, Renaula TL, Garioch JJ, Leonard JN, Fry JS, Collin P, et al. Protective effect of gluten-free diet against development of lymphoma in dermatitis herpetiformis. Br J Dermatol [England]. 1996;135(3):363–7.
47. Bardella MT, Fredella C, Trovato C, Ermacora E, Cavalli R, Saladino V, et al. Long-term remission in patients with dermatitis herpetiformis on a normal diet. Br J Dermatol [England]. 2003;149(5):968–71.
48. Paek SY, Steinberg SM, Katz SI. Remission in dermatitis herpetiformis: a cohort study. Arch Dermatol [Internet]. 2011;147(3):301–5. [cited 2014 Dec 14].
49. McAllister CS, Kagnoff MF. The immunopathogenesis of celiac disease reveals possible therapies beyond the gluten-free diet. Semin Immunopathol [Internet]. 2012;34(4):581–600. [cited 2014 Dec 14].

Chapter 11
Rare Autoimmune Blistering Disorders

Christine S. Ahn and William W. Huang

Abstract The spectrum of autoimmune blistering disorders continues to evolve as previous associations become new entities, and these entities demonstrate distinct clinical, histologic, and immunohistochemical characteristics. The rare autoimmune blistering disorders present both diagnostic and therapeutic challenges to clinicians. Diagnostically, there can be overlapping features between the rare and more common autoimmune diseases. From a therapeutic standpoint, there is a general lack of studies that demonstrate treatment efficacy and outcomes in these entities leading to clinical practice gaps. This chapter will review the clinical and histological features of lichen planus pemphigoides (LPP), bullous lichen planus (BLP), bullous systemic lupus erythematosus (SLE), IgA pemphigus, and subcorneal pustular dermatosis (SPD), and provide an evidence-based review of the treatment options reported in the literature.

Keywords Autoimmune bullous • Lichen planus pemphigoides • Lichen planus • Bullous pemphigoid • IgA pemphigus • Bullous lupus • Subcorneal pustular dermosis • Sneddon-Wilkinson

Abbreviations

BP	Bullous pemphigoid
BMZ	Basement membrane zone
BP180	Bullous pemphigoid 180 antigen
BP230	Bullous pemphigoid 230 antigen
C3	Complement component 3
DIF	Direct immunofluorescence
DEJ	Dermoepidermal junction
Dsc1	Desmocollin-1

C.S. Ahn, MD • W.W. Huang, MD, MPH (✉)
Department of Dermatology, Wake Forest University School of Medicine,
4618 Country Club Road, Winston Salem, NC 27104, USA
e-mail: whuang@wakehealth.edu

N. Sami (ed.), *Autoimmune Bullous Diseases: Approach and Management*,
DOI 10.1007/978-3-319-26728-9_11

Dsg1	Desmoglein-1
Dsg3	Desmoglein-3
EBA	Epidermolysis bullosa acquisita
ELISA	Enzyme-linked immunosorbent assay
H&E	Hematoxylin and eosin
IgA	Immunoglobulin A
IEN	Intraepidermal neutrophilic
IgG	Immunoglobulin G
IIF	Indirect immunofluorescence
LP	Lichen planus
LPP	Lichen planus pemphigoides
NC	Non-collagenous
PUVA	Psoralen plus ultraviolet A
SLE	Systemic lupus erythematosus
SPD	Subcorneal pustular dermatosis
TNF	Tumor necrosis factor

Lichen Planus Pemphigoides

Clinical Features

Lichen planus pemphigoides (LPP) is a rare autoimmune bullous disorder, with less than 100 cases described in the English literature to date. It is characterized by the presence of lesions of lichen planus (LP) as well as vesicles and bullae arising in areas of LP and in uninvolved skin [1, 2]. The vesicles and bullae are subepidermal and demonstrate features of bullous pemphigoid (BP), including the presence of bullous pemphigoid 180 antigen (BP180) [2]. When LPP was first reported, there was controversy over whether it represented two coinciding conditions or a single disease with characteristics of both lichen planus and bullous pemphigoid. It is now understood to be a separate entity that consists of features of LP and BP, and is distinguishable from BP by the nature of the circulating autoantibodies. While BP180 is present in both LPP and BP, autoantibodies react to region 4 within the BP180 non-collagenous (NC)-16a domain in LPP, whereas autoantibodies in BP react to regions 2 and 3 [2]. Diagnostic criteria for LPP used by some authors include: lesions with the clinical appearance of vesicles or bullae arising on both lesions of LP and uninvolved skin, histopathology demonstrating both a subepidermal blister and features of LP, and direct immunofluorescence (DIF) of peri-lesional skin demonstrating linear deposition of complement component 3 (C3) and/or immunoglobulin G (IgG) along the dermoepidermal junction (DEJ) [3].

LPP usually presents in middle-aged adults, with a slight female preponderance and no particular racial predominance [1, 3]. In a review of 78 cases of LPP, the mean age at diagnosis was 54 years, with a peak in incidence among adults in their fifth and sixth decades of life [3]. LPP occurs rarely in children, with less than 20 cases of childhood LPP described to date [4]. In a review of 12 children with LPP, the mean age at diagnosis was 12 years and there was a higher incidence in boys [5]. Clinically, LPP is characterized by the development of lesions typical of lichen planus followed by the development of tense vesicles and bullae, though rare cases have been reported with lichen planus and bullous lesions occurring concomitantly. The lesions of LP are erythematous or violaceous papules and plaques that are classically described as pruritic, polygonal, and planar (Fig. 11.1) [4]. In the following weeks to months, bullous lesions arise in areas of erythema, normal skin, the oral mucosa, or within lichenoid lesions (Fig. 11.2). Similar to the presentation of bullous pemphigoid, the blisters of LPP are tense, dome-shaped, and can be hemorrhagic or contain clear fluid. Bullae tend to develop on the extremities, although they have been reported as generalized eruptions in few patients [3]. Oral mucosal involvement in

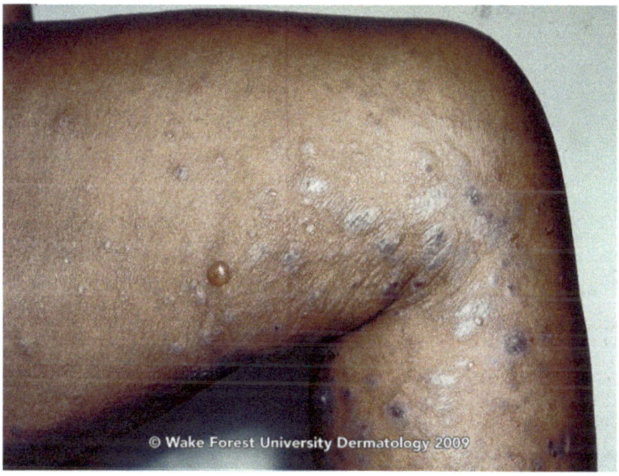

Fig. 11.1 Lichen planus pemphigoides. Violaceous, polygonal, flat-topped lesions of lichen planus on the lower extremity with a tense, dome-shaped blister

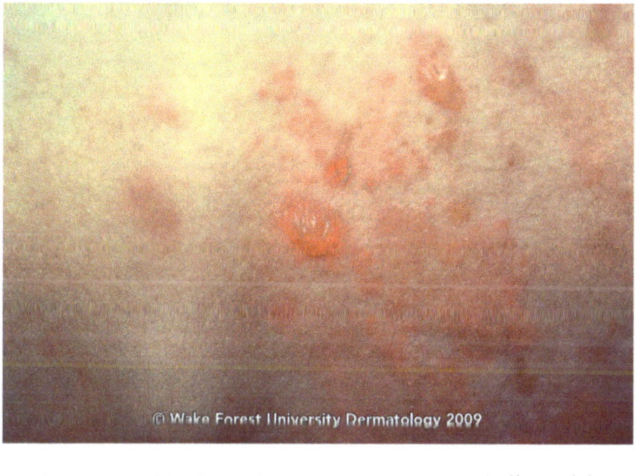

Fig. 11.2 Lichen planus pemphigoides. Clear fluid-filled tense bullae arising on erythematous skin

the form of erosions, white dots, and streaks are also seen in a minority of patients (36 %). On average, the average time elapsed between the development of LP lesions to the development of vesiculobullous lesions of LPP is 8.3 months, while simultaneous appearance of lesions has been observed in up to 6 % of cases [3].

Histologically, the lichenoid lesions of LPP demonstrate classic histopathological features of lichen planus and the bullae demonstrate features of bullous pemphigoid [1]. Biopsy specimens with hematoxylin and eosin (H&E) staining from cutaneous lichenoid lesions demonstrate hyperkeratosis, hypergranulosis, and acanthosis. Colloid bodies of Civatte are seen in some cases, with a band-like lymphocytic infiltrate in the upper papillary dermis. Vesicles and bullae demonstrate a subepidermal blister with associated edema and infiltration of eosinophils, and perivascular mixed inflammatory infiltrates consisting of eosinophils, histiocytes, and lymphocytes [3]. Direct immunofluorescence studies performed on peri-lesional skin biopsies show linear deposition of IgG, C3, and fibrinogen along the basement membrane zone (BMZ) [4]. Indirect immunofluorescence (IIF) studies demonstrate circulating IgG autoantibodies to keratinocyte cell surfaces. When performed, enzyme-linked immunosorbent assay (ELISA) tests often demonstrate positivity for IgG antibodies to desmoglein-1 (Dsg1), BP180, and BP230 [2–4].

The pathogenesis of LPP is not completely understood. Although most cases are idiopathic, there are few reports of LPP developing in association with drugs, phototherapy, and in one case, hepatitis B virus infection [6–9]. The most common culprit medications reported are angiotensin converting enzyme inhibitors such as ramipril and captopril [7–9]. One theory suggests that damage to basal cells in LP can expose sequestered antigens or produce new antigens that lead to autoantibody formation and subsequent bullous lesions. In a study examining circulating antibodies before and after the diagnosis of LPP, autoantibodies to the basement membrane zone were detectable after the development of bullae, but not before. Furthermore, once the bullae were controlled with therapy, anti-BP180 antibodies were no longer detectable [2]. The diagnosis of LPP can be confirmed based on histopathological findings of both LP and subepidermal bullae, and DIF findings of linear deposits of IgG and/or C3 in the BMZ [3].

Systemic Treatment

Systemic Corticosteroids

The use of systemic corticosteroids to treat LPP has been reported most widely in the literature. In greater than half of the cases, systemic corticosteroids alone have been used to successfully treat LPP. In most reports, the bullous eruption resolves within a few weeks of therapy and while there have been relapses reported in patients after several years of disease clearance, the recurrence rate of LPP appears lower than the rate seen in bullous pemphigoid. The recommended dosage is 0.5 mg/kg daily, or 40–60 mg daily for adults [10].

Although systemic corticosteroid therapy is an effective first-line therapy that has demonstrated good clinical response, there are undesirable side effects, particularly in children. In rare reports of LPP in children, different systemic agents were required after difficulty tapering systemic steroid treatment. In one case of LPP in a 2-year-old child, the disease was controlled with systemic corticosteroids at a dose of 2 mg/kg daily. However, attempts to taper the dose below 1 mg/kg daily resulted in recurrent flares of severe bullous disease. The patient was begun on low dose methotrexate and was able to be successfully tapered off systemic steroids [11]. In another case of LPP in a 6-year-old child, topical corticosteroid therapy resulted in no response, and oral prednisolone at 1 mg/kg/day resulted in the cessation of bullae formation within 4 days. However, tapering resulted in flares at 5 and 10 weeks, and again when steroids were stopped. During 2 years of follow-up, the patient had recurrence of LP lesions but not bullous lesions [5].

Dapsone

Dapsone (4,4′-diaminodiphenyl sulphone), traditionally used as an anti-infectious agent, has demonstrated many uses for noninfectious inflammatory dermatologic diseases. There are several cases in adults and children that have documented the successful treatment of LPP with dapsone, either as a single agent or in combination with other systemic agents. In two reports of adults with LPP, dapsone was used in conjunction with oral methylprednisolone and resulted in disease control. After 12 weeks on oral steroids and 16 weeks of dapsone, one patient had no recurrence of any skin lesions after 1 year [12]. In another patient who was previously treated with erythromycin and nicotinamide with little response, dapsone 50 mg daily was used with topical corticosteroids. Within 1 week, bullous lesions began to regress and dapsone was continued for 4 months until complete clearance was achieved. Over 18 months of follow-up there were no recurrences of bullous lesions, although lesions of LP recurred and were managed with topical corticosteroids [13]. There are also reports of poor response to dapsone. In a patient treated with dapsone 100 mg/day, no response was seen after 2 weeks. Once therapy was switched to oral methylprednisolone, there was expedient resolution of skin lesions and steroid therapy was discontinued after only 2 months [12].

In a report of two cases of childhood LPP, both patients were treated successfully with a combination of topical corticosteroids, oral prednisolone, and dapsone. In one patient, clinical remission was achieved within 10 months, and BP180 ELISA remained borderline positive. In another patient, systemic treatment lasted for 19 months, and the patient had mild recurring LP plaques 2 years later that responded to topical steroids, while the BP180 ELISA remained borderline positive [4].

Antibiotics and Nicotinamide

The combined use of antibiotics and nicotinamide (or niacinamide) has been reported in autoimmune bullous diseases. This combination of drugs acts to inhibit neutrophil or eosinophil chemotaxis, inhibit antigen-induced histamine release, suppress antigen responses, and suppress lymphocyte transformation [14]. In the treatment of LPP, therapy with erythromycin and nicotinamide has been reported in children, whereas tetracycline antibiotics have been used in adults, with varying success. In a child diagnosed with LPP, the patient was to begin therapy with dapsone 50 mg daily and topical steroids, but while awaiting the results of glucose-6-phosphatase testing, began treatment with oral erythromycin 30 mg/kg daily in four divided doses and nicotinamide 150 mg three times a day. After 1 week, this was then replaced by dapsone 50 mg daily and topical steroids. The patient had cessation of new bullae within 1 week, and had complete clearance by 4 months. After an 18-month period of follow-up, the patient had no recurrence of bullae, and lesions of LP were treated with topical corticosteroid therapy [13].

In an adult with LPP, initial treatment with oral prednisone induced remission of the disease, but in the presentation of a new flare 3 years later, the patient was treated with tetracycline 500 mg four times daily and nicotinamide 500 mg three times daily. This regimen led to rapid clearance of skin lesions, however, tetracycline was replaced with doxycycline 100 mg twice daily due to the development of renal insufficiency. Bullous eruptions recurred at each attempt to discontinue doxycycline and nicotinamide, and would respond to reinstitution of both drugs [14].

Other Immunosuppressive Agents

Methotrexate has been used as an adjuvant immunosuppressive agent with prednisolone. In one report, a young child with LPP demonstrated response to prednisolone 2 mg/kg daily, but attempts to taper below 1 mg/kg daily resulted in a severe flare of the bullous component of the disease. Methotrexate 0.5 mg/kg daily was initiated and led to disease clearance after 4 weeks of treatment, and prednisolone was tapered over 8 weeks. Follow-up testing of serum anti-BP180 autoantibodies demonstrated decreasing levels along with clinical improvement. After 11 months of treatment with methotrexate, serum level of anti-BP180 autoantibodies decreased from 173 to 42 U/mL and the patient had no recurrence of disease during follow-up [11].

There are sparse reports of azathioprine being used as an adjunctive treatment for LPP. Only one case has been reported in which a patient was treated with combination therapy with prednisolone 40 mg daily, azathioprine 100 mg daily, and topical steroids. Disease control was maintained with prednisolone 25 mg and azathioprine 100 mg daily, although there was no report of subsequent follow-up [10].

In a case of prednisolone-resistant LPP, a patient with extensive lesions involving the soles and oral mucosa was treated with low dose cyclosporine A in combination with prednisolone. After the patient had minimal response to prednisone at 0.4 mg/kg daily, low dose cyclosporine A at 2 mg/kg daily was added and led to improvement of vesicles and bullae. As the patient's clinical lesions improved and the anti-BP180 antibody titer index decreased, cyclosporine A and prednisone were tapered, and the patient remained in remission [15].

Current Opinions

Lichen planus pemphigoides has features of both bullous pemphigoid and lichen planus, which can make treatment with just one modality suboptimal. Based on the severity of the disease, which is defined by the extent of body surface area involvement and severity of symptoms such as pruritus, treatments range from topical therapy to systemic immunosuppressive agents. Topical corticosteroids are an effective and safe first-line treatment in patients with limited cutaneous involvement, as it is used to treat both localized lichen planus and bullous pemphigoid. In cases with extensive cutaneous and/or mucosal involvement requiring systemic treatment, the most studied therapeutic agent for LPP is oral prednisolone. Compared to bullous pemphigoid, LPP has a much younger age of onset and typically follows a less severe clinical course, which makes corticosteroids a reasonable first-line treatment option. However, in patients with contraindications to systemic steroid therapy or in young children, dapsone is the next most commonly reported agent. Dapsone has demonstrated favorable results particularly in younger patients in whom chronic therapy with systemic corticosteroids is undesirable. However, if there are contraindications to dapsone such as glucose-6-phosphatase deficiency or the development of hemolytic anemia, other immunosuppressants such as methotrexate, azathioprine, and cyclosporine can be considered, although the literature reporting on the efficacy of these agents is sparse and anecdotal (Table 11.1). The use of combination therapy with antibiotics and nicotinamide is less favorable due to reports of patients with indefinite treatment duration and disease flares associated with discontinuation.

Deciding whether or not to discontinue a therapy or add an additional therapy can be difficult and depends largely on the extent of clinical response. When treating with systemic corticosteroids, many clinicians use the cessation of new bullae formation within the first 7–14 days as a sign of good clinical response in the initial treatment period. Beyond the initial clinical response, the next challenges are achieving a full clinical response and maintaining disease clearance while tapering medication(s). In the rare cases of extensive disease involvement including the oral mucosa, additional therapeutic measures such as dapsone can be useful adjunct treatments. Once disease control is achieved, tapering must be performed with close monitoring, either with follow-up clinic visits or telephone follow-up at a minimum of weeks 2, 4, 8, and 12. There is wide variability in response to tapering medications, evident by the variable lengths of total treatment periods reported in the literature, ranging between 3 and 18 months, and in some cases, indefinite maintenance therapy. While some patients demonstrate disease stability with no recurrence, other patients demonstrate rapid disease recurrence with medication tapering.

Discussion/Areas of Future Interest

There is limited literature on the efficacy of treatment options for LPP. The lack of evidence for the use of non-steroidal systemic agents is likely reflective of the extent of the typical success of systemic steroids in treating the disease. Few studies report

Table 11.1 Summary of rare autoimmune bullous diseases and treatment algorithm

Disease	Clinical presentation	Histology	Immunofluorescence	1st line treatment	2nd line treatment	3rd line treatment (anecdotal evidence only)
Lichen planus pemphigoides	Lesions of lichen planus with tense vesicles and bullae in areas of LP and normal skin	Hyperkeratosis, hypergranulosis, and band-like lymphocytic infiltrate in the upper papillary dermis, with subepidermal blister with associated edema and eosinophils	**DIF**: Linear deposition of IgG, C3, fibrinogen along BMZ **IIF**: Circulating IgG to Dsg1, BP180, and/or BP230	Systemic steroids (0.5 mg/kg/day)	Dapsone (50–100 mg/day)	Methotrexate Azathioprine Cyclosporine
Bullous lichen planus	Lesions of lichen planus with vesicles and bullae formation over pre-existing papules and plaques	Hyperkeratosis, hypergranulosis, basal vacuolar cell degeneration, with subepidermal blister containing fibrin, eosinophils, and neutrophils	**DIF**: No linear deposition of IgG or C3. Coarse granular deposits of fibrinogen at DEJ only **IIF**: No circulating antibodies	Systemic steroids (0.5 mg/kg/day)	Dapsone (200 mg/day as single therapy) (25–50 mg/day if used as adjuvant therapy) Acitretin (30 mg/day)	Cyclosporine (1–5 mg/kg/day)
Bullous systemic lupus erythematosus	Vesicles and bullae coalescing to form elongated, arciform, or irregular shapes	Subepidermal blister with neutrophils, karyorrhectic debris with occasional lymphocytes, histiocytes, and eosinophils	**DIF**: Granular or linear deposition of IgG, IgA, IgM, and/or C3 in BMZ **IIF**: Circulating IgG to type VII collagen (NC1)	Dapsone (25–50 mg/day)	Methotrexate Mycophenolate mofetil	Rituximab Systemic steroids

IgA pemphigus	Vesicles and bullae that evolve into pustules that coalesce into annular or circinate lesions with central crust	Intraepidermal neutrophilic pustules or vesicles and neutrophilic infiltration in the epidermis	**DIF**: IgA deposition throughout entire epidermis (IEN) or upper epidermis only (SPD). **IIF**: Circulating IgA1 only	Systemic steroids (0.5–1.0 mg/kg/day)	Dapsone (25–125 mg/day) Acitretin	Colchicine (0.5–2 mg/day) Adalimumab
Subcorneal pustular dermatosis	Vesiculopustular lesions that coalesce to form annular or circinate lesions that evolve into crusted lesions with pustules at the periphery	Subcorneal separation with aggregates of keratin and neutrophils within the clef	**DIF**: Negative for IgA and IgM **IIF**: No circulating antibodies	Dapsone (50–200 mg/day)	Colchicine (0.5 mg twice daily) Etretinate/acitretin	Infliximab Etanercept PUVA Systemic steroids

DIF direct immunofluorescence, *IIF* indirect immunofluorescence, *BMZ* basement membrane zone, *Dsg* desmoglein, *BP* bullous pemphigoid, *mg* milligrams, *DEJ* dermoepidermal junction on the level of autoantibody titers throughout the course of the disease, although it can be used as a guide for response to treatment. Further research is needed to evaluate the utility of monitoring autoantibody levels and the correlation between autoantibody titers and disease severity.

Bullous Lichen Planus

Clinical Features

Bullous lichen planus is a variant of lichen planus that presents with typical lesions of LP and vesicles and bullae over pre-existing papules and plaques. Unlike LPP, the bullae are often less extensive, and bullae tend to form only in areas of involved skin with lesions of LP, with few bullae rarely occurring in the adjoining skin (Fig. 11.3) [16]. In contrast, the bullous lesions of LPP form on both lesions of LP and normal skin. The bullous component of bullous LP is most prominent during an LP flare and has a similar distribution to lichen planus, with a predilection for the trunk and extremities. Pruritus is a common presenting symptom, which can precede the development of erythematous or violaceous papules and plaques with bullae forming at the periphery. The bullae are tense, non-hemorrhagic, and can form as a group of numerous vesicles [17, 18]. Oral involvement is uncommon but can occur in this entity. It usually presents as fluid-filled vesicles with surrounding reticular white streaks, often on the buccal mucosa and less commonly on the gingiva and inner aspect of the lips [19–21].

Histologically, bullous LP demonstrates features of lichen planus such as hyperkeratosis, focal hypergranulosis, prominent basal vacuolar cell degeneration, and

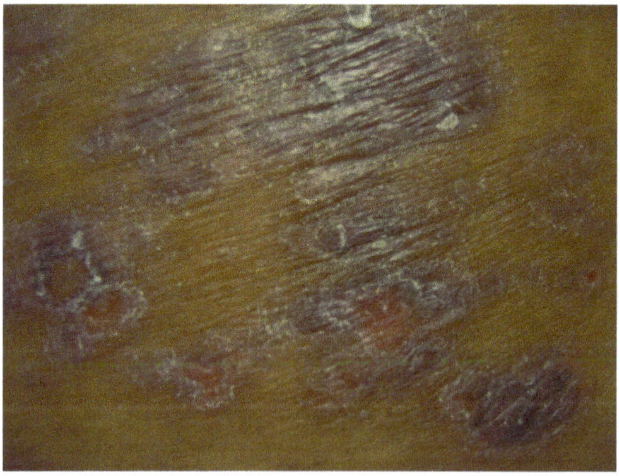

Fig. 11.3 Bullous lichen planus. Erosions where bullae occurred within lesions of lichen planus

band-like lymphohistiocytic cell infiltrates in the upper dermis with few eosinophils that hug the epidermis, leading to the creation of a subepidermal cleft [16]. The subepidermal bullae contain fibrin strands, eosinophils, neutrophils, and occasional histiocytes. Inflammatory cells are also found along the BMZ at the edge of the blister, and perivascular lymphohistiocytic infiltrates can be seen in the papillary and reticular dermis. Although bullous LP can be clinically resemble bullous pemphigoid and LPP, DIF will characteristically lack the linear deposits of immunoglobulins and C3 at the BMZ, and show only reticular and coarse granular deposits of fibrinogen at the dermoepidermal junction. Indirect immunofluorescence will demonstrate immunoglobulins in the stratum granulosum with no circulating antibodies [18, 20].

The pathogenesis of bullae in this entity is thought to be due to upper dermal inflammation, extensive liquefactive degeneration and vacuolation of the basal layer [5]. Few cases have reported bullous LP occurring in response to certain drugs such as intravenous contrast, labetolol, and hepatitis B virus vaccines [22–24]. Theories behind this association suggest that drug-induced lichen planus can be initiated by a cell-mediated immune response to an induced antigenic change in the skin or mucosa. From a diagnostic perspective, bullous LP can clinically be mistaken for bullous pemphigoid or LPP; however, the indirect and direct immunofluorescence assays are distinct in bullous LP and will guide the diagnosis.

Treatment

Systemic Corticosteroids

Corticosteroids are considered the first-line and the most widely used therapeutic agent to treat lichen planus and its variants [25]. Systemic steroids are used in cases of LP that are refractory to topical therapy, extensive in body surface area involvement, or in exanthematous or ulcerative forms. Lichen planus is generally responsive to corticosteroids, and bullous LP appears to have a similar response profile. In case reports that describe the treatment of bullous LP with systemic steroids, the most common doses reported are prednisolone 0.5–1.0 mg/kg daily. In one report of an adult patient, oral prednisolone 40 mg daily was used to treat bullous LP, and was tapered in 6 weeks leading to regression of all skin lesions and with no disease flare or relapse throughout a 6-month follow-up period [16]. Systemic steroids were also reported in a case of a child with bullous LP, at a treatment dose of 20 mg daily. After treatment for approximately 6 weeks, the patient had good response to therapy with no adverse effects. Oral mini-pulse therapy has also been reported in patients, using 5 mg betamethasone orally as a single daily dose on two consecutive days each week, in conjunction with topical betamethasone dipropionate twice daily. This was tapered to 0.5 mg each week, and stopped after 10 weeks. In pulse therapy, potential side effects are decreased and the authors reported adequate disease control with no recurrence after 12 months [26]

Acitretin

Although there are no specific studies or reports that discuss the use of acitretin in patients with bullous LP, it is one of the only treatments for lichen planus that has been studied in a double-blind placebo-controlled trial. In this study, patients with LP were treated with 30 mg acitretin daily for 8 weeks. In 64 % of all patients, there was remission or improvement of symptoms, including pruritus, papulosis, and erythema. Side effects were minimal, with cheilitis and dry mouth being the most commonly reported adverse reactions [25].

Cyclosporine

Cyclosporine has only been studied for the treatment of lichen planus in small uncontrolled case series or case reports. This agent is a systemic treatment that can be used for lichen planus after patients have demonstrated resistance or lack of response to acitretin and/or corticosteroids. Doses used in the literature have been reported between 1 and 5 mg/kg daily, as low doses appear to be sufficient to control the disease [25].

Dapsone

Dapsone has been reported in the treatment of lichen planus and its variants, used alone or more often as an adjunctive agent with corticosteroids. In a review of the use of dapsone as a single agent for lichen planus, 92 patients with any clinical variant of LP were treated with dapsone 200 mg daily for 16 weeks. Complete response was seen in 65 % of patients while 19 % achieved partial response to treatment [25]. In other cases, dapsone was used in combination with prednisone, either if prednisone alone did not achieve complete clearance of disease or as an additional agent during the tapering of steroids. In case reports of patients with LP involving the oral mucosa, dapsone appeared to have increased efficacy in improving oral lesions and in tapering prednisone. Patients were initially treated with 40 mg of prednisone daily, and as prednisone was decreased to 20 mg daily, dapsone at 25 mg daily was added to prevent disease flare. However, in another report, low dose dapsone (25 mg daily) and systemic steroids were sufficient to induce remission in a patient, but tapering to low doses of either dapsone or prednisone resulted in disease flares, which were treated with higher doses of dapsone (50 mg for the first flare, and 100 mg for the second flare) [18].

Current Opinions

There are no reports in the literature beyond anecdotal case reports that specifically evaluate or review the efficacy of different treatment methods for bullous LP. This is likely due to the fact that bullous LP is rare, underreported, and often treated by clinicians under the same guidelines used for treating lichen planus, as this clinical variant does not require a markedly different treatment course. By and large, the main difference between bullous LP and classic lichen planus is the presence of bullae, which can be more concerning to the patient, and rupture and lead to the exposure of more cutaneous sources of entry for infection. Although there are few reports suggesting that bullous LP can be more resistant to treatment than classic LP, this generalization is solely based on anecdotal observations and individual experiences, as the incidence of bullous LP within the population of patients with lichen planus is still not well defined. Corticosteroids and acitretin either alone or in combination are the systemic therapies for lichen planus that have been most extensively used and reported. Adjunctive treatment options include cyclosporine and dapsone, with varying reports of success (Table 11.1) [17]. The approach to the treatment of bullous lichen planus is similar to that of lichen planus, although clinicians should be aware of a possibly higher rate of treatment resistance to the typical first or second-line treatments.

Areas of Future Interest

Further studies on the epidemiology and disease course of bullous LP are warranted. There is limited literature evaluating bullous LP separately from other clinical variants of LP, likely due to the rarity of the disease. Although some authors believe that the clinical course of bullous LP is more recalcitrant to standard therapies for lichen planus, there is scant data to support this notion. Areas of future interest include characterization of the epidemiology of bullous LP, features of the clinical course, and the potential role of other therapeutic options that are used for lichen planus, such as phototherapy.

Bullous Systemic Lupus Erythematosus

Clinical Features

Systemic lupus erythematosus (SLE) is a multi-organ system autoimmune disease that classically presents with cutaneous manifestations such as a malar rash, oral ulcers, discoid lesions, and photosensitivity, seen in up to 76 % of patients during the disease course. Bullous systemic lupus erythematosus is a rare autoantibody-mediated bullous dermatosis that is seen in 1–5 % of patients with SLE [27–29]. In an epidemiologic study in France, the incidence of bullous SLE was reported to be 0.2 cases per million people, and in a series of 67 patients with subepidermal immunobullous disorders, 3 % had bullous SLE [30]. Patients with SLE can also present with a wide range of antibodies that lead to autoimmune bullous dermatoses such as bullous pemphigoid, dermatitis herpetiformis, pemphigus vulgaris, pemphigus foliaceus, linear IgA disease, and epidermolysis bullosa acquisita (EBA). Bullous SLE is a separate autoimmune bullous dermatosis that has been described more recently. It is characterized by a widespread vesiculobullous eruption, with clinical and histological findings resembling bullous pemphigoid or dermatitis herpetiformis. There are at least three different types of bullous SLE based upon the location of the autoantibody in the basement membrane. The most common type of bullous SLE demonstrates antibodies against components of type VII collagen, which can resemble EBA [28].

Clinically, bullous SLE is seen predominantly in African American women in the second and third decades of life. It has only been reported in rare cases in children and adolescents. In relation to SLE, the bullous eruption can occur before the onset of SLE or at any point throughout the disease course; however, patients with bullous SLE tend not to develop other cutaneous manifestations of lupus. Although the onset of bullous SLE eruptions does not necessarily parallel systemic disease activity, there are few reports of bullous flares coinciding with an exacerbation of SLE [31]. The primary lesions are tense vesicles and larger bullae that can be filled with either clear or hemorrhagic fluid and arise in erythematous or normal skin. Multiple vesicles or bullae can form in a cluster, which expand and coalesce to form elongated, arciform, or irregular shapes [30]. Several reports have described erythematous plaques with annular or targetoid erythema multiforme-like configurations. Patients can develop lesions on both sun-exposed and non-sun-exposed skin, but demonstrate a predilection for the flexural and extensor surfaces. Facial and intraoral involvement is relatively common, with common sites including the perioral skin, lip vermillion, oral mucosa, and tongue [32]. Less commonly, the upper trunk and supraclavicular regions are involved [1, 29]. Lesions can be asymptomatic or associated with pruritus or burning sensations. Intraoral lesions initially appear as tense bullae that evolve into painful erosions [33].

On histological examination, the blisters of bullous SLE are subepidermal and contain large numbers of neutrophils and karyorrhectic debris, with occasional lymphocytes, histiocytes, and eosinophils (Fig. 11.4). These findings can appear identical to the histology of dermatitis herpetiformis, which is characterized by subepidermal vesicles and papillary-tip neutrophil microabscesses. In biopsies of nonbullous skin, there are neutrophilic microabscesses in the subepidermis, and marked dermal edema with mixed inflammatory cell infiltrates consisting of neutrophils, eosinophils, lymphocytes, and histiocytes in the upper dermis. On DIF of lesional and perilesional skin, all major classes of immunoglobulins and C3 are often seen in the epidermal basement membrane zone and perivascularly in either granular (60 %) or linear (40 %) patterns [29, 30]. The granular pattern can be differentiated from the pattern seen in dermatitis herpetiformis as the pattern of deposition is not confined to the tips of the dermal papillae as they are in dermatitis herpetiformis. In terms of immunoglobulin deposition, IgG is nearly uni-

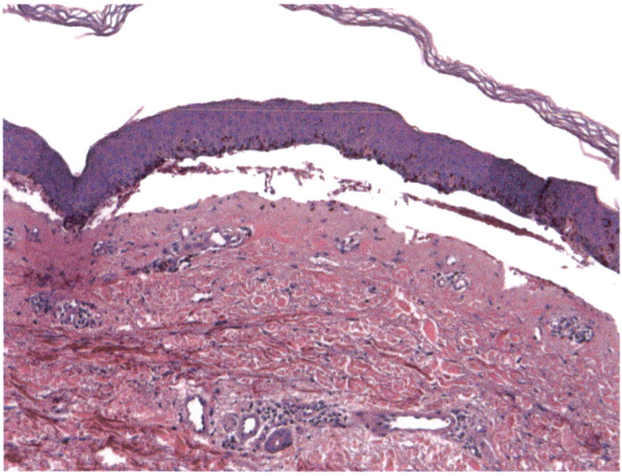

Fig. 11.4 Bullous systemic lupus erythematosus. Subepidermal bulla with neutrophils and karyorrhectic debris. H&E, 10×

versally present, observed in up to 100 % of patients, followed by IgA in 67 % and IgM in 50 %, and complement seen in 77 % of cases [1, 28]. Indirect immunofluorescence is negative for anti-BMZ antibodies [34]. Circulating antibodies are also found in bullous SLE, most commonly to type VII collagen in the NC1 domain.

The major antigenic epitope in bullous SLE is the fibronectin region of the NC1 domain of type VII collagen, which is also seen in patients with EBA. This region plays an important role in mediating the interaction between anchoring fibrils and other matrix proteins. By anchoring fibrils that cross-link the lamina densa and dermal matrix, this region helps to maintain adhesion at the DEJ. In bullous SLE, the presence of circulating antibodies against this epitope prevents interactions between the collagen and extracellular matrix, which leads to the formation of blisters and complement-mediated damage [29].

The diagnosis of bullous SLE can be challenging, as lesions can mimic those of bullous pemphigoid, linear IgA, and the inflammatory variant of EBA. The diagnosis can be made based on criteria that was originally proposed by Camisa and Sharma in 1983, which includes a diagnosis of SLE (according to criteria of the American College of Rheumatology), vesicles and bullae that arise on but are not limited to sun-exposed skin, histopathology compatible with dermatitis herpetiformis, negative IIF for circulating anti-BMZ antibodies, and DIF positive for IgG or IgM, and often IgA at the BMZ [34, 35]. Laboratory testing may reveal positive antinuclear antibody, positive anti-double-stranded DNA antibody, positive anti-Smith antibody, positive antiribonucleoprotein antibody, and/or hypocomplementemia [34].

Treatment

Dapsone

Dapsone is considered the mainstay of the treatment for bullous SLE. The striking response and clearance of lesions in response to dapsone can also be used to confirm the diagnosis, especially in cases where the clinical presentation is difficult to distinguish from EBA. Anecdotally, improvement with initiation of low doses (25–50 mg daily) of dapsone is usually dramatic, with cessation of new blister formation within 24–48 hours and clearance within 1 week. Although there are few studies that evaluate the efficacy of dapsone, in an analysis of 19 patients with bullous SLE, 17 showed improvement within days to weeks of initiation of 50–100 mg daily of dapsone therapy [36]. In one case of a young boy with bullous SLE resistant to systemic corticosteroids and mycophenolate mofetil (MFA), the addition of dapsone at a dose of 200 mg daily for 3 days led to significant regression of disease. The patient was continued on dapsone at decreased doses and tapered over 5 months [34]. Relapse of the disease can be seen with tapering and withdrawal of medication, although flares are rapidly responsive to reinstitution of therapy. Maintenance doses of dapsone between 25 and 50 mg/day are used during the taper process, and in most cases, dapsone can be discontinued with maintained disease control within 12 months [19, 30, 37].

Systemic Corticosteroids

Bullous SLE has demonstrated higher resistance to systemic corticosteroid therapy and other immunomodulators than other manifestations of SLE. High-dose corticosteroids are often used for the treatment of systemic symptoms of SLE, but are relatively ineffective in treating the cutaneous component [30]. However, in eruptions of bullous SLE that occur in the setting of SLE disease flares, treatment with both corticosteroids and other immunosuppressants is prudent [28].

Rituximab

Rituximab is a CD20 chimeric monoclonal antibody that has approved uses for non-Hodgkin lymphomas and rheumatoid arthritis. It has been used off-label in many autoimmune diseases, including SLE. In a report of one case, rituximab was used successfully in a patient with bullous SLE refractory to prednisone and immunosuppressives, including azathioprine and mycophenolate mofetil. After failure with these therapies, the patient was on prednisone and treated with two intravenous infusions of rituximab 1000 mg separated by 2 weeks. Cutaneous bullous lesions improved within 10 days of the first dose of rituximab, and cleared by 2 weeks after the second dose. The patient was subsequently able to be tapered down to 10 mg daily of prednisone [38].

Other Immunosuppressive Agents

Methotrexate has been reported in individual cases in the literature as an effective treatment in the treatment of bullous SLE. In one case report, a patient developed a severe bullous eruption concurrently with a flare of lupus serologies, which had previously been controlled. The patient also had an extensive history of intolerance to numerous drugs in the past, and was thus begun on therapy with oral methotrexate 10 mg weekly. This resulted in rapid and complete clearance of cutaneous lesions, with successful taper and discontinuation of methotrexate [39].

Mycophenolate mofetil is a 2-morpholinoethyl ester of mycophenolic acid that inhibits DNA synthesis by selective inhibition of inosine monophosphate dehydrogenase. It acts as an immunosuppressive agent by targeting T- and B-lymphocytes predominantly, inhibiting T- and B-cell proliferation, inducing apoptosis of T-cells, and inhibiting antibody production by B-cells. In one study of bullous SLE in childhood, MFA and erythromycin were used in combination to treat an eruption of bullous SLE. This combination was found to be an effective therapeutic regimen, with erythromycin acting as an anti-inflammatory agent [40, 41].

Current Opinions

Bullous SLE is a rare bullous cutaneous manifestation of SLE that is typically resistant to treatment with corticosteroids. Due to the rarity of disease, there is only anecdotal evidence upon which therapeutic measures can be guided. Dapsone at low-to-intermediate doses is often enough to induce remission of bullous lesions, as doses higher than 1.5 mg/kg daily tend to increase the risk of hemolytic anemia while not demonstrating any additional treatment efficacy. In cases that are more complex, either due to concurrent systemic and/or visceral symptoms of SLE or resistance to initial treatment, combination treatment with other immunosuppressives such as methotrexate and mycophenolate mofetil appear to have additional effectiveness. Corticosteroid therapy, which is noted to be relatively ineffective in treating bullous SLE as an isolated treatment, may be part of the treatment of bullous SLE when it occurs in the setting of a flare of SLE. Rituximab has only limited anecdotal evidence for its use in bullous SLE, and should be reserved in cases of treatment failure with other agents first (Table 11.1).

Areas of Future Interest

Further studies on the comparative efficacies of second-line immunosuppressive agents such as methotrexate and mycophenolate mofetil, among others, are needed. Currently, individual experiences are the driving force behind which second-line treatments are chosen by clinicians, and it is unclear which may be more effective when bullous SLE occurs in isolation of systemic disease, compared to bullous SLE occurring in the setting of a SLE flare. The ability to distinguish optimal treatment measures in these two settings will likely have a significant impact on the clinical course of patients with this disease.

IgA Pemphigus

Clinical Features

IgA pemphigus is a rare autoimmune intraepidermal bullous entity, with only 70 cases reported in the literature up to 2010 [42]. Although the frequency and racial distribution are unknown due to the rarity of the disease, a review of case reports reveal a slight female predominance, and average age of presentation in the 5th decade of life [43]. There are various other terms that are synonymous to this entity, including intraepidermal neutrophilic IgA dermatosis, intercellular IgA dermatosis, intraepidermal IgA pustulosis, IgA pemphigus foliaceus, and IgA herpetiform pemphigus.

There are two types of IgA pemphigus identified, which include the subcorneal pustular dermatosis (SPD) type and the intraepidermal neutrophilic (IEN) type. Both types have a similar clinical appearance, but can be distinguished by antigen expression. The SPD type demonstrates reactivity against desmocollin-1 (Dsc-1), which is expressed most strongly in the upper epidermis. In the IEN subtype, the autoantigen has been identified as desmoglein-1 and/or desmoglein-3 (Dsg 3) [42]. Clinically, IgA pemphigus presents as a vesiculopustular eruption that can develop on normal or erythematous skin. While other types of pemphigus diseases will be positive for IgG autoantibodies, IgA pemphigus is characterized by the presence of tissue-bound and circulating IgA antibodies that target desmosomal or non-desmosomal cell surface components in the epidermis. The onset of lesions is typically subacute, and they initially present as tense bullae that evolve into flaccid fluid-filled blisters. As neutrophils accumulate, the lesions transform into pustules (Fig. 11.5) [43]. Multiple pustules often form in a group and coalesce into an annular, circinate or serpiginous pattern with a central crust. The areas most commonly involved are the axilla, groin, trunk and proximal extremities. Less commonly, there can be scalp, postauricular, and intertriginous involvement. Mucous membrane involvement is rare in this entity, with only one report of oral mucosal and perianal involvement [44]. Pruritus is reported in approximately 50 % of patients.

On histological examination, the hallmark finding of IgA pemphigus is the presence of intraepidermal neutrophilic pustules or vesicles and neutrophilic infiltration in the epidermis. Acantholysis may be seen, and is often mild when it is present. The extent of acantholysis seen in IgA pemphigus is less than that seen in classic pemphigus. In the subcorneal type, the pustules are located in the upper epidermis, whereas they are suprabasilar and involve the lower or entire epidermis in the intraepidermal type [42]. On DIF of perilesional skin, IgA deposition is seen on the cell surfaces of epidermal keratinocytes (Fig. 11.6). In the SPD type, IgA antibodies are only found in the upper

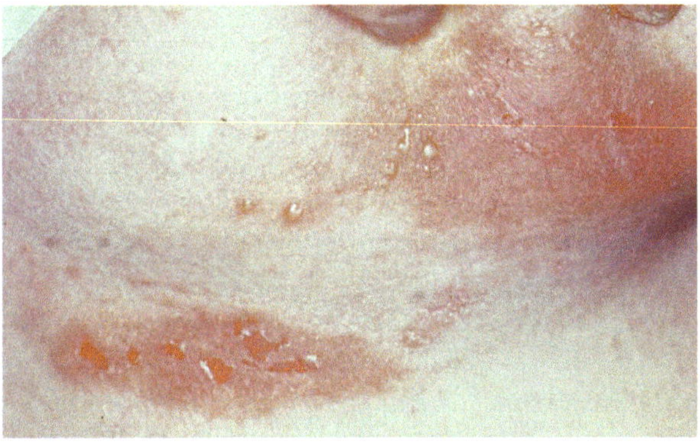

Fig. 11.5 IgA pemphigus. Vesicles and pustules seen in the inframammary region of a woman

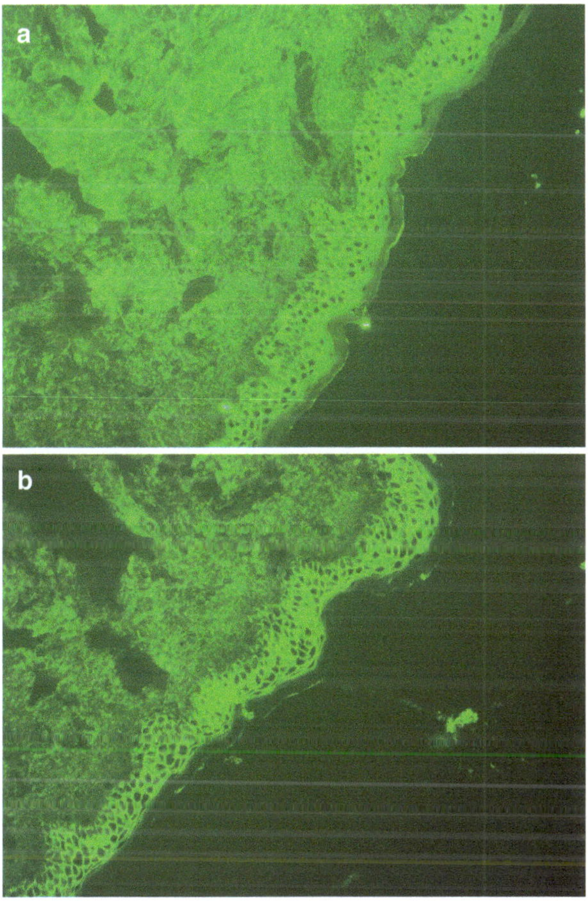

Fig. 11.6 IgA pemphigus. (**a**) DIF showing IgA deposition throughout the entire epidermis. (**b**) IgG deposition, demonstrating weaker staining than IgA

epidermis, whereas they are seen throughout the entire epidermis in the IEN type. Deposition of IgG or C3 may also be seen but will demonstrate weaker staining than IgA [42]. On indirect immunofluorescence, circulating IgA autoantibodies exclusively within the subclass of IgA_1 are seen. In contrast to classic pemphigus, the titers for autoantibodies are lower in IgA pemphigus, and the sensitivity of indirect immunofluorescence is approximately 50 % [43].

The pathogenesis of IgA pemphigus is thought to occur through the reaction of IgA to keratinocyte cell surfaces. The autoimmune targets of the IgA autoantibodies include Dsc1, Dsg1 and Dsg3. Desmocollin and desmoglein glycoproteins are members of the cadherin superfamily, which are calcium-dependent cell adhesion molecules. IgA antibodies bind to keratinocyte cell surface antigens, which leads to the accumulation of neutrophils in the epidermis and leads to intraepidermal blistering [45]. Thus, the gold standard for the diagnosis of pemphigus is demonstration of IgA autoantibodies directed against the cell surface of keratinocytes.

IgA pemphigus has been reported in association with malignancies, including IgA gammopathy, multiple myeloma, and chronic lymphocytic leukemia [42, 46, 47]. However, there are no reports of patients with IgA pemphigus with mortality linked directly as a result of IgA pemphigus, and thus is considered to be less life-threatening than other types of pemphigus [43].

Treatment

Systemic Corticosteroids

Systemic corticosteroids are considered to be the mainstay of treatment of IgA pemphigus, in combination with topical corticosteroids. The suggested dose when initiating steroid therapy is 0.5–1 mg/kg daily. However, few studies have demonstrated the efficacy of systemic steroids in IgA pemphigus in particular. In fact, in a case series of 9 patients with IgA pemphigus, 4 patients were treated with prednisone 0.5–1.5 mg/kg daily, and 3 had no response, while 1 patient had partial remission while on therapy [48].

Dapsone

The main effect of dapsone in the treatment of IgA pemphigus is thought to be through the suppression of neutrophil infiltration. Dapsone as a first-line treatment for IgA pemphigus was studied in a small case series of 6 patients. Patients received doses ranging from 25–125 mg daily. In 1 patient with IEN type disease, complete response was observed. In 2 patients with SPD type, only partial response was achieved. In the 3 remaining patients, dapsone was discontinued due to side effects of methemoglobinemia and hemolysis [48].

Colchicine

Colchicine has been studied in small subsets of patients with IgA pemphigus. The rationale behind colchicine as a potential therapeutic agent is its successes in treating other neutrophilic dermatoses. However, patients with IgA pemphigus have demonstrated limited response to colchicine. In a series of 5 patients treated with colchicine (0.5–2 mg per day), 4 patients did not respond to therapy, and the remaining patient was lost to follow-up [48]. In a report of 2 patients with SPD type IgA pemphigus treated with colchicine, clinical response was achieved within 2–3 weeks of therapy with colchicine 0.5 mg three times daily. However, despite initial responsiveness to therapy, relapses with severe disease exacerbations were noted each time colchicine was discontinued [49].

Retinoids

There are a few case reports that have described the use of retinoids such as isotretinoin and acitretin for the treatment of IgA pemphigus. In one study, isotretinoin, which is a first generation retinoid, was used to treat a patient with subcorneal pustular dermatosis type IgA pemphigus who was not effectively controlled with conventional therapeutic regimens. The patient demonstrated a rapid response to treatment with isotretinoin 20 mg daily, and had complete clearance of skin lesions within 3 weeks [50].

Acitretin, which is a metabolite of etretinate, a second-generation retinoid, has been reported as another second-line treatment option for patients with severe and/or treatment resistant IgA pemphigus. In one report, a patient with severe IgA pemphigus requiring frequent hospitalizations was treated with acitretin, and was only able to achieve partial remission on therapy [48]. In another case report, good response to acitretin in SPD type IgA pemphigus was seen in a patient with a new flare of disease. The patient was treated with 50 mg/day for 3 months with disease control, and then reduced to a maintenance dose of 25 mg every 2 days [51].

Adalimumab

Adalimumab is a recombinant human immunoglobulin antibody that targets tumor necrosis factor (TNF)-α. The mechanism for its effect in IgA pemphigus is thought to be due to the inhibition of TNF-α, which leads to the inhibition of neutrophil infiltration in the epidermis. In one case, adalimumab was used in conjunction with mycophenolate mofetil in a patient who had failed therapy, due to a lack of response to treatment or due to complications associated with alefacept, cyclosporine, acitretin, broadband ultraviolet B therapy, dapsone, methotrexate, and topical and oral corticosteroids [52].

Current Opinions

Similar to the classic autoimmune bullous dermatoses, corticosteroid therapy appears to be the most accepted first-line treatment for IgA pemphigus. As a disease within the pemphigus group, many clinicians may approach the treatment of IgA pemphigus similarly to the treatment approach to pemphigus vulgaris. Although systemic corticosteroid treatment seems to be anecdotally well accepted as first-line, the literature supporting the use of systemic corticosteroids is scant and controversial. Dapsone and colchicine, which demonstrate anti-inflammatory and anti-neutrophil effects, can also be used relatively safely and are treatment options to consider, especially if there are any relative or absolute contraindications to prolonged corticosteroid therapy. Retinoids are a second-line treatment option. However, disease flares are seen once therapy with retinoids is stopped, and long-term maintenance dosing appears to be necessary to maintain disease control. The use of biologics such as adalimumb is still being explored in IgA pemphigus, and should be considered third-line or in cases that have demonstrated resistance or treatment failure to numerous other therapies first (Table 11.1).

Areas of Future Interest

Despite the general acceptance of corticosteroids as first-line therapy, there is little evidence that demonstrates its efficacy in the treatment of IgA pemphigus. Studies that compare the efficacy of corticosteroids to other first-line treatment options such as colchicine and dapsone would be helpful in shedding light on the management of this disease. In treatments such as retinoids where anecdotal evidence is either sparse or mixed, further studies are indicated.

Subcorneal Pustular Dermatosis

Clinical Features

Subcorneal pustular dermatosis (SPD), also known as Sneddon-Wilkinson disease, is a rare chronic pustular dermatosis initially described by Sneddon and Wilkinson in 1956 [53]. It is seen in higher rates among middle-aged or elderly women, and is rarely seen in children or adolescents. It is characterized by a sterile pustular eruption that is often asymptomatic and follows a cyclic and relapsing course [54]. Classically, the pustules are described as half-pustular and half-clear fluid-filled blisters that coalesce to form annular or circinate lesions on normal or erythematous skin, which evolve into crusted lesions within days. The lesions heal centrally while new pustules may appear at the periphery (Fig. 11.7). The distribution of SPD is symmetric, with a predilection for flexural areas such as the axillae, groin, abdominal folds, and inframammary areas. Involvement of the face, palms, soles, and mucous membranes is uncommon [55, 56].

Histological examination of a representative lesion demonstrates subcorneal separation with focal aggregates of keratin and neutrophils in the cleft. In the epidermis, mild spongiosis with focal exocytosis of neutrophils without acantholysis can be seen. In the upper dermis, there are patchy infiltrates composed of lymphocytes, histiocytes, and neutrophils. There can also be perivascular infiltration of neutrophils, and rarely eosinophils and mononuclear cells in the dermis that accompany the pustule formation (Fig. 11.8) [55]. In contrast to the subcorneal type of IgA pemphigus, direct immunofluorescence is negative for IgA and IgM in classic SPD, whereas IgA pemphigus will demonstrate positive immunofluorescence with intercellular IgA deposits against desmocollin-1 [56]. An important component of the diagnosis of SPD is demonstrating sterility of the subcorneal pustule filled with neutrophils, an absence of acantholysis, and negative immunofluorescence. Thus, staining for infectious etiologies are often obtained. Gram stains will be negative for bacteria and periodic acid-Schiff stain negative for fungal organisms.

Although the etiology of SPD is not clear, theories include infectious or autoimmune causes. There are known associations between SPD and other autoimmune-related disorders including pyoderma gangrenosum, rheumatoid arthritis, systemic lupus erythematosus, inflammatory bowel disease, hyperthyroidism, and multiple

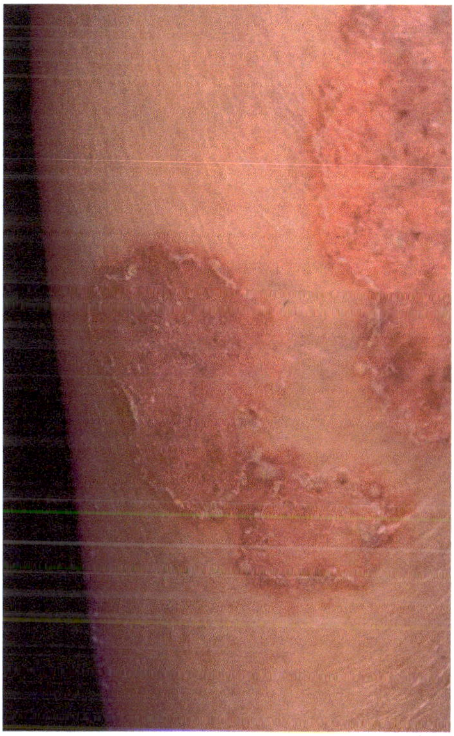

Fig. 11.7 Subcorneal pustular dermatosis. Annular, erythematous lesions with crust and pustules at the periphery

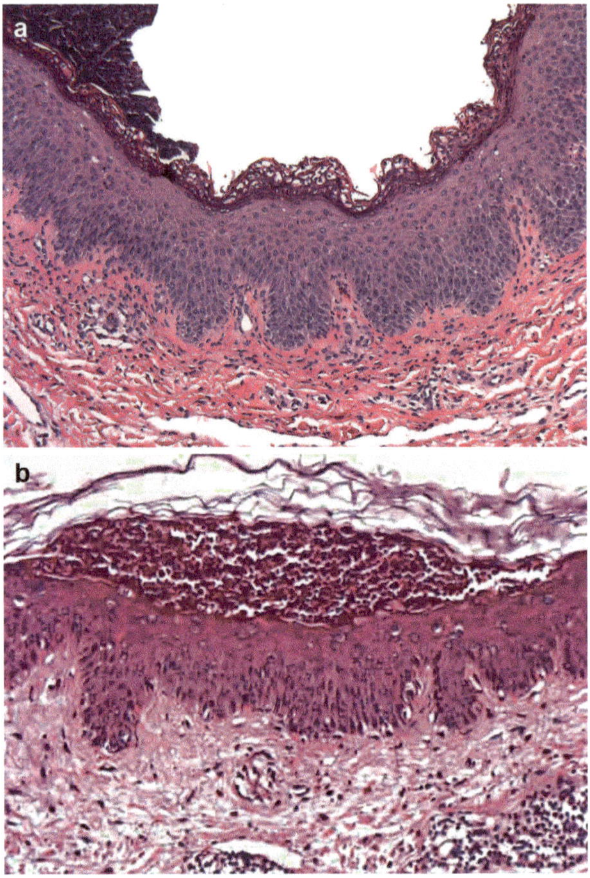

Fig. 11.8 Subcorneal pustular dermatosis. (**a**) Patchy infiltrates of lymphocytes, histiocytes, and neutrophils in the upper dermis. H&E, 10×. (**b**) Subcorneal separation with aggregates of keratin and neutrophils within the clef. H&E, 20×

myeloma, as well as anecdotal associations with mycoplasma pneumonia, Sjogren's syndrome, multiple sclerosis, and malignancies such as IgA myeloma. Some authors recommend basic screening in patients with this disorder for other common autoimmune diseases such as rheumatoid arthritis and monoclonal gammopathy and screening for underlying myeloma by evaluating for urine and serum paraproteinemia [56].

Treatment

Dapsone

Dapsone is considered a first-line agent for the treatment of SPD. Its mechanism of action is through the inhibition of the cytotoxic effects of peripheral neutrophils [58]. Most cases report a dramatic response to dapsone within 4 weeks of treatment, and it is used in doses between 50 and 200 mg/day. In a case report of a child with SPD, dapsone 30 mg daily resulted in nearly complete healing of cutaneous lesions within 2 weeks of therapy. After 4 weeks, treatment was continued on alternate days for another month and then stopped with no recurrence or flare [54]. However, there are cases of refractory SPD or intolerance to dapsone due to methemoglobinemia or hemolytic anemia which can be limiting factors. In one report of resistant SPD, oral dapsone 50 mg daily was used in a patient for 3 months, and then in combination with colchicine for 3 months with no response. The patient had significant side effects of diarrhea and 20-pound weight loss and therapy was discontinued [56]. Furthermore, patients may require a maintenance dose to prevent disease flare [57].

Colchicine

Colchicine has a known inhibitory effect on polymorphonuclear leukocytes, and has known efficacy in the treatment of other dermatologic diseases characterized by leukocyte chemotaxis and neutrophilic infiltration such as Behcet's disease and Sweet's syndrome. In one report of colchicine use for SPD, colchicine was used as an alternative treatment in a patient who developed an allergic reaction to dapsone. The patient was started on oral colchicine 0.5 mg twice daily and the pustular lesions subsided within 1 week, after which the dose was reduced to 0.5 mg daily. The drug was well tolerated and there was no recurrence with discontinuation [59].

Retinoids

In a review of 12 cases of SPD treated with etretinate, almost all cases were initially resistant to dapsone and few had undergone trial with colchicine with no response. In all but two cases, complete response was seen after treatment with etretinate, ranging in dose from 20 to 100 mg daily. In the remaining cases, one patient showed partial response and one patient showed no response and was considered a treatment failure. However, almost all patients who responded to etretinate required continuous maintenance treatment after 15 months of treatment [60].

In another patient who failed treatment with dapsone, acitretin 0.5 mg/kg daily (25 mg/day) was used. The resolution of the pustular eruption was seen within 2 weeks, and the dose of acitretin was decreased to 10 mg daily. After 4 months of disease clearance, acitretin was discontinued, and no relapses were noted up to 30 months after discontinuation [61]. In a case of juvenile SPD, a 10-year old girl was treated with acitretin 0.5 mg/kg daily (10 mg/day). Within 4 weeks, the patient was noted to have almost complete clearance of cutaneous lesions, with the exception of few erythematous plaques on the hands. Treatment was continued with 10 mg acitretin every other day for 1 month, and there were no relapses or significant adverse events reported [55].

Biologics

There are few reports of patients with SPD treated with TNF-α inhibitors. In one case, infliximab was used in a patient with a 7-year history of SPD that was resistant to multiple therapeutic regimens including colchicine, retinoids, systemic glucocorticosteroids, UV phototherapy, azathioprine, and intolerant to dapsone. At one point, the patient initially had good response to acitretin 0.6 mg/kg daily and methylprednisolone 1.3 mg/kg daily used in conjunction, but eventually the clinical response to this regimen was no longer sufficient, and the patient was begun on infliximab. Infliximab was given as a single intravenous dose of 5 mg/kg, infused over 2 hours. Within 24 hours of receiving the first dose, the pustules disappeared within 2 days. Around 12 days after the infusion, pustules began to form again, and another infusion of infliximab was administered at 2 weeks, after which there was another mild relapse of papules without pustules. This minor flare was treated with oral methylprednisolone, and the patient's disease was maintained over 3 months with this treatment and with additional acitretin. The patient remained in remission on maintenance therapy with low dose acitretin [62].

In three cases reported in the literature, patients with recalcitrant SPD were treated with etanercept and achieved excellent disease clearance within 1 year. Two patients had previously failed treatment with dapsone, colchicine, acitretin, methotrexate, mycophenolate mofetil, psoralen plus ultraviolet A (PUVA), and narrowband ultraviolet B phototherapy. Both patients were treated with etanercept 50 mg twice weekly as monotherapy, and had significant improvement within 3–4 months. One patient demonstrated a flare of disease after 8 months, and adjunctive treatment with acitretin 25 mg every other day was sufficient in achieving disease clearance. At 13 months follow-up, patients were clear of disease, while continuing to take etanercept 50 mg twice weekly [63, 64].

Psoralen Plus Ultraviolet A

Psoralen plus ultraviolet A therapy has been used in SPD resistant to treatment with dapsone alone or in combination with colchicine. PUVA was initiated twice weekly for 6 weeks, followed by once weekly for 4 weeks, then once every other week for 2 months, and once a month thereafter. Mild flares of disease were seen with discontinuation of therapy, and maintenance PUVA therapy was required every 3 weeks [56]. There are also instances in which dapsone is initially effective, but after a flare and increase in dapsone dosing, patients continue to have inadequate control of disease. In one such case, the patient was additionally treated with PUVA for three sessions weekly on top of a lower dose of dapsone. Initial dosing was 1.5 J/cm^2. After 10 sessions, there was marked improvement, and after 15 sessions, the patient had almost complete clearance. After 5 weeks, the frequency of exposure was decreased to 2 sessions per week for 2 weeks, then 1 session per week. Six months after the initiation of PUVA, the patient required maintenance with 1 session per week and 50 mg dapsone daily. In other reports, maintenance treatment is required, usually involving 1 session of PUVA per week, and dapsone 50 mg/day [65].

Systemic Corticosteroids

Systemic corticosteroids in conjunction with cyclosporine has achieved disease control in some cases after failure with first-line agents. In one case, treatment with dapsone, sulfapyridine, and acitretin were inadequate in controlling the disease, and upon presentation with a severe flare, the patient was treated with cyclosporine 3 mg/kg/day and prednisolone 1 mg/kg/day. Over 2 weeks the lesions resolved and healed with desquamation after 6 weeks. The patient was stopped on both drugs after 16 weeks, and had no flare, recurrence or complications over 12 months of follow-up [58]. In another case of severe SPD with diffuse cutaneous involvement and systemic symptoms of fever and leukocytosis, the patient was treated with cyclosporine 400 mg/day after developing an adverse reaction to dapsone. After 2 days of treatment, leukocytosis improved. Within 3 weeks, cyclosporine was discontinued as the pustular eruption showed marked improvement, and was clear within 4 weeks. The patient maintained therapy with prednisolone and was tapered over a course of 2 months [66].

Current Opinions

Dapsone is considered to be the first-line treatment for SPD due to its known efficacy in this entity. Despite differences in severity, a trial with dapsone should still be considered as first-line. Another agent to consider for SPD is colchicine, which has a well-established safety profile and efficacy in its use in patients with other neutrophilic dermatoses. Systemic retinoids, which have demonstrated uses in certain pustular dermatoses such as pustular psoriasis and pustulosis palmaris et plantaris, are not typically used in neutrophilic dermatoses, except in SPD. Retinoids show rapid effectiveness, and are usually better tolerated than dapsone, but often require maintenance therapy to avoid relapse of disease [55]. PUVA has demonstrated utility in the treatment of this disease, but requires patient compliance with regular visits and appears to require chronic maintenance therapy for disease control. Prolonged use of PUVA also carries risks of malignancies, which should be kept in mind in patients requiring chronic maintenance therapy. In cases where numerous other treatment agents have been exhausted, including systemic steroid therapy and other immunosuppressive medications TNF-α inhibitors have been used in a few reports with mixed success (Table 11.1). Appropriate laboratory work-up to rule-out occult infection should be performed prior to initiating treatment with anti-TNF-α agents.

Areas of Future Interest

There is a wide range of agents that have demonstrated some evidence of efficacy in the treatment of SPD; however it is difficult for clinicians to choose which agents to use once first-line therapy has failed. Further studies that can report on the efficacy of second-line therapies such as retinoids, PUVA, and steroids would assist in guiding treatment.

References

1. Calonje E, Brenn T, Lazaar A. Inherited and autoimmune bullous diseases. In: Calonje E, Brenn T, Lazar A, Mckee PH, editors. McKee's pathology of the skin. 4th ed. Saint Louis: Elsevier/Saunders; 2012.
2. Sekiya A, Kodera M, Yamaoka T, et al. A case of lichen planus pemphigoides with autoantibodies to the NC16a and C-terminal domains of BP180 and to desmoglein-1. Br J Dermatol. 2014;171(5):1230–5.
3. Zaraa I, Mahfoudh A, Sellami MK, et al. Lichen planus pemphigoides: four new cases and a review of the literature. Int J Dermatol. 2013;52(4):406–12.
4. Goldscheider I, Herzinger T, Varga R, et al. Childhood lichen planus pemphigoides: report of two cases treated successfully with systemic glucocorticoids and dapsone. Pediatr Dermatol. 2013;31(6):751–3.
5. Cohen DM, Ben-Amitai D, Feinmesser M, Zvulunov A. Childhood lichen planus pemphigoides: a case report and review of the literature. Pediatr Dermatol. 2009;26(5):569–74.
6. Maoz KB, Brenner S. Lichen planus pemphigoides triggered by narrowband UVB, paracetamol, and ibuprofen, with autoantibodies to 130 kDa antigen. Skinmed. 2008; 7(1):33–6.
7. Ben Salem C, Chenguel L, Ghariani N, et al. Captopril-induced lichen planus pemphigoides. Pharmacoepidemiol Drug Saf. 2008;17(7):722–4.
8. Zhu YI, Fitzpatrick JE, Kornfeld BW. Lichen planus pemphigoides associated with Ramipril. Int J Dermatol. 2006;45(12):1453–5.
9. Ogg GS, Bhogal BS, Hashimoto T, et al. Ramipril-associated lichen planus pemphigoides. Br J Dermatol. 1997;136(3):412–4.
10. Swale VJ, Black MM, Bhogal BS. Lichen planus pemphigoides: two case reports. Clin Exp Dermatol. 1998;23(3):132–5.
11. Duong B, Marks S, Sami N, Theos A. Lichen planus pemphigoides in a 2-year-old girl: response to treatment with methotrexate. J Am Acad Dermatol. 2012;67(4):e154–6.
12. Demirçay Z, Baykal C, Demirkesen C. Lichen planus pemphigoides: report of two cases. Int J Dermatol. 2001;40(12):757–9.
13. Harjai B, Mendiratta V, Kakkar S, Koranne RV. Childhood lichen planus pemphigoides – a rare entity. J Eur Acad Dermatol Venereol. 2006;20(1):117–8.
14. Fivenson DP, Kimbrough TL. Lichen planus pemphigoides: combination therapy with tetracycline and nicotinamide. J Am Acad Dermatol. 1997;36(4):638–40.
15. Washio K, Nakamura A, Fukuda S, Hashimoto T, Horikawa T. A case of lichen planus pemphigoides successfully treated with a combination of cyclosporine a and prednisolone. Case Rep Dermatol. 2013;5(1):84–7.
16. Verma R, Vasudevan B, Kinra P, et al. Bullous lichen planus. Indian J Dermatol Venereol Leprol. 2014;80(3):279.
17. Wagner G, Rose C, Sachse MM. Clinical variants of lichen planus. J Dtsch Dermatol Ges. 2013;11(4):309–19.

18. Camisa C, Olsen RG, Yohn JJ. Differentiating bullous lichen planus and lichen planus pemphigoides. J Am Acad Dermatol. 1984;11(6):1164–6.
19. Patil A, Prasad S, Ashok L, Sujatha GP. Oral bullous lichen planus: case report and review of management. Contemp Clin Dent. 2012;3(3):344–8.
20. Jindal R, De D, Kanwar AJ. Bullous oral lichen planus: an unusual variant. Indian Dermatol Online J. 2011;2(1):39–40.
21. Unsal B, Gültekin SE, Bal E, Tokman B. Bullous oral lichen planus: report of two cases. Chin Med J (Engl). 2003;116(10):1594–5.
22. Grunwald MH, Halevy S, Livni E, Feuerman EJ. Bullous lichen planus after intravenous pyelography. J Am Acad Dermatol. 1985;13(3):512–3.
23. Gange RW, Jones EW. Bullous lichen planus caused by labetalol. Br Med J. 1978; 1(6116):816–7.
24. Miteva L. Bullous lichen planus with nail involvement induced by hepatitis B vaccine in a child. Int J Dermatol. 2005;44(2):142–4.
25. Cribier B, Frances C, Chosidow O. Treatment of lichen planus: an evidence-based medicine analysis of efficacy. Arch Dermatol. 1998;134:1521–30.
26. Joshi A, Khaitan BK, Verma KK, Singh MK. Generalised and bullous lichen planus treated successfully with oral mini-pulse therapy. Indian J Dermatol Venereol Leprol. 1999;65(6):303–4.
27. dos Santos CE, Velho PH, Marques FM, Werner B, Aragão SC, Rachid Filho A. Bullous systemic lupus erythematosus in a pregnant woman: a case report. Rev Bras Reumatol. 2013;53(5):438–40.
28. Sebaratnam DF, Murrell DF. Bullous systemic lupus erythematosus. Dermatol Clin. 2011;29(4):649–53.
29. Grover C, Khurana A, Sharma S, Singal A. Bullous systemic lupus erythematosus. Indian J Dermatol. 2013;58(6):492.
30. Vassileva S. Bullous systemic lupus erythematosus. Clin Dermatol. 2004;22(2):129–38.
31. Poojary S, Rais S. Bullous systemic lupus erythematosus with lupus nephritis: a rare case of a subepidermal bullous disorder in a child. Cutis. 2012;89(1):17–21.
32. Nico MM, Lourenço SV. Multiple blisters along the lip vermilion are a clue to bullous lupus erythematosus. Acta Derm Venereol. 2012;92(4):404–5.
33. Anyanwu CO, Ang CC, Werth VP. Oral mucosal involvement in bullous lupus. Arthritis Rheum. 2013;65(10):2622.
34. Liu KL, Shen JL, Yang CS, Chen YJ. Bullous systemic lupus erythematosus in a child responding to dapsone. Pediatr Dermatol. 2014;31(4):e104–6.
35. Camisa C, Sharma HM. Vesiculobullous systemic lupus erythematosus. Report of two cases and a review of the literature. J Am Acad Dermatol. 1983;9:924–33.
36. Piette EW, Werth VP. Dapsone in the management of autoimmune bullous diseases. Dermatol Clin. 2011;29(4):561–4.
37. Sirka CS, Padhi T, Mohanty P, et al. Bullous systemic lupus erythematosus: response to dapsone in two patients. Indian J Dermatol Venereol Leprol. 2005;71(1):54–6.
38. Alsanafi S, Kovarik C, Mermelstein AL, Werth VP. Rituximab in the treatment of bullous systemic lupus erythematosus. J Clin Rheumatol. 2011;17(3):142–4.
39. Malcangi G, Brandozzi G, Giangiacomi M, et al. Bullous SLE: response to methotrexate and relationship with disease activity. Lupus. 2003;12(1):63–6.
40. Pehr K. Mycophenolate mofetil and erythromycin for bullous lupus erythematosus of childhood. J Cutan Med Surg. 2012;16(1):50–3.
41. Hamminga EA, Vermeer MH. Bullous systemic lupus erythematosus responding to mycophenolate mofetil. Eur J Dermatol. 2010;20(6):844–5.
42. Porro AM, Caetano Lde V, Maehara Lde S, Enokihara MM. Non-classical forms of pemphigus: pemphigus herpetiformis, IgA pemphigus, paraneoplastic pemphigus and IgG/IgA pemphigus. An Bras Dermatol. 2014;89(1):96–106.
43. Tsuruta D, Ishii N, Hamada T, et al. IgA pemphigus. Clin Dermatol. 2011;29(4):437–42.
44. Erdag G, Qureshi HS, Greer KE, Patterson JW. Immunoglobulin A pemphigus involving the perianal skin and oral mucosa: an unusual presentation. Cutis. 2007;80(3):218–20.

45. Geller S, Gat A, Zeeli T, et al. The expanding spectrum of IgA pemphigus: a case report and a review of the literature. Br J Dermatol. 2014;171(3):650–6.
46. Taintor AR, Leiferman KM, Hashimoto T, et al. A novel case of IgA paraneoplastic pemphigus associated with chronic lymphocytic leukemia. J Am Acad Dermatol. 2007;56:S73–6.
47. Aste N, Fumo G, Pinna AL, Biggio P. IgA pemphigus of the subcorneal pustular dermatosis type associated with monoclonal IgA gammopathy. J Eur Acad Dermatol Venereol. 2003;17(6):725–7.
48. Moreno AC, Santi CG, Gabbi TV, et al. IgA pemphigus: case series with emphasis on therapeutic response. J Am Acad Dermatol. 2014;70(1):200–1.
49. Hodak E, Lapidoth M, David M. Effect of colchicine in the subcorneal pustular dermatosis type of IgA pemphigus. J Am Acad Dermatol. 1999;40(1):91–4.
50. Gruss C, Zillikens D, Hashimoto T, et al. Rapid response of IgA pemphigus of subcorneal pustular dermatosis type to treatment with isotretinoin. J Am Acad Dermatol. 2000; 43(5):923–6.
51. Ruiz-Genao DP, Hernández-Núñez A, Hashimoto T, et al. A case of IgA pemphigus successfully treated with acitretin. Br J Dermatol. 2002;147(5):1040–2.
52. Howell SM, Bessinger GT, Altman CE, Belnap CM. Rapid response of IgA pemphigus of the subcorneal pustular dermatosis subtype to treatment with adalimumab and mycophenolate mofetil. J Am Acad Dermatol. 2005;53(3):541–3.
53. Sneddon IB, Wilkinson DS. Subcorneal pustular dermatosis. Br J Dermatol. 1956; 68(12):385–94.
54. Scalvenzi M, Palmisano F, Annunziata MC, et al. Subcorneal pustular dermatosis in childhood: a case report and review of the literature. Case Rep Dermatol Med. 2013;2013:424797.
55. Yayli S, Bahadir S, Alpay K, et al. A case of juvenile subcorneal pustular dermatosis successfully treated with acitretin. Int J Dermatol. 2006;45(9):1131–3.
56. Khachemoune A, Blyumin ML. Sneddon-Wilkinson disease resistant to dapsone and colchicine successfully controlled with PUVA. Dermatol Online J. 2003;9(5):24.
57. Cheng S, Edmonds E, Ben-Gashir M, Yu RC. Subcorneal pustular dermatosis: 50 years on. Clin Exp Dermatol. 2008;33(3):229–33.
58. Karadoğan SK, Aydoğan K, Başkan EB, Tunali S. A case of subcorneal pustular dermatosis treated successfully with a combination of cyclosporin and prednisolone. J Eur Acad Dermatol Venereol. 2007;21(4):536–7.
59. Pavithran K. Colchicine in the treatment of subcorneal pustular dermatosis. Indian J Dermatol Venereol Leprol. 1995;61(1):56–7.
60. Marlière V, Beylot-Barry M, Beylot C, Doutre M. Successful treatment of subcorneal pustular dermatosis (Sneddon-wilkinson disease) by acitretin: report of a case. Dermatology. 1999;199(2):153–5.
61. Canpolat F, Akpinar H, Cemil BC, et al. A case of subcorneal pustular dermatosis in association with monoclonal IgA gammopathy successfully treated with acitretin. J Dermatolog Treat. 2010;21(2):114–6.
62. Voigtländer C, Lüftl M, Schuler G, Hertl M. Infliximab (anti-tumor necrosis factor alpha antibody): a novel, highly effective treatment of recalcitrant subcorneal pustular dermatosis (Sneddon-Wilkinson disease). Arch Dermatol. 2001;137(12):1571–4.
63. Berk DR, Hurt MA, Mann C, Sheinbein D. Sneddon-Wilkinson disease treated with etanercept: report of two cases. Clin Exp Dermatol. 2009;34(3):347–51.
64. Bedi MK. Successful treatment of long-standing, recalcitrant subcorneal pustular dermatosis with etanercept. Skinmed. 2007;6(5):245–7.
65. Bauwens M, De Coninck A, Roseeuw D. Subcorneal pustular dermatosis treated with PUVA therapy. A case report and review of the literature. Dermatology. 1999;198(2):203–5.
66. Zachariae CO, Rossen K, Weismann K. An unusual severe case of subcorneal pustular dermatosis treated with cyclosporine and prednisolone. Acta Derm Venereol. 2000;80(5):386–7.

Chapter 12
Autoimmune Blistering Diseases in Children

Amy Theos

Abstract The acquired autoimmune bullous diseases are rare in children, but early recognition and prompt treatment are important. A high index of suspicion is necessary to diagnose these conditions that frequently mimic more common childhood diseases. Because there is clinical and histological overlap between these groups of diseases, direct immunofluorescence and/or indirect immunofluorescence are necessary for diagnostic confirmation. The quality of published data regarding the treatment of autoimmune bullous diseases in children is poor, as there are no controlled or comparative trials. This makes it difficult to draw conclusions regarding the best treatment algorithms. Nevertheless, numerous case reports and small, mostly retrospective, case series do suggest treatment options. The goal of treatment is to suppress disease activity and control symptoms with therapies that minimize the potential for serious short and long term adverse effects. Since children may be especially vulnerable to certain medication side effects (e.g., growth retardation from corticosteroids), this makes choosing the best treatment even more important. This chapter will review the most common autoimmune bullous diseases occurring in children: chronic bullous disease of childhood, dermatitis herpetiformis, bullous pemphigoid, epidermolysis bullosa acquisita, and pemphigus.

Keywords Chronic bullous disease of childhood • Linear IgA disease of childhood • Dermatitis herpetiformis • Bullous pemphigoid • Epidermolysis bullosa acquisita • Pemphigus vulgaris • Pemphigus foliaceus • Neonatal pemphigus • Juvenile • Adolescent • Child • Treatment

Abbreviations

BMZ	Basement membrane zone
BP	Bullous pemphigoid
C3	Complement 3

A. Theos, MD
Department of Dermatology, University of Alabama at Birmingham, Birmingham, AL, USA
e-mail: Amy.Theos@childrensal.org

N. Sami (ed.), *Autoimmune Bullous Diseases: Approach and Management*,
DOI 10.1007/978-3-319-26728-9_12

CBC	Complete blood count
CBDC	Chronic bullous disease of childhood
DH	Dermatitis herpetiformis
DIF	Direct immunofluorescence
DPT	Diphtheria pertussis, and tetanus vaccination
EBA	Epidermolysis bullosa acquisita
ELISA	Enzyme-linked immunosorbent assay
FDA	Federal Drug Administration
G6PD	Glucose-6-phosphate dehydrogenase
IgA	Immunoglobulin A
IgG	Immunoglobulin G
IgM	Immunoglobulin M
IIF	Indirect immunofluorescence
IVIG	Intravenous immunoglobulin
PF	Pemphigus foliaceus
PNP	Paraneoplastic pemphigus
PV	Pemphigus vulgaris
TPMT	Thiopurine methyl transferase

Chronic Bullous Disease of Childhood

Introduction

Chronic bullous disease of childhood (CBDC), alternatively referred to as linear IgA bullous disease of childhood, is the most common autoimmune blistering disease occurring in children. It occurs in all ethnic groups and affects males and females equally. Disease onset is usually between 6 months and 10 years of age, with a mean age of onset 4.5 years [1]. Spontaneous remission occurs in the majority of patients within a few months to a few years after disease onset; a minority of patients will have persistence of disease into adulthood [2].

Clinical Presentation

CBDC presents abruptly with localized or generalized tense vesicles or bullae on normal or inflamed skin (Fig. 12.1). The blisters show a predilection for the scalp, around the mouth, ears, lower trunk, perineum and upper thighs. The blisters often elongate or coalesce, forming annular or arcuate configurations. It is common for new blisters to develop around the periphery of crusted erosions (referred to as "string of pearls" or "cluster of jewels"), which, although not pathognomonic, can be a diagnostic clue to CBDC (Fig. 12.2). Pruritus is a frequent complaint and can range from mild to severe. Postinflammatory hyperpigmentation is common after

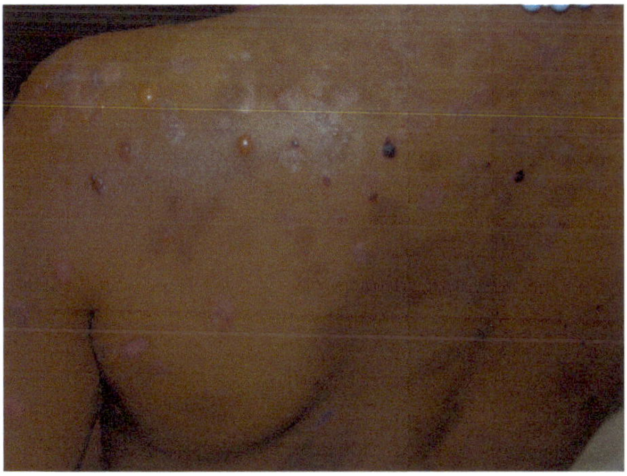

Fig. 12.1 Tense blisters and extensive postinflammatory pigmentary changes in a child with long-standing chronic bullous disease of childhood

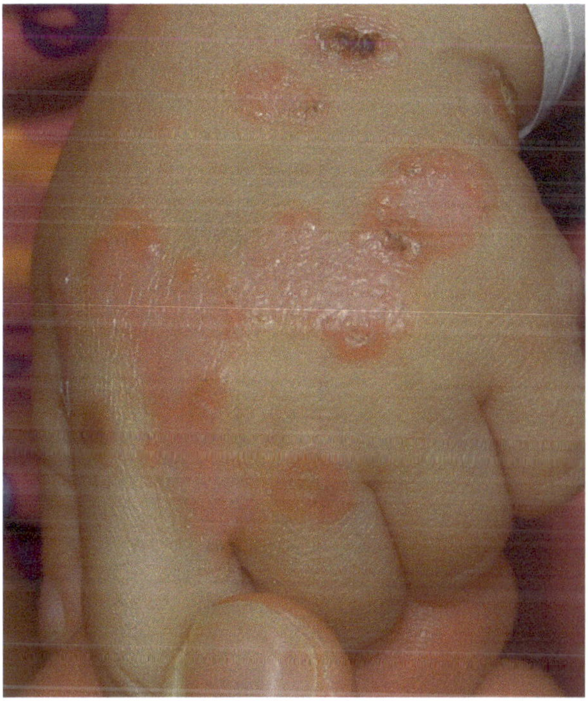

Fig. 12.2 Tense blisters in a "string of pearls" configuration on the dorsal hand of a child with chronic bullous disease of childhood

resolution, but scarring does not occur. The mucous membranes, most commonly the oral and ocular mucosae, may be affected in up to 64 % of patients, but much lower rates have been reported by other authors [1, 3]. Scarring of the ocular and oral mucosae is rare in children, but has been described [4].

Most cases of CBDC in children are idiopathic; but infections (Salmonella enteritis [5], Epstein- Barr virus [6], Group A streptococcal pharyngitis, hepatitis A [7]) and medications (amoxicillin-clavulanic acid [8], trimethoprim-sulfamethoxazole [9], vancomycin [10]) have been reported as possible triggers. It is important to inquire about potential triggers, especially medications, since discontinuation of the medication leads to resolution.

Diagnosis

The diagnosis of CBDC may be suspected clinically in typical cases (young child, lower abdomen and perineal involvement, bullae in "string of pearls" configuration), but direct immunofluorescence (DIF) testing is necessary for confirmation. Histological examination is usually not sufficient for diagnosis in that it can resemble dermatitis herpetiformis or bullous pemphigoid. Hematoxylin-eosin stained biopsy from involved skin demonstrates a subepidermal blister along with a predominantly neutrophilic infiltrate, with or without eosinophils, in the papillary dermis. Papillary neutrophilic microabscesses may be detected, especially if serial sections are studied [11]. Direct immunofluorescence of perilesional skin displays linear deposits of IgA at the dermal-epidermal junction, which is diagnostic for CBDC [12]. Weaker bands of IgG, IgM, and C3 are also occasionally present (some refer to this as mixed bullous disease of childhood) [13]. In equivocal cases, indirect immunofluorescence (IIF) will identify circulating IgA antibodies, usually low titers, in approximately 70 % of children [1, 14].

Treatments

Dapsone and Sulfapyridine

Dapsone or sulfapyridine is the treatment of choice for CBDC. Dapsone is a sulfone antibiotic approved for the treatment of dermatitis herpetiformis and leprosy in pediatric patients (lower age limit not specified). Sulfapyridine is a sulfonamide antibiotic that is no longer available in the United States, but is available in other countries. Although there are no controlled or comparative studies, there is ample anecdotal evidence in the form of case reports and case series to support the use of dapsone or sulfapyridine as monotherapy for the treatment of CBDC [7, 11, 13, 15, 16]. The response to treatment is usually rapid, with resolution of blisters within 2 weeks of starting therapy. Kenani et al. [10] performed a retrospective review of 25 children with CBDC. Nineteen children were treated with dapsone alone (1–2 mg/kg) and 11 of 19 patients achieved disease control after 8–15 days of therapy. Eight patients required the addition of systemic corticosteroids (0.5–1 mg/kg) to control their disease. The duration of treatment ranged from 3 to 60 months. Seventeen patients had achieved remission at the time of publication. Four patients developed methemoglobinemia that necessitated a reduction in dose or withdrawal of medication for a few days, but no other adverse effects were seen. Wojnarowska et al. [1] studied a series of 25 children with CBDC. All children were treated with either dapsone (20–200 mg) or sulfapyridine (0.5–2 g) and all had a response to treatment within 72 hours with relapses when the drug was withdrawn. Sixteen of 25 patients achieved remission over a variable time period of 6 months to 16 years (mean 5.3 years). Eight children were also treated with low dose systemic corticosteroids. Detailed treatment information and side effects were not provided. Marsden et al. [15] reported 20 children with CBDC treated with either dapsone (20–200 mg) or sulfapyridine (0.25–3 g); 12 of 20 children were well controlled with monotherapy and eight children required the addition of corticosteroids.

Corticosteroids

Again the evidence is anecdotal, but it is apparent from the literature that systemic corticosteroids are useful as adjunctive therapy for disease that is resistant to first line treatment and severe disease presentations (e.g., extensive blistering and erosions, severe pruritus, symptomatic mucous membrane involvement), but should be avoided as monotherapy due to the long-term side effects in children [3, 7, 10, 17, 18]. The most frequently used dose is 0.5–1 mg/kg (prednisone/prednisolone). The corticosteroids are continued until the disease is controlled, then they are tapered off, usually over a 3–6 week period. They can then be used intermittently for severe exacerbations if necessary. Wojnarowska et al. [1] used low dose systemic steroids (<10 mg; weight-based dosing not provided) in 8 of 25 children not controlled on dapsone or sulfapyridine and concluded that the value of the addition of low dose systemic corticosteroids is difficult to determine as the effect was neither rapid nor dramatic. If systemic corticosteroids are to be used, it appears at least moderate doses (0.5–1 mg/kg) are necessary.

Medium-potency topical corticosteroids have been reported to be useful as monotherapy for controlling very limited and mild disease [7]. Topical corticosteroids are frequently used as adjunctive therapy with systemic agents for symptom control.

Antibiotics

The semisynthetic penicillins (oxacillin, cloxacillin, dicloxacillin, and flucloxacillin), macrolide antibiotics (erythromycin) and sulfonamides (trimethoprim-sulfamethoxazole) have all been reported to be useful for the treatment of CBDC [3, 10, 19–26]. Alajlan et al. [19] conducted a prospective observational study of seven children with confirmed CBDC treated with flucloxacillin (similar to dicloxacillin). Four of seven patients had a complete response to flucloxacillin and the medication was stopped after 2.5–4 months of therapy with no relapses. The remaining three patients had a complete response, but relapsed when flucloxacillin was stopped and have remained on treatment for 3–6 years. Interestingly, the patients treated within 1 month of disease onset responded better to flucloxacillin then patients with longstanding disease. Periodic monitoring of complete blood count (CBC) and liver function was done and no laboratory abnormalities or adverse effects were seen. An additional nine patients treated with semisynthetic penicillins have been reported with similar results [10, 20–22]. Erythromycin was first reported as an effective treatment by Cooper et al. [23]. A 5-year-old girl with CBDC with + IgA and IgG on DIF and IIF was treated with erythromycin with complete control of her disease within 2 weeks. Discontinuation of erythromycin led to a relapse of blisters and therefore she was on continuous therapy at least 24 months. Other authors have reported similar results [3, 10, 21]. A survey of members of the British Society for Pediatric Dermatology detailed 13 patients treated with erythromycin; used as monotherapy in five children and in combination with other agents (dapsone, prednisolone, nicotinamide, sulfamethoxypyridazine) in eight children. One patient had complete resolution, three had good improvement but relapsed, five patients had some improvement and four patients had minimal response. This data suggests that erythromycin alone is unlikely to produce a sustained remission [24]. Two patients cleared with trimethoprim-sulfamethoxazole within 1 week with no relapse and one cleared within 2 years [3, 25]. Pulimood et al. [26] reported a 2-year-old boy who continued to develop blisters despite dapsone 2.5 mg/kg for 3 weeks. The addition of trimethoprim-sulfamethoxazole led to resolution of blisters in 4 days and complete resolution of disease in 10 months. It is hypothesized that antibiotics are effective due to inherent anti-inflammatory and not antimicrobial properties. Antibiotics have a more favorable side effect profile than dapsone and systemic corticosteroids, require less frequent laboratory monitoring and may be a good alternative in select patients with mild to moderate disease.

Colchicine

Colchicine is an anti-inflammatory drug that is FDA approved in children 4 years and older for the treatment of familial Mediterranean fever. Colchicine appears to be a well-tolerated and effective treatment for CBDC and can be considered an alternative therapy in children with glucose-6-phosphate dehydrogenase deficiency (G6PD) or who develop intolerable side effects from dapsone [27–29]. Banodkar and Al-Suwaid [27] treated eight children with G6PD deficiency or steroid-dependent disease with colchicine 0.5 mg twice a day. Within 4–6 weeks of colchicine therapy, five patients showed a complete response without the need for corticosteroid therapy. Three patients had a good response, but still required corticosteroids, although at lower doses, to maintain remission. Two additional patients were reported with similar responses. One patient developed diarrhea, but overall colchicine was very well tolerated with no other adverse effects. No abnormalities on CBC or liver and renal function tests were seen.

Mycophenolate Mofetil

Mycophenolate mofetil is an immunosuppressive agent that preferentially inhibits T-lymphocytes and has been reported to be an effective steroid-sparing agent in adults with immunobullous disease [30]. It is approved in infants and children for the prevention of renal allograft rejection. There is a single case report describing its use in a child with severe CBDC resistant to dapsone and requiring repeated pulses of corticosteroids for disease control [31]. Mycophenolate mofetil 310 mg/m^2, later decreased to 155 mg/m^2 due to lethargy and decreased oral intake, was initiated and she showed rapid improvement within a few days and was almost clear after 6 weeks of therapy with mycophenolate mofetil and dapsone without the need for additional corticosteroids.

Miscellaneous Treatments

Nicotinamide (30 mg/kg) plus dapsone was helpful in controlling CBDC in a 4-year-old girl who had not responded to high-dose dapsone and systemic corticosteroids over 3 months. Within 2 weeks she had complete resolution of her blisters and was successfully tapered over 12 weeks [32].

Tacrolimus ointment 0.03 % was reported to be helpful in a 4-year-old girl with CBDC who experienced a flare of blisters while on dapsone. The addition of tacrolimus ointment 0.03 % resulted in resolution of blisters within 2 weeks and was used periodically to control flares [33].

Thalidomide was reported in an 8.5-year-old boy with severe CBDC who required systemic steroids for disease control [34]. The patient developed iatrogenic Cushing syndrome after 1 year on corticosteroids. The disease responded to dapsone, but dose-limiting anemia developed. The patient failed to respond to cefadroxil, erythromycin, methotrexate, and azathioprine. Cyclosporine 4 mg/kg induced remission, but was cost prohibitive. Thalidomide 3 mg/kg was started with resolution of disease in 1 month. The thalidomide had to be withdrawn after 1 year of therapy because of the development of leg pain. This patient continues to have disease as an adult.

Intravenous immunoglobulin (IVIG) was reported in a 3-year-old boy with CBDC that initially responded well to dapsone and oral corticosteroids, but due to the development of diabetic ketoacidosis other treatments were sought [35]. His disease was difficult to control despite dapsone 2.5 mg/kg. Erythromycin was not helpful. IVIG 1 mg/kg was given monthly with a reduction in blistering and corticosteroid requirements. He remained clear except for episodic exacerbations during the next year.

Evaluation and Treatment Algorithm

CBDC is a "benign" condition in that it is not fatal and generally resolves spontaneously over a period of months to years with limited sequelae; however it can cause significant morbidity and usually requires systemic treatment to control the disease until spontaneous remission occurs. The goal of therapy in children is to suppress blistering and control pruritus with therapies that minimize the potential for serious adverse effects.

If a child presents with suspected CBDC it is important to obtain a biopsy from involved skin for routine histology along with a biopsy from perilesional skin for DIF. A thorough medication history should be obtained in all cases to rule out the possibility of drug-induced CBDC. The ocular and oral mucosae should be assessed carefully for evidence of involvement and the presence of scarring, which would necessitate more aggressive therapy. If ocular symptoms (pain, discharge, grittiness, redness) are present the child should be referred to an ophthalmologist. If nasal symptoms or hoarseness are present the child should be referred to an otolaryngologist.

There are no grading systems for the assessment of severity so the clinician must use his or her own judgment. Mild disease presents with a few, small localized blisters, often around the mouth and perineum, minimal symptoms and absence of mucosal involvement. Moderate disease probably describes the majority of children and presents with more generalized involvement with vesicles and bullae distributed over the face, trunk, perineum and extremities, mild to moderate pruritus, with or without non-scarring mucosal involvement. Severe disease presents with extensive, generalized involvement, severe and uncontrolled pruritus, and/or symptomatic mucosal involvement, with or without scarring.

Mild disease can often be managed with topical therapy, either a mid to high potency topical corticosteroid or tacrolimus ointment. If topical therapy is ineffective at controlling disease, a macrolide antibiotic (e.g., erythromycin) or semisynthetic penicillin (e.g., dicloxacillin) can be added. The antibiotics and dosing regimens are reported in Table 12.1. If the patient fails to respond to these conservative therapies, dapsone or sulfapyridine can be initiated.

First-line treatment for moderate to severe disease is either dapsone or sulfapyridine. Baseline investigations before starting either treatment include a screening test for the presence of G6PD deficiency, CBC, and liver and renal function tests. Dapsone is usually initiated at a dose of 0.5 mg/kg and titrated up to 2 mg/kg or until disease control is achieved. CBC is checked weekly for the first month, monthly for the next 5 months, then every 6 months. Liver function tests and reticulocyte counts should be monitored monthly for the first 6 months, then every 6 months. Methemoglobin levels should be checked if signs of methemoglobinemia (headache, fatigue, shortness of breath, cyanosis) occur. The response to treatment is generally rapid and response should be seen within 3 weeks. If the disease is not adequately controlled after 3 weeks, adjunctive therapies (most commonly systemic corticosteroids) should be added. Dapsone should be continued at the lowest possible dose as long as necessary to control disease. Periodic treatment withdrawal is necessary to determine if spontaneous remission has occurred. Dose dependent side effects include hemolysis and methemoglobinemia. Idiosyncratic adverse reactions include agranulocytosis, hepatitis, peripheral motor neuropathy, Steven-Johnson syndrome/toxic epidermal necrolysis, and dapsone hypersensitivity syndrome. Dapsone should not be used in patients with G6PD deficiency, severe

Table 12.1 Summary of the antibiotics used to treat pediatric autoimmune bullous diseases

Antibiotic	Pediatric dosing	Side effects	Laboratory monitoring
Dicloxacillin	[a]25–50 mg/kg/day	GI disturbances, allergic reactions, serum-sickness-like reactions, agranulocytosis, leukopenia, thrombocytopenia, hepatitis, nephritis	[b]Periodic CBC, liver and renal function necessary for prolonged therapy
Oxacillin	50 mg/kg/day	GI disturbances, allergic reactions, serum-sickness-like reactions, agranulocytosis, leukopenia, thrombocytopenia, hepatitis, nephritis	Periodic CBC, liver and renal function necessary for prolonged therapy
Erythromycin	30–50 mg/kg/day	GI disturbances, QT prolongation, arrhythmia, rash, hepatitis	None recommended
Trimethoprim-sulfamethoxazole	8 mg/kg/d trimethoprim + 40 mg/kg/day sulfamethoxazole	Rash, SJS/TEN, GI disturbances, agranulocytosis, hemolytic anemia, hepatitis, nephritis	

GI gastrointestinal, *CBC* complete blood cell count, *SJS/TEN* Steven-Johnson syndrome/toxic epidermolysis necrolysis

[a]Four times a day dosing is recommended when treating infection, but twice a day dosing for this indication should be sufficient

[b]Frequency not specified

anemia or hemolysis, or known sensitivity to sulfones or sulfonamides. Dapsone can be compounded in a 2 mg/ml oral suspension that is stable for 90 days; alternatively the 25 mg or 100 mg tablets can be crushed and mixed with jam or honey.

Sulfapyridine is no longer available in the United States, but is available in other countries. It is used by some as an alternative first-line treatment instead of dapsone. It can be combined with dapsone for improved efficacy without additive side effects [36]. The recommended dosing is 60–150 mg/kg and the reported dosing regimens vary from 250 mg to 3 g daily [16, 37]. Adverse effects of sulfapyridine are similar to dapsone, with a lower incidence of hematological side effects, but a higher incidence of cutaneous allergic complications [23].

If the disease is severe or dapsone or sulfapyridine monotherapy is not sufficient to suppress disease activity within 3 weeks, systemic corticosteroids should be added. Doses ranging from 0.5 to 1 mg/kg (sometimes up to 2 mg/kg) are necessary. As soon as the disease is adequately controlled, the corticosteroid should be tapered slowly over 3–6 weeks. If the patient requires frequent courses of systemic corticosteroids, is unable to be tapered off without repeated relapses, or develops unacceptable adverse effects alternative steroid-sparing agents should be sought. Alternative adjunctive treatments include antibiotics (Table 12.1), nicotinamide, mycophenolate mofetil, azathioprine, cyclosporine, intravenous immunoglobulin, or thalidomide (roughly in that order, but individualized to patient and disease severity).

In patients with G6PD deficiency alternative first-line therapies are colchicine and antibiotics. Colchicine can be used as monotherapy or in combination with corticosteroids. The recommended dose is 0.5 or 0.6 mg twice a day (only the 0.6 mg tablets are available in the US). Response should be seen within 2–6 weeks. Once disease control is obtained colchicine should be tapered to the lowest dose that controls disease. Baseline investigation includes CBC, liver and renal function, and urinalysis. These should be repeated periodically. Gastrointestinal disturbance (diarrhea, nausea, vomiting, abdominal pain) is the most common side effect and is dose dependent. Less common side effects include anemia, bone marrow suppression and peripheral nephropathy. Colchicine should not be used in patients with hepatic or renal impairment. See Table 12.2 for summary of treatment algorithm.

Table 12.2 Treatment algorithm for pediatric autoimmune bullous diseases

Disease	Severity	First line treatment	Second line treatment	Third line treatment
Chronic bullous disease of childhood	Mild	Moderate to high potency topical CS or tacrolimus ointment	Antibiotic (see Table 12.1), dapsone (0.5–2 mg/kg)	Colchicine (0.6 mg BID), nicotinamide (30 mg/kg)
	Mod/Severe	Dapsone (0.5–2 mg/kg) or sulfapyridine (60–150 mg/kg)	Oral CS[a] (0.5–2 mg/kg)	Mycophenolate mofetil (35 mg/kg), azathioprine (2 mg/kg), cyclosporine (3–5 mg/kg), IVIG (2 g/kg q 2–4 weeks), thalidomide
Dermatitis herpetiformis		Gluten free diet and dapsone (0.5–2 mg/kg)	Sulfapyridine (60–150 mg/kg) or sulfasalazine	
Bullous pemphigoid	Mild	Moderate to high potency topical CS	Oral CS (0.5–2 mg/kg) or dapsone (0.5–2 mg/kg)	
	Mod/Severe	Oral CS (0.5–2 mg/kg)	Add dapsone (0.5–2 mg/kg) or sulfapyridine (60–150 mg/kg)	Mycophenolate mofetil (35 mg/kg), azathioprine (2 mg/kg), cyclosporine (3–5 mg/kg), methotrexate (0.3–0.5 mg/kg), rituximab (375 mg/m^2 q week × 2–4 doses), IVIG (2 g/kg q 2–4 weeks)
Epidermolysis bullosa acquisita		Oral CS (1–2 mg/kg) and dapsone (1–2 mg/kg)	Mycophenolate mofetil (35 mg/kg)	Azathioprine (2 mg/kg), cyclosporine (3–5 mg/kg), methotrexate (0.3–0.5 mg/kg), IVIG (2 mg/kg q 2–4 weeks)

(continued)

Table 12.2 (continued)

Disease	Severity	First line treatment	Second line treatment	Third line treatment
Pemphigus vulgaris	Mild	Moderate to high potency topical CS[b]	Oral CS (1–2 mg/kg)	
	Mod/ Severe	Oral CS (2–3 mg/kg)	Azathioprine (2 mg/kg) or mycophenolate mofetil (35 mg/kg) or Methotrexate (0.3–0.5 mg/kg)	[c]Rituximab (375 mg/m^2 q week × 2–4 doses), IVIG (2 mg/kg q 2–4 weeks), cyclosporine (3–5 mg/kg), cyclophosphamide
Pemphigus foliaceous	Mild	Moderate to high potency topical CS	Oral CS (1–2 mg/kg), dapsone (0.5–2 mg/kg), hydroxychloroquine (3–5 mg/kg)	
	Mod/ Severe	Oral CS (1–2 mg/kg)	Azathioprine (2 mg/kg), mycophenolate mofetil (35 mg/kg), Methotrexate (0.3–0.5 mg/kg)	[c]Rituximab (375 mg/m^2 q week × 2–4 doses), IVIG (2 mg/kg q 2–4 weeks), cyclosporine (3–5 mg/kg), cyclophosphamide

Mod moderate, *CS* corticosteroid, *IVIG* intravenous immunoglobulin
[a]Oral CS (prednisone/prednisolone)
[b]Monitor closely for disease progression and advance therapy if that occurs
[c]Consider as second line treatment in patients with severe disease

Dermatitis Herpetiformis

Introduction

Like CBDC, dermatitis herpetiformis (DH) is an IgA-mediated disease that in certain populations may be more common than CBDC. DH is rare before puberty, but in one analysis of childhood onset the mean age was 7.5 years [15]. DH has been reported to occur as young as 8 months of age [38]. DH is more common in Europe and unusual in Africa and Asia [39]. Without treatment, the disease usually persists indefinitely. All children with DH have an underlying gluten-sensitive enteropathy.

Clinical Presentation

The disease classically presents with symmetrically-distributed, intensely pruritic, grouped urticarial papules and vesicles, due to the intense pruritus erosions and excoriations may be the most abundant sign. DH most frequently involves the elbows, knees, scapulae, shoulders, sacrum, buttocks, hairline and scalp. Acral petechiae or purpura have been reported more frequently in children [40]. The mucous membranes are generally spared.

Diagnosis

Histology of an intact vesicle shows subepidermal clefting with a predominantly neutrophilic infiltrate and dermal papillary microabscesses. DIF from perilesional skin shows the presence of a granular deposition of IgA within the dermal papillae, which is diagnostic for DH.

Treatments

Gluten-Free Diet

A gluten-free diet is the treatment of choice for DH because it improves both the cutaneous and gastrointestinal pathology. A review by Ermacora et al. [41] evaluated 76 children treated with a gluten-free diet alone. Cutaneous lesions resolved in 82 % of the children within 1–3 months. Because the onset of action is somewhat slow and strict adherence to the diet may be difficult, dapsone is usually used in conjunction with a gluten-free diet, at least initially.

Dapsone

Dapsone is FDA approved for the treatment of DH in pediatric patients (lower age limit not specified). The standard starting dose is 0.5 mg/kg increasing to 2 mg/kg until disease control is achieved. Although there are no controlled trials documenting the efficacy of dapsone as a treatment of childhood DH there is convincing evidence in the literature to support its use. Marsden [15] reported 25 children with DH; 15 were treated with dapsone and all 15 had rapid improvement in pruritus and skin lesions, often within 48 h. The monitoring and side effects of dapsone are discussed under CBDC.

Sulfapyridine

Sulfapyridine is an option, although less effective, in patients who can't tolerate dapsone [15]. Sulfapyridine is no longer available in the US, having been replaced by its prodrug, sulfasalazine. Sulfasalazine is metabolized into sulfapyridine and is used in the treatment of inflammatory bowel disease. There are a few patients with suspected DH, including adolescents that have responded to treatment with sulfasalazine [42, 43].

Evaluation and Treatment Algorithm

The diagnosis of suspected DH in children should be confirmed with histology and DIF. If confirmed, referral to a gastroenterologist is warranted. A gluten-free diet is the treatment of choice and should be attempted in all patients. Dapsone is indicated for the rapid relief of pruritus and treatment of skin lesions. Once the patient is on a gluten free diet and skin lesions are controlled, dapsone should be tapered gradually to the lowest possible dose that controls the disease. In patients compliant with a gluten-free diet it can eventually be discontinued. If the patient is not controlled or cannot adhere to a gluten-free diet and is intolerant of dapsone, sulfapyridine or sulfasalazine can be tried. Moderate to high potency topical steroids can be used adjunctively on localized lesions.

Childhood Bullous Pemphigoid

Introduction

Bullous pemphigoid (BP) is another one of the more common immunobullous disease to occur in children. According to the cases reported in the literature it is much more common in Caucasians (61 % white versus 17 % black, 17 % Asian, 6 % Hispanic) and slightly more common in females (60 % of reported cases) [44]. There are two peaks of incidence in childhood BP: before age one (infantile BP) and again at 8 years of age [45]. A subtype of BP in children has been labeled localized vulval pemphigoid [46, 47]. Childhood BP has a very good prognosis, with remission occurring in most patients several weeks to a year after onset, with infrequent relapses. Despite the good prognosis, generalized disease can be life-threatening and should be treated appropriately [48, 49]. Childhood bullous pemphigoid has been reported to occur a few hours to 3 weeks after vaccination with DPT/polio alone or in conjunction with vaccines against pneumococcus, *H. influenza*, hepatitis B, or meningococcus. There are three cases that recurred with subsequent vaccinations, although the recurrence was less severe than the initial outbreak [50].

Clinical Presentation

BP presents with the abrupt onset of large, tense bullae on normal-appearing, red or urticarial skin, frequently accompanied by erosions and crusting (Fig. 12.3). Infantile BP more commonly involves the palms, soles, and face while childhood BP more commonly involves the genital region. Localized vulval pemphigoid involves only the vulva or scrotum [46, 47]. Mucous membranes are involved in approximately half of patients [51]. The blisters can be localized or disseminated. Pruritus is frequently present. The lesions heal without scarring.

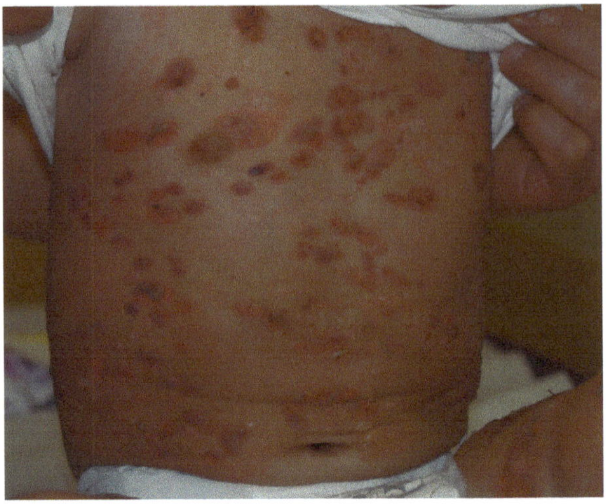

Fig. 12.3 Tense blisters, erythema and erosions on the trunk of a child with bullous pemphigoid

Diagnosis

Nemeth et al. [52] proposed the following criteria for diagnosis: (1) onset prior to 18 years of age; (2) tense blisters with typical histology (subepidermal blister with eosinophils); (3) DIF from perilesional skin showing a linear deposition of IgG and/or C3 as the major immunoreactant at the BMZ or a positive IIF showing circulating IgG antibodies directed against the BMZ. IIF on salt split skin reveals binding of IgG autoantibodies to the epidermal side and can be used to differentiate BP from epidermolysis bullosa acquisita (EBA); although rare cases with epidermal and dermal as well as pure dermal patterns have been reported [53]. Immunoblot assay or ELISA reveals circulating IgG autoantibodies directed against BP180/230 and can be useful for confirmation of diagnosis in uncertain cases. Eosinophilia is a frequent finding on CBC and may provide an early clue to diagnosis [54].

Treatments

Corticosteroids

Corticosteroids, systemic and/or topical, are the preferred treatment for childhood BP. Most cases reported have responded to moderate doses of systemic corticosteroids (0.5–2 mg/kg) that are able to be tapered off after a period of time without relapses. Topical corticosteroids have shown similar efficacy for localized disease. Waisbourd-Zinman et al. [45] described seven infants with BP. All infants were treated with prednisone 1–2 mg/kg and five infants responded with resolution of blisters within a few days to 3 months. They also summarized 71 additional cases from the literature. Twenty-five infants and children were treated with only systemic corticosteroids and almost all were reported to have a rapid response. Thirteen children were treated with only topical corticosteroids (ranging from low to high potency) with a varying rate of response. These children with localized disease, with the exception of one, had disease either localized to the palms and soles or vulva. Nineteen patients were not adequately controlled on systemic corticosteroids alone and adjunctive therapy with dapsone, sulfapyridine, IVIG, mycophenolate mofetil and/or cyclosporine was required. Intravenous pulsed methylprednisolone has also been reported to be effective at inducing remission [55].

Dapsone or Sulfapyridine

Dapsone and sulfapyridine have both been reported to be effective either as monotherapy or in combination with other medications, most commonly systemic corticosteroids. Marsden et al. [17] reported five patients (3 months to 14 years) with disseminated BP. Two patients were treated with dapsone (50–100 mg) and one patient was treated with sulfapyridine with a rapid response. Motegi et al. [56] reported a 14 year old girl with BP localized to hands and feet who was successfully treated with dapsone. Treatment with dapsone 1.5 mg/kg resulted in complete healing in 1 month and remission by 1 year. However, there have been several other reports that have not substantiated the beneficial effect of sulfones alone for BP in children [52].

Dapsone and sulfapyridine are more commonly used as adjuvant therapies for patients with generalized disease. There are numerous reports in the literature documenting the use of dapsone or sulfapyridine in conjunction with corticosteroids, but details are limited [45]. Petronius et al. [57] reported a 3.5 month old female with generalized BP that did not respond adequately to methylprednisolone 0.75 mg/kg. The addition of dapsone 1 mg/kg titrating up to 4 mg/kg resulted in a complete response within a few weeks. There are reports of two infants and a 3-year-old with generalized BP showing a complete and rapid response to corticosteroids and dapsone [55, 58]. It is difficult to interpret what effect the dapsone had on the response to treatment because the patients were treated with both medications simultaneously. Dapsone has also been used in combination with erythromycin and niacinamide [59].

Immunosuppressants

There are three case reports describing the use of mycophenolate mofetil for children with BP. A 16-year-old with severe disseminated BP was treated with prednisolone 1 mg/kg and mycophenolate mofetil 2 g daily [60]. She showed an excellent response within 3 weeks and was successfully tapered off of her steroids in 4 months. Two infants were treated with myclophenolate mofetil. One was an 8-month-old girl treated with mycophenolate mofetil 20 mg/kg, which allowed her prednisone to be tapered from 2 to 1 mg/kg, fair control of her disease [44]. The second was treated with mycophenolate mofetil 500–600 mg/m^2, in addition to corticosteroids and bimonthly IVIG [45]. Mycophenolate mofetil may have steroid-sparing properties in childhood BP. There are also isolated reports describing the use of azathioprine, cyclosporine, and methotrexate as steroid-sparing agents [45].

Intravenous Immunoglobulin

IVIG has shown varying results in children with severe or refractory BP. Xiao et al. [61] reported a 3.5 month old boy who responded to high dose IVIG (5 g/day) for 4 days. Only one course was given and no other medications were used. He continued to have mild flares not requiring treatment. Ister et al. [62] reported a 3-month-old boy with disease unresponsive to prednisolone (2 mg/kg). IVIG (1 g/kg) was administered every 2–3 weeks with immediate improvements followed by relapses for 11 months, when remission was obtained. Other infants have been treated with varying response: one infant did not respond to an unspecified dose of IVIG [55]; two infants were temporarily controlled with IVIG (200 mg/kg × 5 days and 2 g/kg every 4 weeks), but eventually required rituximab for disease control [63, 64]; another infant was treated with IVIG (2 g/kg every 2 weeks) in addition to mycophenolate mofetil and pulsed methylprednisolone [45].

Rituximab

Rituximab is an anti-CD20 antibody that depletes B lymphocytes and has been widely used in children to treat a variety of pediatric autoimmune disorders. There are four individual reports of it being used to treat refractory BP in children [63–66]. Rituximab 375 mg/m^2 was given weekly for 2–4 infusions in patients that had disease refractory to high-dose systemic steroids and other immunosuppressants. Treatment with rituximab resulted in improvement that corresponded to the decrease in CD20 cell count and allowed for significant reduction in immunosuppressant medications. One patient required addition of daclizumab [65] and one patient died 3 months after the last dose of rituximab of an unknown cause [63].

Miscellaneous

Erythromycin was first reported by Fox in 1982 [67] as a successful treatment for BP in two patients. Since then it has been reported in isolated case reports, usually in combination with prednisone, dapsone, or nicotinamide, to be a safe and potentially useful treatment for childhood BP [59].

Tacrolimus ointment 0.1 % was reported as useful for controlling localized vulval pemphigoid in an 8-year-old girl [68].

Plasma exchange and extracorporeal photochemotherapy was used successfully in one pediatric patient with associated inflammatory bowel disease without any adverse effects [69].

Evaluation and Treatment Algorithm

BP generally has a very good prognosis in infants and children, with the majority of cases resolving within a few weeks to 1 year after onset. Occasionally the disease can have a more severe and protracted course. A number of cases have been reported to occur shortly after routine childhood vaccinations, but there is no evidence that future vaccinations should be avoided. If a child presents with suspected BP it is necessary to confirm the diagnosis with histopathologic examination of a fresh blister and DIF of perilesional skin and/or IIF.

Corticosteroids are the first-line treatment for childhood BP. Localized disease, which most commonly involves acral sites, face, and genitals, can be treated with moderate to high potency topical corticosteroids with or without occlusion. Tacrolimus ointment could be tried as an alternative topical therapy if corticosteroids are not effective or contraindicated. If localized disease fails to respond to topical therapy, a trial of systemic corticosteroids (prednisone/prednisolone 0.5–2 mg/kg) can be initiated. Alternative treatments include dapsone (1–2 mg/kg), sulfapyridine (60–150 mg/kg), or erythromycin (50 mg/kg) alone or in combination with nicotinamide (30–40 mg/kg). Medications should be slowly tapered once a complete response is achieved.

Moderate to severe generalized disease should be treated initially with systemic corticosteroids at 1 mg/kg, increasing to 2 mg/kg if needed. If a complete response is achieved the corticosteroid can be slowly tapered over several weeks to months. If the disease is resistant or relapses upon taper, adjuvant therapy with dapsone or sulfapyridine is recommended (see CBDC for specifics). If response to corticosteroid and sulfone therapy is inadequate or contraindicated, other immunosuppressants such as mycophenolate mofetil (35 mg/kg), azathioprine (2 mg/kg), cyclosporine (3–5 mg/kg) or methotrexate (0.3–0.5 mg/kg) can be considered. All immunosuppressants require regular laboratory monitoring. Screening for thiopurine methyl transferase (TPMT) levels prior to initiation of azathioprine is necessary. The evidence is limited and anecdotal, and it is currently not possible to recommend one agent over another. IVIG can be considered as an alternative treatment in patients with disease refractory to the above treatments. The dosing regimens varied widely so specific recommendations regarding optimum dose is not possible. A dose of 2 g/kg every 2–4 weeks seems reasonable. The need for intravenous delivery, cost and repeated infusions are disadvantages. Rituximab (375 mg/m^2 weekly for 2–4 weeks) is an alternative therapy for refractory BP.

Childhood Epidermolysis Bullosa Aquisita

Introduction

Epidermolysis bullosa aquisita (EBA) is extremely rare in children, with fewer than 50 reported cases. EBA has been reported in children 3 months to 12 years [70–72]. A single case was reported in a newborn caused by vertical transfer of maternal autoantibodies [73]. EBA in children appears to respond more readily to treatment compared to EBA in adults. Most childhood cases remit in 1–4 years. Scarring of mucosal surfaces can cause significant morbidity.

Clinical Presentation

There are three main subtypes of EBA: (1) a noninflammatory type that mimics dystrophic epidermolysis bullosa and presents with trauma-induced blisters primarily on extensor surfaces, atrophic scarring, milia and nail dystrophy; (2) an inflammatory type that can mimic CBDC or BP with widespread erythema, pruritus and tense blisters; and (3) a predominantly mucous membrane form that mimics cicatricial bullous pemphigoid with erosions and scarring of oral, genital and conjunctival mucosae [39]. The inflammatory type is the most common in children [70]. Mucous membrane involvement is seen in the majority of children with EBA and can resolve with or without scarring. Scarring of the mucous membranes can cause diminished oral intake, malnutrition, symblepharon, and blindness.

Diagnosis

EBA can mimic several other bullous diseases and diagnosis is difficult. Skin biopsy will reveal subepidermal blisters with an inflammatory cell infiltrate composed mostly of neutrophils and eosinophils. DIF shows linear deposition of IgG, occasionally with weak IgM and IgA, along the BMZ. IIF of serum using salt split skin will reveal IgG binding to the dermal side of the blister. This helps distinguish EBA from BP. A few cases in children have been reported to have IgA-mediated EBA [74]. Immunoblotting and ELISA will identify IgG antibodies directed against various portions of collagen VII [70, 75].

Treatments

Corticosteroids with Dapsone

Based on the limited reports, systemic corticosteroids (prednisone/prednisolone 1 mg/kg) with dapsone (2 mg/kg) are the most effective treatment [53, 76–79]. Edwards et al. reported the largest series of five patients. Two patients treated with dapsone and prednisone were in remission by 10 and 24 months. One patient treated with dapsone then sulfapyridine was in remission in 4 years. Two patients treated with prednisone had partial remission at 1 and 2 years. Su et al. reported an 11-year-old girl with severe generalized disease. She did not respond to intravenous methylprednisolone 1 mg/kg, but did improve within a week of adding dapsone 1.2 mg/kg.

Miscellaneous

Tran et al. [74] reported childhood IgA-mediated EBA responding to mycophenolate mofetil. A 2-year-old girl developed disease that required moderate doses of corticosteroids and dapsone for disease control. The addition of mycophenolate mofetil allowed tapering of her corticosteroid over a 9 month period and clearing of her steroid-induced Cushingoid habitus.

Caux et al. [80] reported a child with IgA-mediated EBA that was resistant to treatment with corticosteroids, dapsone, azathioprine, and cyclosporine. Blindness resulted from her disease.

Evaluation and Treatment Algorithm

It is important to establish an accurate diagnosis of EBA in children. First-line treatment is prednisone 1 mg/kg in combination with dapsone 2 mg/kg. Once a response is noted the corticosteroid can be tapered slowly over several weeks to months; if no relapse is noted, dapsone can also be gradually tapered. Topical corticosteroids can be used as adjunctive therapy. Adjuvant or alternative treatments, based primarily on adult data, include mycophenolate mofetil, azathioprine, colchicine, cyclosporine, and IVIG. IgA-mediated EBA may require more aggressive therapy, especially if severe mucosal involvement is apparent.

Pemphigus in Children

Introduction

Although pemphigus is extremely rare in children, all subtypes have been reported to occur, including pemphigus vulgaris (PV), pemphigus foliaceus (PF) and paraneoplastic pemphigus (PNP). With the exception of endemic PF, PV is the most common subtype in children. PV affects males and females equally; it affects all races [39]. The mean age of onset of PV is 12 years [81]. With the exception of neonatal pemphigus, PV is extremely rare before 3 years of age. The course of PV in children is chronic, characterized by relapses often requiring long-term treatment with immunosuppressive agents [82]. The mortality rate is 2.9 % in children ≤12 years and 4 % in adolescents [83]. Neonatal pemphigus is observed in up to

10 % of children born to mothers with PV, and occasionally PF, and is caused by transplacental passage of maternal antibodies. Neonatal has an excellent prognosis and the lesions heal spontaneously, often within 2–3 weeks, with or without topical corticosteroids [81].

Sporadic PF is very uncommon in children. In contrast, endemic PF (fogo selvagem), which occurs in rural areas of Brazil, Columbia, and Tunisia, primarily affects children and young adults. A review of sporadic cases of PF in children found that it is slightly more common in males (1.33:1) and has an average age at presentation of 7.7 years [84]. Sunlight and infections have been implicated as possible triggers. PF appears to follow a benign course, with most children free of disease within a year.

PNP generally affects children between 8 and 18 years of age. It shows no gender preference and appears to more frequently affect Hispanic children [85]. It occurs almost exclusively in association with undiagnosed Castleman's disease (angiofollicular lymphoid hyperplasia). The mortality rate is high despite treatment of the underlying neoplasm and is generally attributed to bronchiolitis obliterans.

Clinical Presentation

PV presents with blisters and painful mucosal erosions, affecting the mouth in almost all patients, followed by the genital, ocular, and nasal mucosae [86]. Flaccid blisters on normal-appearing skin along with painful superficial erosions and crusts appear on the skin surface. The Nikolsky sign is positive. The mucosal lesions generally precede the cutaneous lesions. Mucosal lesions may cause pain, decreased oral intake and weight loss, and dysuria.

PF presents with crusted red plaques, erosions and superficial flaccid blisters preferentially affecting the scalp and face, followed by the trunk and upper extremities. The lesions can be arcuate or polycyclic and photodistributed. Rare cases present as erythroderma. The mucous membranes are spared.

PNP presents as an intractable, painful stomatitis, frequently in conjunction with genital and conjunctival involvement. Cutaneous involvement can be varied with blisters, erosions or lichenoid lesions. In children, unlike in adult disease, the mucocutaneous lesions are most often lichenoid and not blistering [85].

Diagnosis

All diseases are diagnosed through a combination of clinical, histological and immunofluorescence findings. PV is characterized histologically by suprabasilar acantholysis and tombstoning of basal keratinocytes. Acantholytic and inflammatory cells can be present in the blister cavity. DIF reveals intercellular IgG and/or C3 throughout the epidermis in a chicken-wire pattern. IIF using monkey esophagus demonstrates IgG autoantibodies that bind epidermis in 90 % of patients; titers correlate with disease activity in some patients [81]. PF closely resembles PV except that the findings are more superficial resulting in a subcorneal or intragranular blister [84]. ELISA can demonstrate antibodies against desmoglein 1 or 3 in PV and desmoglein 1 in PF. PNP histologically shows either a lichenoid/interface infiltrate with variable degree of cell necrosis, intraepithelial acantholysis, or most frequently a combination of the two patterns. DIF of perilesional skin shows IgG and C3 in the intercellular spaces and variable staining of the BMZ. IIF using monkey esophagus shows antibodies binding to the epidermis and BMZ. IIF using bladder substrate shows epithelium binding in all cases. A key diagnostic feature of PNP is the presence of IgG autoantibodies against desmoplakin I, envoplakin, and periplakin on immunoprecipitation [85].

Treatments

The treatments for PV, PF and PNP are similar and will be described primarily for PV. In general, PF is milder and responds readily to treatment with oral and/or topical corticosteroids and infrequently requires aggressive therapy in children. In contrast, PNP is extremely difficult to treat and is poorly response to a number of immunosuppressive agents, along with treatment of the underlying neoplasm. Neonatal pemphigus is mild and does not require treatment other than supportive therapy.

Corticosteroids

Systemic corticosteroids are the primary treatment for PV in children. A retrospective analysis [86] of 33 patients ≤12 years old found that 90 % of patients were treated with systemic corticosteroids of varying formulations and dosing regimens. Weight-based dosing was not provided, but the average initial dose was 88 mg. The duration of therapy ranged from 1 to 10 years (average 3.7 years). Thirty-six percent of patients received a variety of adjuvant therapies. Only 18 % of patients achieved a complete recovery off of treatments. Importantly, 66.7 % of patients treated with systemic corticosteroids developed adverse effects, including Cushingoid features, growth retardation and systemic infections. The authors concluded that children are especially vulnerable to the side effects of high-dose, long-term corticosteroids. A similar report in adolescents with PV (13–18 years) showed similar results [83]. Almost all (90 %) patients were treated with corticosteroids and 50 % of patients this was the only treatment. Nineteen percent of patients experienced adverse effects, primarily related to corticosteroids. Infection, weight gain, and Cushingoid appearance were the most common. A small number of patients with limited disease responded to the long-term use of topical corticosteroids.

Azathioprine

Azathioprine is the most commonly reported adjuvant therapy for PV in children. The suggested dose is 2 mg/kg assuming normal TPMT levels. Bjarnason et al. [81] reviewed the literature and found 7 children treated with azathioprine and corticosteroids without any adverse effects. Popadic et al. [82] described two adolescents treated similarly with good results.

Intravenous Immunoglobulin

Asarch et al. [87] reported 8 juvenile patients with PV treated with IVIG (2 g/kg/cycle given over three consecutive days). In four patients it was used as monotherapy and in the other four patients it was initially combined with corticosteroids that were tapered. An average of 28.5 cycles was given over an average period of 43 months. Seven out of eight patients achieved long term clinical remission. No serious adverse effects were noted.

Rituximab

Vinay et al. [88] published the largest retrospective case series, which included 10 patients <18 years of age with either PV (7) or PF (3). Patients received rituximab as a fixed-dose of 500 mg or 375 mg/m^2 twice, 15 days apart. All patients had resistant disease, severe disease or contraindications to standard treatments. All patients showed a clinical response; eight patients achieved complete remission. Six patients relapsed/flared an average of 13 months after last infusion. Relapse was mild and controlled with standard treatment in four patients and two patients required a second cycle of rituximab. At the end of the study period five patients were in complete remission and off of therapy. Infusion reactions and angioedema were the only reported adverse effects. Fuertes et al. [89] reported an adolescent with a 14-year history of refractory PV who responded dramatically to 4 weekly cycles of rituximab 375 mg/m^2. He maintained clinical remission off of therapy for at least 18 months after treatment. Fuertes summarized six other cases reported in the literature. Four patients achieved clinical remission 2–9 months after treatment and a follow up period of 8–18 months.

Miscellaneous Treatments

Dapsone has been used in combination with corticosteroids in patients with mild to moderate disease [81].

Other immunosuppressant agents including cyclophosphamide, cyclosporine, mycophenolate mofetil, and methotrexate have been used as adjuvant therapy. Data is limited to one or two case reports so definitive conclusions regarding these agents cannot be made.

Hydroxychloroquine and chloroquine have been reported as useful in children with PF and may be helpful especially in photodistributed eruptions [84, 90].

Evaluation and Treatment Algorithm

The diagnosis of suspected pemphigus should be confirmed with skin or mucosal biopsies from lesional skin for routine histology and perilesional skin for DIF. If available, serum for IIF to obtain pemphigus antibodies is helpful. A recent medication history should be obtained to rule out the remote possibility of drug-induced pemphigus. Secondary bacterial infections, which can delay healing, should be treated. A thorough evaluation for Castleman's disease is required for patients with PNP.

Very mild and limited disease can be treated with moderate to high potency topical corticosteroids and/or intralesional corticosteroids. These patients should be followed closely to assess response to treatment and disease progression.

The first line treatment for patients with moderate or severe disease is systemic corticosteroids. Prednisone or prednisolone (2–3 mg/kg) is a standard starting dose; the dose can be increased if needed. About 50 % of children with pemphigus can be treated with corticosteroids as monotherapy, but prolonged treatment with moderate or high dosages or short repeated courses should be avoided due to the high risk of complications in children (e.g., growth retardation, infection). Once disease control is achieved the corticosteroid should be tapered very slowly over several months. Alternate day therapy is preferable if this maintains response. Topical and/or intralesional corticosteroids can be used as adjuvant therapy for localized, persistent disease. High dose intravenous pulsed corticosteroids can be considered in severe recalcitrant disease, especially in patients with a high antibody titer.

Adjuvant therapy is necessary if disease is not controlled within 3 weeks on high dose corticosteroids, relapses upon taper or adverse effects develop. Based on the literature, the addition of azathioprine (2 mg/kg) has been the most frequently used steroid-sparing agent in children with PV. Other steroid-sparing treatments for PV are methotrexate, cyclosporine, mycophenolate mofetil and cyclophosphamide. Because of the limited reports it is not possible to recommend one over another and the choice of treatment should be individualized to the patient and disease severity. Dapsone could be considered as an adjuvant in patients with mild disease, but not enough evidence is available to recommend this in patients with more significant disease.

In refractory cases, rituximab or IVIG can be considered. Based on a limited number of patients IVIG appears to be effective and may be effective as monotherapy. The main advantage of this treatment is that it is not immunosuppressive, but numerous infusions are often necessary to attain remission. Rituximab is becoming a first or second line treatment in adults with pemphigus. Based on the literature is appears to be effective for childhood disease and should be considered in patients with refractory disease.

Future Areas of Concentration: Therapeutic Questions and Deficiencies

Unfortunately, all of the current evidence regarding the treatment of autoimmune bullous diseases in children is limited and retrospective, likely due to the rarity of these diseases. Prospective studies, preferably multi-center comparative trials would be welcome. Identifying factors that predict response to treatment are important. Evaluating the actual efficacy of some of the reported more "benign" treatments (e.g., antibiotics, colchicine, nicotinamide) would be advantageous. The long term effects of both the disease and the treatments need to be better defined in children. Disease severity scores would be helpful in determining treatment choices as well as assessing response to therapy. Quality of life and the effects that these diseases have on the psychosocial development of the child need to be performed.

References

1. Wojnarowska F, Marsden RA, Bhogal B, Black MM. Chronic bullous disease of childhood, childhood cicatricial pemphigoid, and linear IgA disease of adults. A comparative study demonstrating clinical and immunopathologic overlap. J Am Acad Dermatol. 1988;19:792–805.
2. Burge S, Wojnarowska F, Marsden A. Chronic bullous dermatosis of childhood persisting into adulthood. Pediatr Dermatol. 1988;5:246–9.
3. Monia K, Aida K, Amel K, et al. Linear IgA bullous dermatosis in Tunisian children: 31 cases. Indian J Dermatol. 2011;56:153–9.
4. Edwards S, Wojnarowska F, Armstrong LM. Chronic bullous disease of childhood with oral mucosal scarring. Clin Exp Dermatol. 1991;16:41–3.
5. Simon JC, Dietrich A, Kapp A, Schopf E. Chronic bullous dermatosis in childhood. Association with salmonella enteritis. Hautarzt. 1995;46:485–9.
6. Baldari U, Raccagni AA, Celli B, Righini MG. Chronic bullous disease of childhood following Epstein-Barr virus seroconversion: a case report. Clin Exp Dermatol. 1996;21:123–6.
7. Nanda A, Dvorak R, Al-Sabah H, Alsaleh QA. Linear IgA bullous disease of childhood: an experience from Kuwait. Pediatr Dermatol. 2006;23:443–7.
8. Ho JC, Ng PL, Tan SH, Giam YC. Childhood linear IgA bullous disease triggered by amoxicillin-clavulanic acid. Pediatr Dermatol. 2007;24:E40–3.
9. Nantel-Battista M, Al Dhaybi R, Hatami A, et al. Childhood linear IgA bullous disease induced by trimethoprim-sulfamethoxazole. J Dermatol Case Rep. 2010;3:33–5.
10. Kenani N, Mebazaa A, Denguezli M, et al. Childhood linear IgA bullous dermatosis in Tunisia. Pediatr Dermatol. 2009;26:28–33.
11. Chorzelski TP, Jablonska S. IgA linear dermatosis of childhood (chronic bullous disease of childhood). Br J Dermatol. 1979;101:535–42.
12. Prystowsky S, Gilliam JN. Benign chronic bullous dermatosis of childhood. Linear IgA and C3 deposition on the basement membrane. Arch Dermatol. 1976;112:837–8.
13. Powell J, Kirtschig G, Allen J, et al. Mixed immunobullous disease of childhood: a good response to antimicrobials. Br J Dermatol. 2001;144:769–74.
14. Willsteed E, Bhogal BS, Black MM, et al. Use of 1 M NaCl split skin in the indirect immunofluorescence of the linear IgA bullous dermatoses. J Cutan Pathol. 1990;17:144–8.
15. Marsden RA, McKee PH, Bhogal B, et al. A study of benign chronic bullous dermatosis of childhood and comparison with dermatitis herpetiformis and bullous pemphigoid occurring in childhood. Clin Exp Dermatol. 1980;5:159–76.

16. Rogers M, Bartlett B, Walder B, Cains G. Chronic bullous disease of childhood –aspects of management. Aust J Derm. 1982;23:62–9.
17. Marsden RA. The treatment of benign chronic bullous dermatosis of childhood, and dermatitis herpetiformis and bullous pemphigoid beginning I childhood. Clin Exp Dermatol. 1982;7:653–63.
18. Ang P, Goh BK, Giam YC. Case reports of linear IgA bullous dermatosis of childhood. Ann Acad Singapore. 1999;28:849–54.
19. Alajlan A, Al-Khawajah M, Al-Sheikh O, et al. Treatment of linear IgA bullous dermatosis of childhood with flucloxacillin. J Am Acad Dermatol. 2006;54:652–6.
20. Siegfried EC, Sirawan S. Chronic bullous disease of childhood: successful treatment with dicloxacillin. J Am Acad Dermatol. 1998;39:797–800.
21. de las Heras MN. Linear IgA bullous dermatosis of childhood: good response to antibiotic treatment. Clin Exp Dermatol. 2014;39:395–7.
22. Skinner Jr RB, Rotondo CK, Schneider MA, et al. Treatment of chronic bullous dermatosis of childhood with oral dicloxacillin. Pediatr Dermatol. 1995;12:65–6.
23. Cooper SM, Powell J, Wojnarowska F. Linear IgA disease: successful treatment with erythromycin. Clin Exp Dermatol. 2002;27:677–9.
24. Farrant P, Carley C, Carmichael A. Is erythromycin an effective treatment for chronic bullous disease of childhood? A national survey of members of the British Society for Paediatric Dermatology. Pediatr Dermatol. 2008;25:479–82.
25. Piamphongsant T, Sirimachan S, Himmunknan P. Juvenile blistering diseases: the problems of diagnosis and treatment. Asian Pac J Allergy Immunol. 1986;4:133–7.
26. Pulimood S, Ajithkumar K, Jacob M, et al. Linear IgA bullous dermatosis of childhood: treatment with dapsone and co-trimoxazole. Clin Exp Dermatol. 1997;22:90–1.
27. Banodkar DD, Al-Suwaid AR. Colchicine as a novel therapeutic agent in chronic bullous dermatosis of childhood. Int J Dermatol. 1997;36:213–6.
28. Ang P, Tay YK. Treatment of linear IgA bullous dermatosis of childhood with colchicine. Pediatr Dermatol. 1999;16:50–2.
29. Zeharia A, Hodak E, Mukamel M, et al. Successful treatment of chronic bullous dermatosis of childhood wit colchicine. J Am Acad Dermatol. 1994;30:660–1.
30. Nousari HC, Sragovich A, Kimyai-Asadi A, et al. Mycophenolate mofetil in autoimmune and inflammatory skin disorders. J Am Acad Dermatol. 1999;40:265–8.
31. Farley-Li J, Mancini AJ. Treatment of linear IgA bullous dermatosis of childhood with mycophenolate mofetil. Arch Dermatol. 2003;139:1121–4.
32. Khanna N, Pandhi RK, Gupta S, Singh MK. Response of chronic bullous dermatosis of childhood to a combination of dapsone and nicotinamide. J Eur Acad Dermatol Venereol. 2001;15:368.
33. Dauendorffer JN, Mahe E, Saiag P. Tacrolimus ointment, an interesting adjunctive therapy for childhood linear IgA bullous dermatosis. J Eur Acad Dermatol Venereol. 2008;22:364–5.
34. Madnani NA, Khan KJ. Linear IgA bullous dermatosis of childhood: response to thalidomide. Indian J Dermatol Venereol Leprol. 2010;76:427–9.
35. Moleiro S, Santos V, Calha M, Pessoa G. Atypical response to treatment in linear IgA bullous dermatosis of childhood: Revision of literature. Dermatol Online J. 2011;17:5.
36. Mintz EM, Morel KD. Treatment of chronic bullous disease of childhood. Dermatol Clin. 2011;29:699–700.
37. Esterly NB, Furey NL, Kirschner BS, et al. Chronic bullous dermatosis of childhood. Arch Dermatol. 1977;113:42–6.
38. Lemberg D, Day AS, Bohane T. Coeliac disease presenting as dermatitis herpetiformis in infancy. J Paediatr Child Health. 2005;41:294–6.
39. Sansaricq F, Stein SL, Petronic-Rosic V. Autoimmune bullous diseases in childhood. Clin Dermatol. 2012;30:114–27.
40. Heinlin J, Knoppke B, Kohl E, et al. Dermatitis herpetiformis presenting as digital petechiae. Pediatr Dermatol. 2012;29:209–12.
41. Ermacora E, Prampolini L, Tribbia G, et al. Long-term follow-up of dermatitis herpetiformis in children. J Am Acad Dermatol. 1986;15:24–30.

42. Willsteed E, Lee M, Wong LC, Cooper A. Sulfasalazine and dermatitis herpetiformis. Australas J Dermatol. 2005;46:101–3.
43. Lowney ED. Use of sulfasalazine in dermatitis herpetiformis in young people. Arch Dermatol. 1978;114:1553.
44. Fisler RE, Saeb M, Liang MG, et al. Childhood bullous pemphigoid. A clinicopathologic study and review of the literature. Am J Dermatopathol. 2003;25:183–9.
45. Waisbourd-Zinman O, Ben-Amitai D, Cohen A, et al. Bullous pemphigoid in infancy: clinical and epidemiologic characteristics. J Am Acad Dermatol. 2008;58:41–8.
46. Schumann H, Amann U, Tasanen K, et al. A child with localized vulval pemphigoid and IgG autoantibodies targeting the C-terminus of collagen XVII/BP180. Br J Dermatol. 1999;140:1133–8.
47. Saad RW, Domloge-Hultsch N, Yancey KB, et al. Childhood localized vulvar pemphigoid is a true variant of bullous pemphigoid. Arch Dermatol. 1992;128:807–10.
48. Kuenzli S, Grimaitre M, Irischer J, et al. Childhood bullous pemphigoid: report of a case with life-threatening course during homeopathy treatment. Pediatr Dermatol. 2004;21:160–3.
49. Trueb RM, Didierjean L, Fellas A, et al. Childhood bullous pemphigoid: report of a case with characterization of the targeted antigens. J Am Acad Dermatol. 1999;40:338–44.
50. de la Fuente S, Hernandez-Martin A, de Lucas R, et al. Postvaccination bullous pemphigoid in infancy: report of three new cases and literature review. Pediatr Dermatol. 2013;30:741–4.
51. Oranje AP, van Joost T. Pemphigoid in children. Pediatr Dermatol. 1989;6:267–74.
52. Nemeth AJ, Klein AD, Gould EW, Schachner LA. Childhood bullous pemphigoid. Arch Dermatol. 1991;127:378–86.
53. Edwards S, Wakelin SH, Wojnarowska F, et al. Bullous pemphigoid and epidermolysis bullosa acquisita: presentation, prognosis, and immunopathology in 11 children. Pediatr Dermatol. 1998;15:184–90.
54. Marcus KA, Halbertsma FJ, van Steensel MA. A case of juvenile bullous pemphigoid – successful treatment with diaminodiphenylsulfone and prednisone. Pediatr Dermatol. 2009;26:55–8.
55. Osawa M, Ueda-Hayakawa I, Isei T, et al. A case of childhood bullous pemphigoid with IgG and IgA autoantibodies to various domains of BP180. J Am Acad Dermatol. 2014;70:129–31.
56. Motegi S, Abe M, Tamura A, et al. Childhood bullous pemphigoid successfully treated with diaminodiphenyl sulfone. J Dermatol. 2005;32:809–12.
57. Petronius D, Bergman R. Bullous pemphigoid in two young infants. Pediatr Dermatol. 2002;19:119–21.
58. Chimanovitch I, Hamm H, Georgi M, et al. Bullous pemphigoid of childhood: autoantibodies target the same epitopes within the NC16A domain of BP180 as autoantibodies in bullous pemphigoid of adulthood. Arch Dermatol. 2000;136:527–32.
59. Oranje AP, Vuzevski VD, van Joost T, et al. Bullous pemphigoid in children. Report of three cases with special emphasis on therapy. Int J Dermatol. 1991;30:339–42.
60. Fox JC, Kenkare S, Petronic-Rosic V, et al. Bullous pemphigoid in late childhood successfully treated with mycophenolate mofetil as an adjuvant therapy. Pediatr Dermatol. 2010;27:537–9.
61. Xiao T, Li B, Wang YK, et al. Childhood bullous pemphigoid treated by i.v. Immunoglobulin. J Dermatol. 2007;34:650–3.
62. Ister M, Pouessel G, Ythier H, et al. Postvaccinal, corticosteroid-resistant bullous pemphigoid in infancy: treatment with intravenous immunoglobulin. Pediatr Dermatol. 2014;31:e94–5.
63. Fuertes I, Luelmo J, Leal L, et al. Refractory childhood pemphigoid successfully treated with rituximab. Pediatr Dermatol. 2013;30:e96–7.
64. Schulze J, Bader P, Henke U, et al. Severe bullous pemphigoid in an infant—successful treatment with rituximab. Pediatr Dermatol. 2008;25:462–5.
65. Szabolcs P, Reese M, Yancey KB, et al. Combination treatment of bullous pemphigoid with anti-CD20 and anti-CD25 antibodies in a patient with chronic graft-versus-host disease. Bone Marrow Transplant. 2002;30:327–9.

66. Schmidt E, Seitz CS, Benoit S, et al. Rituximab in autoimmune bullous diseases: mixed responses and adverse effects. Br J Dermatol. 2007;156:352–6.
67. Fox BJ, Odom RB, Findlay RF. Erythromycin therapy in bullous pemphigoid: possible anti-inflammatory effects. J Am Acad Dermatol. 1982;7:504–10.
68. Lebeau S, Mainetti C, Masouye I, et al. Localized childhood vulval pemphigoid treated with tacrolimus ointment. Dermatology. 2004;208:273–5.
69. Tripodi G, Risso M, Tenerini L, et al. Drug-resistant bullous pemphigoid and inflammatory bowel disease in a pediatric case successfully treated by plasma exchange and extracorporeal photochemotherapy. J Clin Apher. 2007;22:26–30.
70. Mayuzumi M, Akiyama M, Nishie W, et al. Childhood epidermolysis bullosa acquisita with autoantibodies against the noncollagenous 1 and 2 domains of type VII collagen: case report and review of the literature. Br J Dermatol. 2006;155:1048–52.
71. Baican A, Chiriac G, Torio-Padron N, Sitaru C. Childhood epidermolysis bullosa acquisita associated with severe dental alterations: a case presentation. J Dermatol. 2013;40:410–1.
72. Yang B, Wang C, Wang N, et al. Childhood epidermolysis bullosa acquisita: report of a Chinese case. Pediatr Dermatol. 2012;29:614–7.
73. Abrams ML, Smidt A, Benjamin L, et al. Congenital epidermolysis bullosa acquisita: vertical transfer of maternal autoantibody from mother to infant. Arch Dermatol. 2011;147:337–41.
74. Tran MM, Anhalt GJ, Barrett T, Cohen BA. Childhood IgA-mediated epidermolysis bullosa responding to mycophenolate mofetil as a corticosteroid-sparing agent. J Am Acad Dermatol. 2006;54:734–6.
75. Schmidt E, Hopfner B, Chen M, et al. Childhood epidermolysis bullosa acquisita: a novel variant with reactivity to all three structural domains of type VII collagen. Br J Dermatol. 2002;147:592–7.
76. Trigo-Guzman FX, Conti A, Aoki V, et al. Epidermolysis bullosa acquisita in childhood. J Dermatol. 2003;30:226–9.
77. Su JC, Varigos GA, Dowling J. Epidermolysis bullosa acquisita in childhood. Australas J Dermatol. 1998;39:38–41.
78. Callot-Mellot C, Bodemer C, Caux F, et al. Epidermolysis bullosa acquisita in childhood. Arch Dermatol. 1997;133:1122–6.
79. Park SB, Cho KH, Youn JL, et al. Epidermolysis bullosa acquisita in childhood—a case mimicking chronic bullous dermatosis of childhood. Clin Exp Dermatol. 1997;22:220–2.
80. Caux F, Kirtschig G, Lemarchand-Venencie F, et al. IgA-epidermolysis bullosa acquisita in a child resulting in blindness. Br J Dermatol. 1997;137:270–5.
81. Bjarnason B, Flosadottir E. Childhood, neonatal, and stillborn pemphigus vulgaris. Int J Dermatol. 1999;38:680–8.
82. Popadic S, Medenica L, Skiljevic D, et al. Pemphigus vulgaris in three adolescents: The course of the disease. Australas J Dermatol. 2011;52:e3–7.
83. Asarch A, Gurcan HM, Ahmed AR. A current review of juvenile pemphigus vulgaris: analysis of data on clinical outcomes. Am J Clin Dermatol. 2010;11:21–33.
84. Metry DW, Hebert AA, Jordon RE. Nonendemic pemphigus foliaceus in children. J Am Acad Dermatol. 2002;46:419–22.
85. Mimouni D, Anhalt GJ, Lazarova Z, et al. Paraneoplastic pemphigus in children and adolescents. Br J Dermatol. 2002;147:725–32.
86. Mabrouk D, Ahmed R. Analysis of current therapy and clinical outcome in childhood pemphigus vulgaris. Pediatr Dermatol. 2011;28:485–93.
87. Asarch A, Ahmed AR. Treatment of juvenile pemphigus vulgaris with intravenous immunoglobulin therapy. Pediatr Dermatol. 2009;26:197–202.
88. Vinay K, Kanwar AJ, Sawatkar GU, et al. Successful use of rituximab in the treatment of childhood and juvenile pemphigus. J Am Acad Dermatol. 2014;71:669–75.
89. Fuertes I, Guilabert A, Mascaro JM, Iranzo P. Rituximab in childhood pemphigus vulgaris: a long-term follow-up case and review of the literature. Dermatology. 2010;22:13–6.
90. Petratos MA, Andrade R. Pemphigus erythematosus. Report of a case in a child less than 6 year of age. Am J Dis Child. 1967;113:394–7.

Chapter 13
Systemic Corticosteroids

Henry B. Townsend, Anthony M. Turkiewicz, and Xena A. Whittier

Abstract Corticosteroids play an essential role in the treatment of many inflammatory autoimmune diseases and often are the first line treatment option for rapid clinical response. The significant therapeutic effects, however, are often accompanied by adverse side effects. The most common and serious complication is glucocorticoid-induced osteoporosis, remaining a potentially preventable but often poorly treated side effect. Although a rarer complication, osteonecrosis is more debilitating and occurs most commonly in patients taking higher doses of corticosteroids. Metabolic and endocrine side effects, including hyperglycemia and diabetes mellitus, are potential complications, even at low dosing. Hypothalamic-pituitary adrenal suppression with secondary adrenal insufficiency can be observed more rapidly at higher dosing or longer treatment duration, although has been observed with shorter duration and lower dosing of corticosteroids as well. Corticosteroid treatment may also induce or exacerbate psychiatric disorders such as anxiety, depression, and, less commonly, psychosis. Cardiovascular side effects may also occur with corticosteroid use including hypertension, dyslipidemia and atherosclerosis. Perhaps most notably and well-described is the increased susceptibility to infections accompanying corticosteroid use, thought to occur largely through several alterations in host defenses. Ophthalmologic side effects including cataract development and increased intraocular pressure require close monitoring in the setting of long-term glucocorticoid use. In addition, several adverse GI side effects including reflux disease, gastritis and peptic ulcers have been noted with corticosteroid use. Strategies for prevention of these adverse events remain an important component during corticosteroid management.

H.B. Townsend, MD (✉)
Rheumatology Associates PC, Birmingham, AL, USA
e-mail: hbtownsend@aol.com

A.M. Turkiewicz, MD
Clinical Research Unit, Rheumatology Associates, Birmingham, AL, USA
e-mail: aturkiewicz@charter.net

X.A. Whittier, MD
Rheumatology, University of Alabama at Birmingham, Birmingham, AL, USA
e-mail: xwhittier@gmail.com

N. Sami (ed.), *Autoimmune Bullous Diseases: Approach and Management*,
DOI 10.1007/978-3-319-26728-9_13

Keywords Corticosteroids • Glucocorticoids • Inflammation • Glucocorticoid-induced osteoporosis • Osteonecrosis • Hyperglycemia • Cataracts

Introduction

Corticosteroids have played an integral role in the treatment of autoimmune diseases since their Nobel Prize-winning discovery in 1948 by Hench and colleagues. Corticosteroids continue to be the first line treatment option for rapid improvement of many inflammatory autoimmune diseases. Despite great therapeutic advances in the past several years, there still exist many cases in which long-term treatment with steroids is necessary. Unfortunately, the tremendous therapeutic effects of steroids are frequently accompanied by several adverse side effects [1]. In addition, the steroid associated side effects may occur rapidly with high doses, or gradually with chronic low dose treatment. Therefore, clinicians should think about potential corticosteroid associated adverse effects during every patient encounter and utilize proactive preventative guidelines and chronic monitoring measures in order to minimize steroid associated morbidity.

Mechanism of Action of Glucocorticoids

Inflammation is caused by a myriad of cells and mediators that are encoded by inflammatory genes. Corticosteroids affect several pathways in the inflammatory process and ultimately decrease both production of inflammatory mediators as well as the function and numbers of T-cells, B-cells, and macrophages [2].

The major mechanism for immunosuppression is through inhibition of nuclear factor kappa beta (NF-κB) [2]. NF-κB is a critical transcription factor involved in the synthesis of many cytokines and adhesion proteins that promote the immune response [3]. Inhibition of this transcription factor alone therefore significantly reduces the capacity of the immune system to mount a response.

Glucocorticoids suppress T-cell mediated immunity by inhibiting genes that code for several inflammatory cytokines including IL-1, IL-2, IL-6, IL-8, TNF-alpha, and IFN-γ [2, 3]. Reduced inflammatory cytokine production reduces T-cell proliferation and numbers. Glucocorticoids also induce T-cell apoptosis. Glucocorticoid induced apoptosis is most prominent in immature T cells inside in the thymus, but peripheral T cells are also affected [2]. In addition, glucocorticoids suppress the humoral (B-cell mediated) immune response. Glucocorticoids reduce IL-2 synthesis which leads to diminished B cell clonal expansion and antibody synthesis. Macrophage function is inhibited by glucocorticoids via down-regulation of the expression of Fc receptors on macrophages, resulting in decreased phagocytosis of opsonized cells [3].

Glucocorticoids also inhibit inflammation via upregulation of the production of endogenous anti-inflammatory proteins. One of the major proteins involved is lipocortin, which is upregulated by glucocorticoids due to its anti-inflammatory effects. Lipocortin reduces inflammation by inhibition of Phospholipase A2. Phospholipase A2 produces prostaglandins, leukotrienes and oxygen radicals by converting membrane-bound phospholipids to arachadonic acid [3]. Additionally, several other proinflammatory cytokines are inhibited by lipocortin including IL-1, IL-2, IFN-γ and TNF-alpha [3].

As our understanding of glucocorticoids and their anti-inflammatory effects continues to evolve, there is hope for future development of novel glucocorticoids with improved efficacy and reduced side effects [4].

Glucocorticoid-Induced Osteoporosis

Glucocorticoid-induced osteoporosis (GIOP) is probably the most common, yet one of the most poorly treated and potentially preventable, serious complications of glucocorticoid therapy [5]. A review of several studies over the past 10 years reveals that less than 50 % of patients receiving long-term glucocorticoids have been evaluated for osteoporosis, and less than 25 % have been treated. There is great variability among clinicians in both the awareness of glucocorticoid-induced osteoporosis and the importance of prevention and treatment as the standard of care [6]. The specialty of physician providing care was associated with receipt of both testing and treatment, with odds of receiving a bone mass measurement and antiosteoporotic medication three to four times higher in patients of rheumatologists compared with internists or family practitioners [7].

Bone loss and fractures occur most commonly in postmenopausal women, but men and premenopausal women are also at risk. Bone loss is estimated to occur in 50 % of patients treated with glucocorticoids for greater than 6 months. Studies have shown loss of 15–20 % of bone mineral density (BMD) in the first 6 months after starting treatment with glucocorticoids, followed by a slower rate of 1–3 % per year thereafter [6]. Initial bone loss is primarily trabecular bone from sites such as the lumbar spine and greater trochanter [8]. Cortical bone loss from the femoral neck and shaft occurs at a slower rate.

Glucocorticoids exert negative effects on bone health via multiple mechanisms [8]. GIOP occurs primarily due to decreased bone formation and, secondarily, as a result of increased bone resorption. Glucocorticoid inhibition of bone formation occurs by an overall decrease in osteoblast number and function [8]. Osteoblast reduction is secondary to a decrease in osteoblastic cell replication and differentiation as well as the increased apoptosis of mature osteoblasts. Also, glucocorticoids inhibit osteoblast synthesis of type I collagen, the major component of the bone extracellular matrix [8]. The increased bone resorption which occurs in GIOP appears to involve the receptor of the activator of the nuclear factor-kB ligand (RANK-L) and osteoprotegerin. RANK-L is an osteoblastic signal that binds to an osteoclast receptor and, in association with colony stimulating factor (CSF)-1, induces osteoclastogenesis [8]. Osteoprotegerin is a decoy receptor that binds RANK-L, preventing it from binding to the osteoclast receptor and subsequent osteoclastogenesis. Glucocorticoids increase the expression of RANK-L and CSF-1 and decrease osteoprotegerin production by osteoblasts, ultimately resulting in bone resorption [8].

Glucocorticoids also induce osteoporosis by increasing renal calcium excretion and decreasing intestinal calcium absorption, leading to a negative calcium balance. Lastly, treatment with glucocorticoids causes reduced sex steroid hormone production. Reported mechanisms by which this occurs include decreased gonadotropin and ACTH release from the pituitary gland, resulting in reduced production of adrenal androgens and the direct inhibition of testicular and ovarian steroidogenesis. Recommendations for the prevention and treatment of GIOP have recently been published by the American College of Rheumatology (ACR) in an effort to improve awareness and increase the rate of GIOP treatment [9]. The updated recommendations from the prior 2001 recommendations include the use of serial bone density assessments in addition to a 10-year probability of fracture screening tool, as well as incorporating newer therapeutic options for the prevention and treatment of GIOP. While a detailed discussion of these recommendations is beyond the scope of this discussion, a summary of pertinent preventative strategies is outlined in Tables 13.1 and 13.2.

Osteonecrosis

Osteonecrosis is a rarer but more insidious and debilitating complication of treatment with corticosteroids. Osteonecrosis occurs most commonly in patients taking prednisone doses of greater than 15 mg/day. High dose pulsed intravenous steroids, steroid dose packs, and intra-articular steroid injections have also been associated with the development of osteonecrosis [10]. Other risk factors for osteonecrosis include vitamin D deficiency, high alcohol consumption, history of venous or arterial thrombosis, chronic treatment with anticoagulant and anti-convulsant medications, and treatment with Depo-Provera. Osteonecrosis occurs most commonly in the hip, knee, and ankle joints. Osteonecrosis should be suspected in any patient being treated with glucocorticoids who complains of chronic joint pain. Plain radiographs are frequently normal in patients with osteonecrosis, thus MRI scanning may be necessary to make the diagnosis.

Metabolic and Endocrine Side Effects

Hyperglycemia and diabetes mellitus are potential complications of even low dose corticosteroids. Persons at the highest risk for these adverse effects include those with existing glucose intolerance, obese persons, the elderly, and patients with a

Table 13.1 Strategies for the prevention of glucocorticoid adverse events

Adverse effects	Diagnostic studies	Preventative intervention
Glucocorticoid-induced osteoporosis	Dual Energy Absorptiometry (DXA scan)[a]	Calcium, vitamin D Risk factor modification[b] Bisphosphonates Denosumab Teriparitide Raloxifene Hormonal therapy Calcitonin
Osteonecrosis	X-rays MRI	Early diagnosis and reduced weight bearing
Endocrine (Diabetes mellitus)	Regular glucose monitoring Hemoglobin A1c	Diet and weight control Oral anti-diabetic medications and insulin
Endocrine (HPA suppression)	Cosyntropin stimulation test	Slow tapering of glucocorticoids
Psychiatric	Discussion with patient/family	Antidepressants Anxiolytics Sleep aids
Cardiovascular (dyslipidemia, atherosclerosis, hypertension)	Lipid profile Monitor blood pressure	Lipid-lowering agents Anti-hypertensives
Infectious	PPD, Chest radiograph	Vaccinations
Ophthalmologic	Annual eye examination	None known
Gastrointestinal	Monitor CBC Stool occult blood testing Endoscopy	Chewable calcium carbonate with vitamin D supplement Proton-pump inhibitor H2-blocker

HPA hypothalamic pituitary axis
[a]Weight bearing exercise, smoking cessation, moderation of alcohol and caffeine intake
[b]Recommend Baseline testing at the onset of glucocorticoid therapy in women and men age 50 or older with repeat testing every 2 years

Table 13.2 Medications for the prevention and treatment of glucocorticoid-induced osteoporosis

Medication	Dosage	Route of administration
Alendronate (Fosamax)	70 mg/week	Oral
Risedronate (Actonel)	35 mg/week or 150 mg/month	Oral
Ibandronate (Boniva)	150 mg/month 3 mg/3 months	Oral Intravenous
Zolendronic acid (Reclast)	5 mg/12 months	Intravenous
Denosumab (Prolia)	60 mg/6 months	Subcutaneous injection
Teriparitide (Forteo)	20 mcg/day	Subcutaneous injection

significant family history of diabetes. Corticosteroid –induced diabetes usually responds to steroid dose reduction and may fully reverse after cessation of glucocorticoid use. In general, all patients in whom treatment with corticosteroids is expected to last greater than 30 days, should have their glucose levels checked prior to initiation of corticosteroid therapy and periodically thereafter. Fasting glucose levels greater than 125 mg/dl or random glucose levels greater than 200 mg/dl warrant hemoglobin A1c testing [11].

Long-term corticosteroid treatment also commonly causes hypothalamic-pituitary-adrenal (HPA) suppression with secondary adrenal insufficiency. Although not fully understood, this has been observed to occur after the use of as little as 10 mg/day of prednisone for 4–6 weeks [11]. HPA suppression may occur more rapidly with higher doses of corticosteroids or with twice-a-day dosing. Symptoms of adrenal insufficiency after corticosteroid use include arthralgias, myalgias, fatigue, nausea, vomiting, and hypotension. In cases of suspected glucocorticoid-induced adrenal insufficiency, a cosyntropin stimulation test may help confirm the diagnosis [11].

Psychiatric Side Effects

Treatment with corticosteroids frequently induces or exacerbates many psychiatric conditions including depression, anxiety, and disrupted sleep. Psychosis is also an uncommon but well described potential complication of corticosteroids [12]. Memory impairment, particularly in older patients, can occur at doses as low as 5 mg/day. Psychiatric side effects are significantly more likely to occur with twice daily dosing and with dosages above 30 mg/day [13]. Given the fact that depression, anxiety, and disrupted sleep are already very common in patients with chronic autoimmune diseases, clinicians may need to add or intensify treatment with antidepressants, anxiolytics, and sleep aids during treatment with corticosteroids.

Cardiovascular Side Effects

Corticosteroid use is associated with an increased risk of serious cardiovascular events and hypertension. Treatment with prednisone doses ≥7.5 mg/day was associated with a greater than 2.5-fold increased risk of cardiovascular events in a population-based study of more than 150,000 persons [14].

Chronic corticosteroid use has been associated with dyslipidemia and atherosclerosis in several conditions including systemic lupus erythematosus (SLE), asthma, and organ transplant recipients [15–17]. In lupus patients, the adverse lipid profile effects appear to occur at prednisone doses greater than 10 mg/day [15].

Increased hypertension has been observed in about 30 % of patients using glucocorticoids [18]. Fluid retention has been postulated to partially account for this observation. As with dyslipidemia, the risk of hypertension with glucocorticoid use appears to be greatest with doses greater than 10 mg/day. Lipids and blood pressure should be monitored and aggressively treated in patients being treated with chronic glucocorticoids with either a personal or family history of hypertension, cardiac disease, or renal disease.

Infectious Disease Side Effects

Corticosteroids increase susceptibility to many types of infectious agents. This issue has been well researched in patients with rheumatic diseases. Using the National Data Bank for Rheumatic Diseases in the USA, over 16,000 patients were followed for 3.5 years and observed for hospitalized pneumonia. Patients receiving glucocorticoid therapy had hospitalized pneumonia rates 1.7 times greater than those not receiving glucocorticoids. The study even identifies risk at doses less than 5 mg/day (hazard ratio 1.4) and even higher risk at 10–15 mg/day (hazard ratio 2.3). The increased rate of serious infections was more pronounced during the first 90 days after initiation of treatment with glucocorticoids [relative risk (RR) 2.99] [19]. A cohort study of 15,597 RA patients from a Medicare beneficiary database found that glucocorticoid use doubled the rate of serious bacterial infections compared with methotrexate use (RR 2.1), with a dose–response relationship for doses greater than 5 mg/day: (5 mg/day, RR 1.34; 6–9 mg/day, RR 1.53; 10–19 mg/day, RR 2.97; 20 mg/day, RR 5.48) [20].

Infections with tuberculosis, atypical organisms and herpes zoster also occur more commonly in persons taking glucocorticoids. A large, case-controlled epidemiological study of all cases of tuberculosis in the UK from 1990 to 2000, found patients with tuberculosis were nearly five times more likely to have been using glucocorticoids at the time of their diagnosis [21]. *Pneumocystis jiroveci* infection has been observed to occur more frequently in patients taking prednisone doses higher than 15 mg/day [22].

The increased risk of infections is believed to occur through multiple alterations in host defenses including altered cellular and humoral immunity, decreased phagocytosis and intracellular killing, and inhibition of cytokine release [3]. In the current era of inflammatory autoimmune disease treatments, patients are often receiving other immunosuppressive agents in addition to glucocorticoids, making it imperative that one maintain a high index of clinical suspicion for infection in patients with unusual symptoms.

Ophthalmologic Side Effects

The development of cataracts is a well-recognized complication of long-term corticosteroids [23]. Early cataract formation has been reported with both oral and inhaled steroids and with dosages as low as 5 mg/day [24, 25]. Increased intraocular pressure with secondary visual disturbance may also occur with chronic corticosteroid use. Corticosteroids may also hasten the onset of glaucoma in persons at risk for this ocular disease [26]. In light of the ocular risks, it is advisable that all long-term glucocorticoid users have periodic eye examinations.

Gastrointestinal Side Effects

Corticosteroid use has also been associated with an increased risk of adverse gastro-intestinal effects (GI) including gastroesophageal reflux disease, gastritis, peptic ulcers, bleeding, and gastrointestinal perforation [27, 28]. GI side effects are significantly more common at doses greater than 15 mg/day and in persons who are also being treated with a non-steroidal anti-inflammatory drug or oral bisphosphonate medication [28]. Daily treatment with a chewable calcium carbonate with vitamin D supplement can be an effective means of preventing and treating both corticosteroid associated GI adverse side effects and osteoporosis.

Conclusions

Glucocorticoids remain an important and highly prescribed component of the treatment regimen for patients with autoimmune diseases. An increasing body of literature supports the efficacy of glucocorticoids for both short-term symptomatic relief and as disease-modifying agents. Basic science research is also yielding increasing insights regarding the mechanisms by which glucocorticoids cause both beneficial and deleterious effects. One of the most serious and well-described adverse effects of glucocorticoids is osteoporosis. Unfortunately, this also remains the most undertreated of potential complications. Strategies for the prevention of this complication along with other glucocorticoid adverse events exist as summarized (Table 13.1). Balancing the benefits of symptomatic improvement and disease modification with the true risk of side effects remains the major challenge of glucocorticoid use. Proactive utilization of such prevention strategies can serve to significantly decrease the well-documented adverse effects associated with prolonged glucocorticoid use.

References

1. Curtis JR, Westfall AO, Allison J, et al. Population-based assessment of adverse events associated with long-term glucocorticoid use. Arthritis Rheum. 2006;55:420–6.
2. Barnes P. How corticosteroids control inflammation: Quintiles Prize Lecture. Br J Pharmacol. 2006;148:245–54.
3. Rhen T, Cidlowski J. Antiinflammatory action of glucocorticoids – new mechanisms for old drugs. N Engl J Med. 2005;353:1711–23.
4. Schacke H, Berger M, Rehwinkel H, Asadullah K. Selective glucocorticoid receptor agonists (SEGRAs): novel ligands with an improved therapeutic index. Mol Cell Endocrinol. 2007;275:109.

5. Maricic M. Update on glucocorticoid-induced osteoporosis. Rheum Dis Clin North Am. 2011;37:415–31.
6. Saag KG. Bone safety of low-dose glucocorticoids in rheumatic diseases. Ann N Y Acad Sci. 2014;1318:55–64.
7. Saag KG, Gehlbach SH, Curtis JR, et al. Trends in prevention of glucocorticoid-induced osteoporosis. J Rheumatol. 2006;33:1651–7.
8. Natsui K, Tanaka K, Suda M, et al. High-dose glucocorticoid treatment induces rapid loss of trabecular bone mineral density and lean body mass. Osteoporos Int. 2006;17:105–8.
9. Canalis E, Delany AM. Mechanisms of glucocorticoid action in bone. Ann N Y Acad Sci. 2002;966:73–81.
10. Grossman J, Gordon R, Ranganath V, et al. American College of Rheumatology 2010 recommendations for the prevention and treatment of glucocorticoid-induced osteoporosis. Arthritis Care Res. 2010;62(11):1515–26.
11. Weinstein RS. Glucocorticoid-induced osteonecrosis. Endocrine. 2012;41:183–90.
12. Lansang MC, Hustak LK. Glucocorticoid-induced diabetes and adrenal suppression: how to detect and manage them. Cleve Clin J Med. 2011;78:748–56.
13. Warrington TP, Bostick JM. Psychiatric adverse effects of corticosteroids. Mayo Clin Proc. 2006;81:1361–7.
14. Kenna HA, Poon AW, et al. Psychiatric complications of treatment with corticosteroids: review with case report. Psychiatry Clin Neurosci. 2011;65:549–60.
15. Petri M, Perez-Gutthann S, Spence D, et al. Risk factors for coronary artery disease in patients with systemic lupus erythematosus. Am J Med. 1992;93:513–9.
16. El-Shaboury AH, Hayes TM. Hyperlipidemia in asthmatic patients receiving long-term steroid therapy. Br Med J. 1973;2:85–6.
17. Becker DM, Chamberlain B, Swank R, et al. Relationship between corticosteroid exposure and plasma lipid levels in heart transplant recipients. Am J Med. 1988;85:632–8.
18. Whitworth JA. Mechanisms of glucocorticoid-induced hypertension. Kidney Int. 1987;31:1213–24.
19. Wolfe F, Caplan L, Michaud K. Treatment for rheumatoid arthritis and the risk of hospitalization for pneumaonia: associations with prednisone, disease-modifying antirheumatic drugs, and antitumor necrosis factor therapy. Arthritis Rheum. 2006;54:628–34.
20. Schneeweiss S, Setoguchi S, Weinblatt ME, et al. Antitumor necrosis factor alpha therapy and the risk of serious bacterial infections in elderly patients with rheumatoid arthritis. Arthritis Rheum. 2007;56:1754–64.
21. Jick SS, Lieberman ES, Rahman EU, Choi HK, et al. Glucocorticoid use, other associated factors, and the risk of tuberculosis. Arthritis Rheum. 2006;55:19–26.
22. Yale SH, Limper AH. Pneumocystis carinii pneumonia in patients without acquired immunodeficiency syndrome: associated illnesses and prior corticosteroid therapy. Mayo Clin Proc. 1996;71:5–13.
23. Townsend HB, Saag KG. Glucocorticoid use in rheumatoid arthritis: benefits, mechanisms, and risks. Clin Exp Rheumatol. 2004;22 Suppl 35:S77–82.
24. Cumming RG, Mitchell P, Leeder SR. Use of inhaled corticosteroids and the risk of cataracts. N Engl J Med. 1997;337:8–14.
25. Skalka HW, Prchal JT. Effect of corticosteroids on cataract formation. Arch Ophthalmol. 1980;98:1773–7.
26. Garbe E, LeLorier J, Boivin JF, Suissa S. Risk of ocular hypertension or open-angle glaucoma in elderly patients on oral glucocorticoids. Lancet. 1997;350:979–82.
27. Piper JM, Ray WA, Daugherty JR, Griffin MR. Corticosteroid use and peptic ulcer disease: role of nonsteroidal anti-inflammatory drugs. Ann Intern Med. 1991;114:735–40.
28. Garcia-Rodriguez LA, Hernandez-Diaz S. The risk of upper gastrointestinal complications associated with nonsteroidal anti-inflammatory drugs, glucocorticoids, acetaminophen, and combinations of these agents. Arthritis Res. 2001,3:98–101.

Chapter 14
Local Treatments and Supportive Care

Salma Faghri de la Feld and Naveed Sami

Abstract While the primary treatment of autoimmune blistering diseases (ABD) has been systemic therapy, it is important to be aware of the value of several non-systemic treatments. Topical corticosteroids (both as monotherapy and adjuvant therapy), intra-lesional corticosteroids and corticosteroid elixirs can play an important role in treatment. In addition, non-steroidal treatments such as topical calcineurin inhibitors and non-steroidal elixirs have also been reported in treatment of ABD. Furthermore, it is important to be aware of exogenous factors contributing to ABD (including food and nutrition, iodine, poor oral hygiene and ultraviolet light). Treatment of ABD is not complete without consideration of infection control and vaccination guidelines. Systemic antihistamines are also helpful in controlling symptoms of pruritus. A variety of local treatment options have proven to be beneficial in mild as well as moderate and severe disease as an adjuvant. Patients should be constantly encouraged and reminded that these measures may help reduce the dosage and duration of their systemic treatments, and in some mild cases provide remission of the ABD.

Keywords Local treatments in autoimmune blistering diseases • Adjuvant treatments in autoimmune blistering diseases • Topical corticosteroids • Intralesional corticosteroids • Side effects of local corticosteroids • Non-steroidal topical therapies • Elixirs • Infection control • Vaccines • Ultraviolet light • Food and nutrition • Antihistamines

S.F. de la Feld, MD, FAAD (✉)
Department of Dermatology, Emory University School of Medicine,
1525 Clifton Road, 1st Floor, Suite 105, Atlanta, GA 30322, USA
e-mail: salma.faghri@emory.edu

N. Sami, MD, FAAD
Department of Dermatology, University of Alabama – Birmingham,
Birmingham, AL 35294, USA
e-mail: nsderm@gmail.com; nsami@uabmc.edu

N. Sami (ed.), *Autoimmune Bullous Diseases: Approach and Management*,
DOI 10.1007/978-3-319-26728-9_14

Introduction

The primary treatment of autoimmune blistering diseases (ABD) has been systemic therapy. However, supportive treatment measures are also helpful in controlling these disorders. This includes local treatments, eliminating possible culprit medications, and controlling any exacerbating factors. These supportive measures are often considered adjunctive treatment recommendations and have been derived from treating other inflammatory dermatosis with similar issues.

In this chapter, we will attempt to provide a literature review regarding topical treatments in the various diseases along with some anecdotal recommendations based on our observations.

Topical Corticosteroids

Most patients with autoimmune blistering diseases have been prescribed local corticosteroid therapy. It has been used both as monotherapy and as adjunctive treatment to other systemic conventional treatments. The vehicle has varied depending on the disease and the area of involvement.

Topical Corticosteroids as Monotherapy

Topical corticosteroid therapy has been a mainstay of treatment for inflammatory skin diseases. The most common ABD for which topical steroids have been reported is bullous pemphigoid (BP). BP tends to be localized in the majority of cases to the skin and classically presents in the elderly. Topical corticosteroids were first reported in 1976 for use in BP as monotherapy in four patients and as adjuvant therapy in five patients (combined with either a steroid-sparing agent or a short course of systemic steroids). Six of these patients had only localized BP [1]. A recent survey of dermatologists in the United Kingdom found that the majority used topical steroids alone for localized pemphigoid [2].

One of the dilemmas surrounding the use of topical steroids has been the potency of the topical steroid. In 1989, an open label study treated ten patients with BP with topical clobetasol cream twice daily. Improvement was seen between 4 and 17 days. Then patients were discharged on maintenance therapy with less potent topical steroids, and tapered off topical steroids over 5 weeks to 13 months. One patient was unable to tolerate the transition to less potent topical steroids [3].

Another common clinical dilemma is initiating a topical steroid as monotherapy versus as an adjuvant with systemic steroids. In 2002, Joly et al. attempted to answer this question in a randomized, multi-center, non-blinded trial on 341 newly-diagnosed patients with BP [4]. The study compared clobetasol cream (40 g/day) to oral prednisone (0.5–1.0 mg/kg dosing), with patients stratified based on disease severity. Both treatments were continued until 15 days after disease control was established, and then gradually decreased. The 1-year survival rate of patients with extensive BP using clobetasol cream was higher (at 76 %) than the oral prednisone group (at 58 %). There were more severe complications in the oral prednisone group (at 54 %) than the clobetasol cream group (at 29 %) in patients with extensive BP. Of patients with severe BP, there was increased mortality in the oral prednisone group (41 %) when compared with the clobetasol cream group (24 %). Of note, patients with moderate BP did not have a significant difference between the two treatment arms when looking at clearance of skin lesions, overall survival and severe complications [4]. Limitations of this study include lack of follow-up past 1 year, lack of details on the extent of nursing assistance needed for topical therapy and lack of details on extent of striae with topical therapy. It is also unclear if better survival is from fewer side effects or from better control of underlying disease [5]. The authors hypothesize that the benefits are due to both local and systemic effects of clobetasol cream [4], but the extent of systemic absorption from clobetasol cream is unclear [5]. The mortality rates discussed by Joly et al. may also be higher than some American and British studies making it difficult to extrapolate their findings to all patients with BP [6]. Another reported limitation of topical steroid use is cost [7].

A follow-up randomized control trial was published in 2009 of 312 BP patients, comparing lower doses and shorter duration to their standard regimen used previously. Patients either received a milder regimen of clobetasol cream 10–30 g/day (based on weight and disease severity) or their standard regimen of 40 g/day of clobetasol cream. Clobetasol cream was tapered over 4 months in the milder regimen and over 12 months in the standard regimen. Results for disease control and relapse rates between the two regimens were similar, but again showed benefits from superpotent topical corticosteroids. The milder regimen used 70 % less total cumulative dose of clobetasol cream. Adjusted analyses of the data suggested that the milder regimen had an almost two-fold decreased risk of potentially fatal side effects or mortality in patients with moderate BP [8].

Many additional papers have also examined the benefits of topical corticosteroids in BP [9–14]. One review on wet dressings (also called "wet wraps") observed four out of five BP patients had marked improvement and one of five patients had moderate improvement with triamcinolone "wet wraps" (approximately 5–6 times each day while inpatient) [15]. Use of superpotent topical steroids alone (most with clobetasol propionate cream 20–30 g daily during the first month, then tapered starting 2 weeks after disease control) for a mean duration of 9–12 months has also been reported to decrease serum BPAG 180 and BPAG 230 autoantibody levels [16].

Topical steroids can have beneficial effects in pemphigus (both pemphigus vulgaris and pemphigus foliaceus), but are only used as monotherapy in a few patients with mild disease. Improvement from clobetasol propionate cream has been reported in seven patients after 15 days (with cutaneous lesions) and 1 month (with mucosal lesions). Four of these patients stayed clear with topical steroids alone after a mean of 19 months. Three patients required systemic therapy due to exacerbations which could not be controlled with topical treatments after a mean duration of 2–11 months [17].

Topical Corticosteroids as an Adjuvant

Additional studies have reported topical corticosteroids to be a useful adjuvant in the treatment of BP with systemic therapy including methotrexate [18], minocycline [9], miocamycin [19] and oral tetracycline and niacinamide with topical 0.5 % gentian violet [20]. There seem to be two methods of using topical steroids with systemic treatments. Some studies suggest starting a systemic agent simultaneously with a topical steroid [18], while others recommend starting with a topical steroid initially, and then adding a systemic agent if the patient does not improve [9].

An open, clinical, records-based, retrospective, multicenter study reviewed 70 patients with BP, who were treated initially with super potent topical steroids (most with clobetasol) and methotrexate (for a mean of 12.3 weeks) followed by maintenance treatment with methotrexate alone at an average dose of 10 mg/week (for a mean of 8.45 months). All 70 patients showed initial complete remission (after a mean of 21.9 days). Seventy-six percent of patients stayed in remission with methotrexate alone, and 24 % of patients had at least one flare [18]. Stockman et al. performed an open prospective trial of ten patients with BP over 24–72 months. In this study, patients with BP were initially treated with topical corticosteroids, and if an optimal treatment response was not observed, then a systemic agent (such as systemic tetracycline, oral corticosteroids and azathioprine) was added. Patients with less than 25 % body surface area were successfully treated with potent class I topical steroids alone (five patients) or in combination with oral minocycline (two patients). Three patients (with 22 %, 42 % and 51.5 % body surface area) required systemic corticosteroids [9].

Topical corticosteroids are an important treatment modality for ABDs. These can help both with symptomatic treatment for pruritus along with providing localized disease control. For mild disease, these can initially be used as monotherapy. However, for progressive disease, it is best used as an adjuvant. The optimal choice for the potency of the topical steroid can be difficult and is often determined by severity of disease (extent and progression) and the use of a systemic adjuvant therapy. If the clinician is uncertain, medium potency topical steroids such as triamcinolone 0.1 % cream can be initiated twice a day to affected areas (not including the face or body folds) since this is less costly and can be available in a larger quantity to cover a larger surface area. However, if there is localized disease which is not progressive, a class 1 topical steroid such as clobetasol and halobetasol can be considered for a short duration to avoid the use of systemic agents, especially in the elderly.

Topical Corticosteroids for Mucosal Bullous Disease

Topical corticosteroids have been reported in the literature for mucous membrane pemphigoid in various formulations, including fluocinonide 0.05 % in an adhesive base [21] as well as in a modified custom fluoride carrier [22], clobetasol ointment in orabase [23], triamcinolone in orabase [24], and clobetasol propionate plus nystatin in orabase paste applied in a gingival tray [25] as well as elixirs (which will be described in a separate section below). One study suggests that beclomethasone inhaler and nasal sprays can be helpful in patients with nasal, pharyngeal or esophageal mucous membrane pemphigoid [26].

Use of triamcinolone in orabase has been reported to help treat mucous membrane pemphigoid, both alone (5 patients) and as an adjuvant to dapsone (15 patients). Of the five patients with mild to moderate disease treated with topical steroid monotherapy, one patient had complete resolution, one patient had over 75 % improvement and three patients had over 50 % improvement. Of the 17 patients with moderate to severe disease treated with topical steroid and systemic dapsone, 10 patients had complete resolution, five patients had over 75 % improvement and 2 patients had to stop dapsone due to systemic side effects of anemia after 2 weeks [24]. Triamcinolone acetonide 0.1 % in an adhesive dental paste (in a pediatric patient) has been reported as a helpful adjuvant treatment in one patient with oral pemphigus vulgaris [27].

Topical steroids in a gel-based vehicle can be more adherent to oral mucosa than triamcinolone acetonide in orabase. Topical steroids under occlusion using a dental tray can also help local absorption and possibly improve efficacy. It has been suggested that in elderly patients this can be accomplished using their dentures. Dentures also provide a protective barrier [26]. A double-blind cross-over study examined fluocinonide 0.05 % in an adhesive base as monotherapy in three women with mucous membrane pemphigoid and one woman with pemphigus. It was used 5–6 times per day on erosions for 2 weeks (with no eating or drinking after applications for at least 30 min). Two mucous membrane pemphigoid patients and the one pemphigus patient had partial remission with fluocinonide 0.05 % in an adhesive base, and one mucous membrane pemphigoid patient had complete remission [21].

Of note, a double-blind clinical trial has compared clobetasol 0.05 % ointment in orabase to fluocinonide ointment in orabase in patients with oral vesiculoerosive disease (which included three patients with benign mucous membrane pemphigoid and three patients with pemphigus vulgaris). While both were effective, the study suggests that clobetasol ointment was faster at decreasing pain [23].

Clobetasol propionate 0.05 % (0.1 g) plus 100,000 IU/cc nystatin (3.846 g) in orabase paste (200 g) applied in a gingival tray has been studied in 22 patients with mucous membrane pemphigoid. It was applied three times per day after meals. Eleven additional patients with oral erosions were included in the study (with either oral lichen planus or localized gingival erosions). Results were reported collectively as showing a decrease in pain and ulceration after 2 weeks of treatment in half of the patients [25].

Commercially available topical steroids are used by clinicians for mucosal involvement, especially the oral cavity. Triamcinolone dental paste is an oral specific formulation which can be applied to the affected areas in the mouth, and is most effective if left on affected areas overnight. Patients should also be advised to thoroughly rinse their mouth with water the next morning to avoid secondary Candida infections. Some patients have also found gels to be beneficial, including fluocinonide and clobetasol gel. These may be harder to hold in place on affected areas in the mouth and caution should be exercised since these may initially cause burning on oral lesions.

Intralesional Corticosteroids

Intralesional triamcinolone injections (5.0–7.5 mg/mL with a maximum of 40 mg triamcinolone acetonide in one session) every 2–4 weeks have also been reported to help oral mucous membrane pemphigoid, especially on the tongue, palate and buccal mucosa as reported in a review by Ahmed, Rogers and colleagues. This review provides several practical recommendations summarized here. The beveled edge of the needle should face the epithelium and the injection should be close to the dermatoepidermal junction (in order to provide targeted therapy and to avoid atrophy from deep injections). Topical hygiene is highly recommended prior to injection. Changing the injection needle frequently can help prevent transmitting infections. Viscous lidocaine or Cetacaine spray can serve as local anesthesia [28].

A small study has suggested that oral intralesional triamcinolone injections in pemphigus may help decrease the amount of time to remission and decrease the amount of systemic therapy, but early findings were not statistically significant [29]. Endoscopic intralesional steroid injections have also been reported to help treat esophageal involvement of epidermolysis bullosa acquisita in conjunction with thermoplastic dilators [30]. Topical and intralesional steroids have also been reported to be used in a patient with both HIV and mucous membrane pemphigoid [31].

Intralesional steroids are beneficial to help facilitate healing both for oral mucosal and cutaneous lesions. These are usually most helpful in "stubborn" lesions (such as slow to heal lesions in areas of constant trauma). In most such areas, multiple rounds of monthly injections can be required before resolution is observed. Recent guidelines recommend using intralesional injections to treat new lesions during the maintenance phase, but not for "relapse/flare" (which would require modifying systemic treatments). Care must be taken to avoid injecting near an area of infection. As such, it is better to use intralesional steroids as an adjuvant during maintenance treatment [32].

Corticosteroid Elixirs

Several oral elixirs have also been studied in mucous membrane pemphigoid [26, 33].

Rotating between rinsing the mouth only (and not swallowing) with hydrogen peroxide, elixir of dexamethasone and elixir of diphenhydramine separately and diluted with tap water (to 1:4 or 1:6 concentration, as tolerated) has been reported.

Timing should involve using hydrogen peroxide rinse and then diphenhydramine rinse before meals for its analgesic effects. Unlike viscous lidocaine, hydrogen peroxide and diphenhydramine do not affect the patient's ability to taste their meal. Timing should also involve using hydrogen peroxide rinse followed by elixir of dexamethasone after meals, between meals and once before bedtime (for a total of six to seven mouth rinses per day) [26].

Clobetasol 0.05 % mouthwash with 100,000 IU/cc nystatin in aqueous solution has been reported effective in three patients with oral mucous membrane pemphigoid. Five minutes of rinsing 10 cc of clobetasol mouthwash solution was used three times per day after meals (with no swallowing). Overall, the majority of patients in the study had improvement in pain and ulceration [33].

In the United States, "magic mouth wash" is often prescribed. The general principle of any elixir should be to contain a potent topical steroid in combination with an anesthetic. These can be used up to three times per day before meals since the purpose of these elixirs is to reduce pain and inflammation to allow patients to be able to eat and maintain adequate nutrition.

Side Effects of Local Corticosteroids

One study measured morning urine cortisol levels in three patients after 3 days of 30 g of whole body topical steroid use. They found no change with the use of triamcinolone 0.1 % cream, but did find a drop in morning urine cortisol to 5.0 nmol/L with 3 days of clobetasol cream. This study also found a drop in morning urine cortisol levels in two patients after six consecutive days of using 20 g of whole body clobetasol cream [10]. Similarly, studies looking at the use of superpotent topical steroids in psoriasis have also shown decreases in serum and urine cortisol levels [34–36].

Given the risk of systemic side effects from oral corticosteroids, different vehicles and routes of local administration of corticosteroids can be an alternative for treating exacerbations of disease. While daily compliance can be a potential issue, it can be best concluded that such usage is individualized to each patient's situation by the treating clinician.

Non-steroidal Topical Therapies

In addition to topical steroids, several studies have looked at topical therapy with steroid-sparing agents to treat ABDs, which include immune modulators (such as topical tacrolimus, pimecrolimus and cyclosporine) as well as topical antibiotics (tetracycline ointment and mouthwash).

In the setting of BP, there have been a few case reports of topical tacrolimus being an effective adjuvant to help decrease the doses of systemic therapies. Effects have been noted as early as 2 weeks after starting to apply topical tacrolimus [37–39]. Specifically, topical tacrolimus has been used in pretibial pemphigoid [40], vesicular pemphigoid [38], and localized pemphigoid [39]. One case reported that a patient with vesicular pemphigoid was able to stop systemic steroids after 2 weeks of topical therapy and was maintained on topical tacrolimus 0.1 % ointment alone [38].

In the setting of mucous membrane pemphigoid, topical tacrolimus has been reported to be helpful as an adjuvant for genital lesions [41], as well as alone for oral lesions [42–44] and ocular lesions [45]. Specifically, tacrolimus 0.1 % ointment was used once daily to genital mucous membrane pemphigoid as an effective adjuvant to oral prednisone 40 mg/day. The prednisone was ultimately stopped and the patient was maintained on tacrolimus 0.1 % ointment alone, which resulted in complete clearance of erosions after 3 months [41]. Two reports of tacrolimus 0.1 % ointment alone for oral mucous membrane pemphigoid reported complete response after 2–3 months [42] and moderate response after 6 weeks [43], respectively. In addition tacrolimus 0.03 % oral suspension (used alone as a twice daily oral 5 minute rinse) has been reported helpful in one case of oral mucous membrane pemphigoid, with complete response after 2 months [44]. Tacrolimus 0.03 % ointment has been reported effective and well tolerated in one patient with ocular cicatricial pemphigoid. The patient was also treated initially with dexamethasone-tobramycin ophthalmic ointment twice daily, which was stopped 1 week after starting tacrolimus 0.03 % ointment daily. The patient remained asymptomatic 3 months later on tacrolimus ointment alone [45].

Tacrolimus ointment has been used as an adjuvant in ocular pemphigus [45] as well as pemphigus foliaceus [46]. One patient with ocular pemphigus was treated with tacrolimus 0.03 % ointment twice daily in addition to mycophenolate mofetil, oral prednisone and prednisolone acetate 1 % eye drops, and was able to tolerate tapering off of oral prednisone [45]. One patient with pemphigus foliaceus who was also being treated with dapsone 100 mg/day was given tacrolimus 0.1 % ointment to lesions on half of his face and clobetasone butyrate 0.05 % ointment to the other half of his face. There was no difference in the response to clobetasone butyrate ointment versus tacrolimus ointment [46].

In addition, eleven patients with cutaneous pemphigus vulgaris were treated with pimecrolimus 1 % cream or placebo as an adjuvant to oral prednisone and azathioprine. Patients treated with pimecrolimus cream showed significant improvement after 15 days [47].

The benefits of topical therapy in linear IgA disease have also been examined. One case report examined using clobetasol ointment on half of the body and tacrolimus ointment on the other half of the body. Only the side treated with clobetasol showed improvement in vesicles and bullae within 1 month, but unfortunately it also showed extensive striae in that time as well [48]. Since then, there has been a case report on the benefit of tacrolimus ointment as an adjuvant to systemic dapsone [49].

Dapsone gel has been reported in the treatment of acne, granuloma faciale, idiopathic follicular mucinosis, erythema elevatum diutinum. Although oral dapsone has been reported to have effects in the treatment of bullous disease, topical dapsone gel has not yet been reported in the treatment of bullous disease.

Non-steroidal Elixirs

Several non-steroidal oral elixirs have also been studied in mucous membrane pemphigoid, including tetracycline mouthwash [50] and 5 mL of cyclosporine 100 mg/mL swish [51], each of which is described in further detail below. Of note, topical sirolimus mouthwash has also been used in oral pemphigus, but without benefit [52]. As mentioned above, tacrolimus 0.03 % oral suspension (used alone as a twice daily oral 5 min rinse) has also been reported helpful in one case of oral mucous membrane pemphigoid, with complete response after 2 months [44].

One patient with oral and perianal pemphigoid has been reported to show beneficial effects within weeks of using topical tetracycline. Specifically, he used tetracycline mouthwash (250 mg in 5–10 mL of water) four times per day (for 5 min each) as well as tetracycline 3 % ointment to perianal lesions. The oral lesions (unlike the perianal lesions) did recur, requiring oral minocycline for control during exacerbations [50].

Topical cyclosporine 100 mg/mL swish (5 mL) without swallowing has been reported to help patients with oral bullous disease [53, 54]. One case report found that cyclosporine mouthwash three times per day for 5-minutes each helped improve oral pemphigus within 6 months in one patient on oral prednisolone who had failed several other systemic agents [54]. Another study looked at using 5 mL of cyclosporine 100 mg/mL swish three times per day for 8 weeks in patients with bullous disease. They found that two patients with oral mucous membrane pemphigoid showed improvement with topical cyclosporine alone (with clearance of five oral ulcers in one patient and with notable improvement but not complete clearance of gingival erythema and pain). One patient with BP showed moderate improvement in erythema, pain and erosions with this regimen. Relapse occurred in two of the preceding patients upon stopping the cyclosporine swish. In addition, two of three patients with oral pemphigus vulgaris who used cyclosporine swish as an adjuvant showed some improvement [53].

Non-steroidal formulations for topical agents and elixirs can be helpful in providing a localized steroid-sparing effect (Table 14.1). These may not be covered by insurance carriers since these are being used as "off label" treatments. While these can often be more expensive, they should still be considered as possible alternatives for chronic local treatment.

Table 14.1 Oral elixirs

Tetracycline mouthwash (250 mg in 5–10 mL of water) four times per day (5 min each)
Tacrolimus 0.03 % oral suspension, oral rinse for 5 min twice daily
Rotating between rinsing the mouth with hydrogen peroxide, elixir of dexamethasone and elixir of diphenhydramine separately
Clobetasol 0.05 % mouthwash with 100,000 IU/cc nystatin in aqueous solution for 5 min three times per day after meals
5 mL of cyclosporine 100 mg/mL swish for 5 min three times per day

Exogenous Factors That May Cause Blistering Disease

Exogenous factors have been reported to cause pemphigus. In 2003, Brenner reported three categories causing pemphigus as follows: (1) thiols (sulfhydryl group), (2) phenol (including topical phenol), (3) other (non-thiol and non-phenol). She reported that thiol-induced acantholysis has been noted *in vitro* by directly interfering with cell adhesion, whereas phenol-induced acantholysis may occur by keratoinocytes inducing IL-1alpha and TNF-alpha [55]. Phenol containing drugs reported to cause pemphigus include cephalosporins and rifampin as well as levodopa, heroin, phenobarbital, pentachlorophenol and aspirin [56].

One study interviewed 126 pemphigus patients and 173 healthy controls to identify potential risk factors in environmental exposures. Patients exposed to metal vapor (occupationally) and pesticides had an increased risk of pemphigus. This multi-site study found the highest risk for exposure to pesticides and related materials to be in patients from Bulgaria and Israel (as compared to Brazil, India, Italy, Spain and the United States) [57]. Theories for the mechanism of pemphigus due to pesticides include its pro-estrogenic effect [57] and allergic contact dermatitis [58].

Interestingly, it has also been observed that former smokers or current smokers had a lower risk for developing pemphigus than those who never smoked [57]. However, subsequent studies have found contrary results [59]. In 2008, a study of 10 smokers with pemphigus and 60 non-smokers with pemphigus found no baseline difference in the extent of pemphigus, but did find that after 1 year of treatment, smokers more frequently developed partial remission [60]. While a recent review on pemphigus associations suggests that smoking is not contraindicated in pemphigus [61], the authors do not advocate the use of tobacco since long term health risks far outweigh the possible benefits.

Food and Nutrition

While there are no specific studies that suggest foods to be an etiology of blistering lesions in the mouth, there are certain foods that have been suggested as being possible culprits in exacerbating disease or preventing lesions from healing. These include mango, cassava, mustard, coconut and areca nut [62]. While there has been some suggestion of an association between a higher intake of spices with pemphigus [63], it is important to note that spicy foods can be difficult to tolerate in patients with oral blistering disease and may potentially lead to more oral lesions.

Exacerbations of oral bullous disease have been reported in association with certain foods and trauma in the setting of oral lichen planus. Examples of triggers include tomatoes, spicy foods, and citrus as well as dental work and heavy alcohol and tobacco use [51]. These triggers likely have similar effects in ABDs with oral involvement, given the potential for mechanical trauma and irritation. Hence, physicians should emphasize at the initial visit the importance of ideally avoiding or minimizing certain foods, including citrus, spicy, cinnamon, and hard, crunchy foods.

In addition, BP patients with poor nutrition (measured by low albumin) have been associated with poorer outcome in the first year after hospitalization [64]. Hence, patients should be advised to eat chicken and fish, which would provide increased amounts of protein and be less traumatic for the oral cavity.

Dermatitis herpetiformis improves with dietary avoidance of gluten. It has also been suggested that a gluten-free diet can possibly help prevent the risk of lymphoma [65, 66]. Gluten is a protein that can be found in wheat, barley, rye and many processed foods and some medications. It is particularly important that patients pay attention to food labeling as some foods, such as oats (which are generally considered safe) may at times be processed with gluten (making them unsafe). Patients should additionally pay attention to prescription and over-the-counter medications and topical therapies (including lip balms, toothpastes, mouthwashes) [67]. Gluten can also be found in beer and whiskey. Many supermarkets have a separate section for gluten-free products. While gluten-free labeling is accurate in the United States about 95 % of the time [68], trace amounts of gluten may be found in several gluten-free labelled products [69]. Mulder et al. provides a helpful table of safe foods, which may be practical to give to patients [70]. Several additional resources are available online for patients including: The Gluten Intolerance Group (www.gluten.net), Academy of Nutrition and Dietetics (www.eatright.org), and National Foundation for Celiac Awareness (www.celiaccentral.org). Patients will need to maintain a well-balanced diet, while also avoiding gluten completely [71]. Of note, dermatitis herpetiformis can additionally flare with exposure to iodine, including radiocontrast material [72–74].

Poor oral hygiene has also been reported in gingival lichen planus [51]. Mucous membrane pemphigoid patients have been reported to have worse periodontal status compared to a control population in two studies [75, 76], but no statistically significant decrease in one small study [77]. Given the potential risk for periodontal disease, a detailed protocol for oral hygiene has been reported as helpful in a small study of 12 patients [78]. However, patients should be cautioned against elective dental procedures due to the risk of exacerbation from potential trauma. Anesthesiologists should also be made aware of potential traumatic lesions developing in the oral, pharyngeal, and laryngeal areas from intubations in ABD patients.

Ultraviolet Light

Ultraviolet light has been reported to exacerbate multiple ABDs [79–88]. Cases have been reported to both UVB [80, 81, 86, 87] as well as UVA [85, 87, 88]. BP has also been reported to occur after exposure to red light of photodynamic therapy (peak 636 nm) [89] used to treat biopsy-proven Bowen's disease on the lower legs. In addition, low level laser therapy (including the 980 nm diode laser) has been reported as a treatment in mucous membrane pemphigoid [90–92].

It is important to remind all patients with ABDs to use sun protection to help prevent a photo-exacerbation of their disease. Sunscreens with an SPF of at least 30 and ideally containing physical blockers such as zinc oxide and titanium dioxide should be strongly encouraged. Clothing with UPF (ultraviolet protective factor) should be emphasized as part of the treatment since photo-protection could prevent both relapse of the disease along with preventing potential skin cancers from prolonged immune suppression.

Infection Control

Patients with ABDs have experienced decreased mortality from the disease itself with the introduction of steroid-sparing systemic agents. Unfortunately, these treatments also increase the risk for opportunistic infections. These infections are often a major cause of morbidity in ABDs, either secondary to the breakdown of the skin barrier or immune suppression [93].

A prospective study of 172 patients with newly-diagnosed pemphigus found that 14 patients developed opportunistic infections after a mean of 4 months following their diagnosis (while on systemic treatments for pemphigus). The risk of developing an opportunistic infection within the first year of diagnosis of pemphigus was found to be 9.3 %, with increased risk in older patients and possibly diabetic patients [94]. Infections reported in bullous patients include bacterial, viral and fungal sources. Reported bacterial infections include Staphylococcus aureus (including methicillin-resistant cases) and Streptococcus A [95], as well as Nocardia, Cytomegalovirus, Legionella and Listeria [94]. Nocardia has been reported in both pemphigus vulgaris [81, 96, 97] and BP [98]. Studies have found sepsis to be one of the highest causes of mortality in both pemphigus [99] and BP [100].

Given the risk of opportunistic infections while on chronic immunosuppressives, three studies have examined the role of routine prophylaxis for pneumocystis pneumonia. Overall, less than 2 % of their examined cases developed pneumocystis pneumonia, and study sizes range from 198 to 334 patients [101–103]. As such, it is recommended that physicians consider pneumocystis prophylaxis in high risk patients and to have a high suspicion in patients developing pulmonary symptoms while on immunosuppressive agents.

Viral or herpetic lesions can mimic immunobullous disease, especially in patients on immunosuppressive therapy. Viral infections include recurrent oral herpes simplex [104], genital herpes simplex [105], severe herpetic gingivostomatitis [106], generalized herpes simplex [107] and varicella zoster [108], and can be potentially fatal [109, 110]. One study suggests ABD patients may have occult herpes simplex colonization [111]. Viral-specific studies should be performed of any recalcitrant blisters.

Scabies can mimic pruritus in ABD, and if not diagnosed can mistakenly be treated with increased immunosuppression [112]. In addition, some new patients may initially be misdiagnosed with ABD when they actually have bullous scabies [113–117].

A variety of fungal infections have also been reported. One case reported a flare of local BP associated with concomitant dermatophyte infection (identified on culture and potassium hydroxide preparation) [118]. Rare reported infections in ABD patients include Cryptococcal cellulitis [119], primary cutaneous Blastomycosis [120] and various presentations of Nocardia [94, 96–98, 121].

Patients may often observe increased pain in mucosal areas of involvement including the oral cavity, esophagus, and genital area. This can often be secondary to the presence of Candida infection, which can present from the usage of corticosteroids and systemic immunosuppressants. Patients should be examined if they report an exacerbation, as increasing systemic medications may lead to progression of mucosal Candidiasis.

Prevention of infections is a key factor in the overall clinical outcome. Patients should be encouraged not to "pop" or drain blisters since this could provide a route for infection. Fluid filled blisters can be soaked up to three times per day with an aluminum acetate solution which has both anti-infectious and astringent properties. In the United States, a common available brand is *Domboros*.

There are other over-the-counter antibacterial products which can also be used for topical hygiene and can help clear and possibly prevent infections. Topical therapies with antibacterial properties include the following: benzoyl-peroxide soap or creamy wash (mostly gram positive coverage), acetic acid (vinegar) diluted with water in solution (gram negative coverage) as well as hydrogen peroxide solution (diluted 1:4) with antiseptic mouthwash, and chlorhexidine (coverage against both gram positive and negative bacteria). While iodine solutions also have anti-septic properties, these would not be preferred due to potential local irritant reactions and risk of exacerbating dermatitis herpetiformis.

Since most patients will be on long term immune suppression, screening for certain infections (including tuberculosis and hepatitis serologies) is crucial at the initial visit. If any of the screening tests are found to be positive, infectious disease and hepatology should be consulted before proceeding with systemic treatment.

Vaccinations are an extremely important modality for the prevention of infection. It is recommended that patients continue with their vaccination schedules and vaccines, unless contraindicated. Live vaccines are contraindicated in patients on immunosuppression. These contraindicated live vaccines include zoster, live influenza, measles, mumps and rubella [93, 122].

Antihistamines

Antihistamines are used commonly to control pruritus in many dermatological disorders. Many of the ABDs can have intense pruritus during the initial onset or during a relapse of the disease. While these can be acutely controlled in most instances with topical and systemic steroids, some patients may require the addition of an antihistamine as an adjuvant anti-pruritic agent. Since there are no studies evaluating the role and efficacy of anti-histamines in controlling pruritus in ABDs, both first and second generation anti-histamines may be considered as anti-pruritic agents in the appropriate patient. Antihistamines are generally avoided in pregnancy due to the risk of teratogenicity in the first trimester. However, specific first and second generation antihistamines, classified by the FDA as Category B, can sometimes be considered as adjuvant anti-pruritic treatments for pemphigoid gestationis since this presents later in pregnancy. These can include chlorpheniramine, dexchlorpheniramine, loratidine, and cetirizine, pending prior consultation with and approval by the patient's obstetrician [123].

Conclusions

In this chapter, the authors have tried to emphasize non-systemic measures which can help improve outcomes. A variety of topical and local treatment options have proven to be beneficial in mild as well as moderate and severe ABDs as an adjuvant. The regimen will often be determined by many clinical and non-clinical factors and must be individualized by the treating physician. Clinicians should constantly remind patients to minimize the risk of infection, excessive sun exposure, and trauma, including direct contact from the water of high-pressure showers. Appropriate nutritional recommendations should also be emphasized since compliance can be difficult. Patients should be constantly encouraged and reminded that while these measures may not provide a "cure," such precautions may help reduce the dosage and duration of their systemic treatments.

References

1. Person JR, Rogers RS, Perry HO. Localized pemphigoid. Br J Dermatol. 1976;95(5):531–4.
2. Taghipour K, Mohd Mustapa MF, Highet AS, Venning VA, Kirtschig G. The approach of dermatologists in the UK to the treatment of bullous pemphigoid: results of a national survey. Clin Exp Dermatol. 2013;38(3):311–3.
3. Westerhof W. Treatment of bullous pemphigoid with topical clobetasol propionate. J Am Acad Dermatol. 1989;20(3):458–61.
4. Joly P, Roujeau J-C, Benichou J, Picard C, Dreno B, Delaporte E, et al. A comparison of oral and topical corticosteroids in patients with bullous pemphigoid. N Engl J Med. 2002;346(5):321–7.
5. Gelfand JM, Werth VP. Treatment of bullous pemphigoid with topical corticosteroids: review of a randomized controlled trial. Arch Dermatol. 2002;138(9):1236–7.
6. Korman NJ. Oral and topical corticosteroids in bullous pemphigoid. N Engl J Med. 2002;347(2):143–5; author reply 143–5.
7. Spigel GT. Oral and topical corticosteroids in bullous pemphigoid. N Engl J Med. 2002;347(2):143–5; author reply 143–5.
8. Joly P, Roujeau J-C, Benichou J, Delaporte E, D'Incan M, Dreno B, et al. A comparison of two regimens of topical corticosteroids in the treatment of patients with bullous pemphigoid: a multicenter randomized study. J Invest Dermatol. 2009;129(7):1681–7.
9. Stockman A, Beele H, Vanderhaeghen Y, Naeyaert JM. Topical class I corticosteroids in 10 patients with bullous pemphigoid: correlation of the outcome with the severity degree of the

disease and review of the literature. J Eur Acad Dermatol Venereol JEADV. 2004;18(2):164–8.
10. Terra JB, Potze WJB, Jonkman MF. Whole body application of a potent topical corticosteroid for bullous pemphigoid. J Eur Acad Dermatol Venereol JEADV . 2014;28(6):712–8.
11. Claudy A. Evaluation of the safety and efficacy of a potent topical cortico-steroid in the treatment of bullous pemphigoid. Clin Dermatol. 2001;19(6):778–80.
12. Zimmermann R, Faure M, Claudy A. Prospective study of treatment of bullous pemphigoid by a class I topical corticosteroid. Ann Dermatol Venereol. 1999;126(1):13–6.
13. Paquet P, Richelle M, Lapiere CM. Bullous pemphigoid treated by topical corticosteroids. Acta Derm Venereol. 1991;71(6):534 5.
14. Muramatsu T, Iida T, Shirai T. Pemphigoid and pemphigus foliaceus successfully treated with topical corticosteroids. J Dermatol. 1996;23(10):683–8.
15. Bingham LG, Noble JW, Davis MDP. Wet dressings used with topical corticosteroids for pruritic dermatoses: a retrospective study. J Am Acad Dermatol. 2009;60(5):792–800.
16. Fichel F, Barbe C, Joly P, Bedane C, Vabres P, Truchetet F, et al. Clinical and immunologic factors associated with bullous pemphigoid relapse during the first year of treatment: a multicenter, prospective study. JAMA Dermatol. 2014;150(1):25–33.
17. Dumas V, Roujeau JC, Wolkenstein P, Revuz J, Cosnes A. The treatment of mild pemphigus vulgaris and pemphigus foliaceus with a topical corticosteroid. Br J Dermatol. 1999;140(6):1127–9.
18. Du-Thanh A, Merlet S, Maillard H, Bernard P, Joly P, Estève E, et al. Combined treatment with low-dose methotrexate and initial short-term superpotent topical steroids in bullous pemphigoid: an open, multicentre, retrospective study. Br J Dermatol. 2011;165(6):1337–43.
19. Mervic L, Dragos V, Pavlović MD. Linear IgA bullous dermatosis of childhood: successful treatment with miocamycin and topical corticosteroid. Clin Exp Dermatol. 2009;34(7):e391–2.
20. Hornschuh B, Hamm H, Wever S, Hashimoto T, Schröder U, Bröcker EB, et al. Treatment of 16 patients with bullous pemphigoid with oral tetracycline and niacinamide and topical clobetasol. J Am Acad Dermatol. 1997;36(1):101–3.
21. Lozada F, Silverman S. Topically applied fluocinonide in an adhesive base in the treatment of oral vesiculoerosive diseases. Arch Dermatol. 1980;116(8):898–901.
22. Aufdemorte TB, De Villez RL, Parel SM. Modified topical steroid therapy for the treatment of oral mucous membrane pemphigoid. Oral Surg Oral Med Oral Pathol. 1985;59(3):256–60.
23. Lozada-Nur F, Miranda C, Maliksi R. Double-blind clinical trial of 0.05 % clobetasol propionate (corrected from proprionate) ointment in orabase and 0.05 % fluocinonide ointment in orabase in the treatment of patients with oral vesiculoerosive diseases. Oral Surg Oral Med Oral Pathol. 1994;77(6):598–604.
24. Arash A, Shirin L. The management of oral mucous membrane pemphigoid with dapsone and topical corticosteroid. J Oral Pathol Med Off Publ Int Assoc Oral Pathol Am Acad Oral Pathol. 2008;37(6):341–4.
25. Gonzalez-Moles MA, Ruiz-Avila I, Rodriguez-Archilla A, Morales-Garcia P, Mesa-Aguado F, Bascones-Martinez A, et al. Treatment of severe erosive gingival lesions by topical application of clobetasol propionate in custom trays. Oral Surg Oral Med Oral Pathol Oral Radiol Endod. 2003;95(6):688–92.
26. Ahmed AR, Rogers RS. Bullous pemphigoid. Therapy and management. Clin Dermatol. 1987;5(1):146–54.
27. Hempstead RW, Marks JG. Pediatric pemphigus vulgaris. Treatment with topical adrenal steroids. Arch Dermatol. 1984;120(7):962–3.
28. Ahmed AR, Kurgis BS, Rogers RS. Cicatricial pemphigoid. J Am Acad Dermatol. 1991;24(6 Pt 1):987–1001.
29. Mignogna MD, Fortuna G, Leuci S, Adamo D, Dell'Aversana Orabona G, Ruoppo E. Adjuvant triamcinolone acetonide injections in oro-pharyngeal pemphigus vulgaris. J Eur Acad Dermatol Venereol JEADV. 2010;24(10):1157–65.

30. Moura EG, Couto-Júnior DS, Alvarado-Escobar H, da Costa-Martins B, Sallum RA, Artifon EL, et al. Epidermolysis bullosa acquisita complicated by esophageal stenosis. Endoscopic treatment with thermoplastic dilators and intralesional steroid injection. Rev Gastroenterol Méx. 2011;76(3):279–85.
31. Singh AP, Chaitra TR, Ravishankar TL, Singh SP, Mohapatra AK. HIV patient with mucous membrane pemphigoid: a case report. Ethiop J Health Sci. 2014;24(2):179–82.
32. Fortuna G, Mignogna MD. Clinical guidelines for the use of adjuvant triamcinolone acetonide injections in oro-pharyngeal pemphigus vulgaris: the oral medicine point of view. J Oral Pathol Med Off Publ Int Assoc Oral Pathol Am Acad Oral Pathol. 2011;40(4):359–60.
33. Gonzalez-Moles MA, Morales P, Rodriguez-Archilla A, Isabel IR-A, Gonzalez-Moles S. Treatment of severe chronic oral erosive lesions with clobetasol propionate in aqueous solution. Oral Surg Oral Med Oral Pathol Oral Radiol Endod. 2002;93(3):264–70.
34. Gilbertson EO, Spellman MC, Piacquadio DJ, Mulford MI. Super potent topical corticosteroid use associated with adrenal suppression: clinical considerations. J Am Acad Dermatol. 1998;38(2 Pt 2):318–21.
35. Walsh P, Aeling JL, Huff L, Weston WL. Hypothalamus-pituitary-adrenal axis suppression by superpotent topical steroids. J Am Acad Dermatol. 1993;29(3):501–3.
36. Weston WL, Fennessey PV, Morelli J, Schwab H, Mooney J, Samson C, et al. Comparison of hypothalamus-pituitary-adrenal axis suppression from superpotent topical steroids by standard endocrine function testing and gas chromatographic mass spectrometry. J Invest Dermatol. 1988;90(4):532–5.
37. Chu J, Bradley M, Marinkovich MP. Topical tacrolimus is a useful adjunctive therapy for bullous pemphigoid. Arch Dermatol. 2003;139(6):813–5.
38. Chuh AA. The application of topical tacrolimus in vesicular pemphigoid. Br J Dermatol. 2004;150(3):622–3.
39. Ko M-J, Chu C-Y. Topical tacrolimus therapy for localized bullous pemphigoid. Br J Dermatol. 2003;149(5):1079–81.
40. Calcaterra R, Carducci M, Franco G, Mussi A, Morrone A. Topical tacrolimus treatment for localized pretibial bullous phemphigoid. J Eur Acad Dermatol Venereol JEADV. 2009;23(2):177–9.
41. Günther C, Wozel G, Meurer M, Pfeiffer C. Topical tacrolimus treatment for cicatricial pemphigoid. J Am Acad Dermatol. 2004;50(2):325–6.
42. Assmann T, Becker J, Ruzicka T, Megahed M. Topical tacrolimus for oral cicatricial pemphigoid. Clin Exp Dermatol. 2004;29(6):674–6.
43. Suresh L, Martinez Calixto LE, Radfar L. Successful treatment of mucous membrane pemphigoid with tacrolimus. Spec Care Dentist Off Publ Am Assoc Hosp Dent Acad Dent Handicap Am Soc Geriatr Dent. 2006;26(2):66–70.
44. Lee HY, Blazek C, Beltraminelli H, Borradori L. Oral mucous membrane pemphigoid: complete response to topical tacrolimus. Acta Derm Venereol. 2011;91(5):604–5.
45. Hall VC, Liesegang TJ, Kostick DA, Lookingbill DP. Ocular mucous membrane pemphigoid and ocular pemphigus vulgaris treated topically with tacrolimus ointment. Arch Dermatol. 2003;139(8):1083–4.
46. Cohen SN, Lim RPR, Paul CJ, Abdullah A. Equal efficacy of topical tacrolimus and clobetasone butyrate in pemphigus foliaceus. Int J Dermatol. 2006;45(11):1379.
47. Iraji F, Asilian A, Siadat AH. Pimecrolimus 1 % cream in the treatment of cutaneous lesions of pemphigus vulgaris: a double-blind, placebo-controlled clinical trial. J Drugs Dermatol JDD. 2010;9(6):684–6.
48. Hull CM, McKenna JK, Zone JJ. Topical corticosteroids and bullous pemphigoid. Arch Dermatol. 2003;139(2):225–6.
49. Dauendorffer JN, Mahé E, Saiag P. Tacrolimus ointment, an interesting adjunctive therapy for childhood linear IgA bullous dermatosis. J Eur Acad Dermatol Venereol JEADV. 2008;22(3):364–5.
50. Bauco van der Wal V, Jonkman MF. Topical tetracycline in cicatricial pemphigoid. J Am Acad Dermatol. 1997;36(3 Pt 1):492–3.

51. Eisen D. The clinical features, malignant potential, and systemic associations of oral lichen planus: a study of 723 patients. J Am Acad Dermatol. 2002;46(2):207–14.
52. Poot AM, Jonkman MF. Topical sirolimus for oral pemphigus vulgaris: 3 unresponsive cases. J Am Acad Dermatol. 2012;67(5):e228–9.
53. Eisen D, Ellis CN, Voorhees JJ. Topical cyclosporine for oral bullous disorders. J Am Acad Dermatol. 1990;23(5 Pt 1):936–7.
54. Gooptu C, Staughton RC. Use of topical cyclosporin in oral pemphigus. J Am Acad Dermatol. 1998;38(5 Pt 2):860–1.
55. Brenner S, Srebrnik A, Goldberg I. Pemphigus can be induced by topical phenol as well as by foods and drugs that contain phenols or thiols. J Cosmet Dermatol. 2003;2(3–4):161–5.
56. Goldberg I, Kashman Y, Brenner S. The induction of pemphigus by phenol drugs. Int J Dermatol. 1999;38(12):888–92.
57. Brenner S, Tur E, Shapiro J, Ruocco V, D'Avino M, Ruocco E, et al. Pemphigus vulgaris: environmental factors. Occupational, behavioral, medical, and qualitative food frequency questionnaire. Int J Dermatol. 2001;40(9):562–9.
58. Brenner S, Wolf R, Ruocco V. Contact pemphigus: a subgroup of induced pemphigus. Int J Dermatol. 1994;33(12):843–5.
59. Fawzy MM, Hegazy RA, Abdel Fattah AF. Ear, nose, and throat involvement in Egyptian patients with pemphigus vulgaris: a step towards a better management. Int J Dermatol. 2013;52(10):1268–73.
60. Valikhani M, Kavusi S, Chams-Davatchi C, Hallaji Z, Esmaili N, Ghandi N, et al. Impact of smoking on pemphigus. Int J Dermatol. 2008;47(6):567–70.
61. Ruocco E, Wolf R, Ruocco V, Brunetti G, Romano F, Lo Schiavo A. Pemphigus: associations and management guidelines: facts and controversies. Clin Dermatol. 2013;31(4):382–90.
62. Tur E, Brenner S. Contributing exogenous factors in pemphigus. Int J Dermatol. 1997;36(12):888–93.
63. Wohl Y, Brenner S. Pemphigus in Israel--an epidemiologic analysis of cases in search of risk factors. Isr Med Assoc J IMAJ. 2003;5(6):410–2.
64. Rzany B, Partscht K, Jung M, Kippes W, Mecking D, Baima B, et al. Risk factors for lethal outcome in patients with bullous pemphigoid: low serum albumin level, high dosage of glucocorticosteroids, and old age. Arch Dermatol. 2002;138(7):903–8.
65. Hervonen K, Salmi TT, Ilus T, Paasikivi K, Vornanen M, Laurila K, et al. Dermatitis herpetiformis refractory to gluten-free dietary treatment. Acta Derm Venereol. 2016;96(1):82–86.
66. Lewis HM, Renaula TL, Garioch JJ, Leonard JN, Fry JS, Collin P, et al. Protective effect of gluten-free diet against development of lymphoma in dermatitis herpetiformis. Br J Dermatol. 1996;135(3):363–7.
67. Gainor CL. Celiac disease: helping patients live gluten free. Nurse Pract. 2011;36(9):14–9; quiz 19–20.
68. Thompson T, Simpson S. A comparison of gluten levels in labeled gluten-free and certified gluten-free foods sold in the United States. Eur J Clin Nutr. 2015;69(2):143–6.
69. Collin P, Thorell L, Kaukinen K, Mäki M. The safe threshold for gluten contamination in gluten-free products. Can trace amounts be accepted in the treatment of coeliac disease? Aliment Pharmacol Ther. 2004;19(12):1277–83.
70. Mulder CJJ, van Wanrooij RLJ, Bakker SF, Wierdsma N, Bouma G. Gluten-free diet in gluten-related disorders. Dig Dis. 2013;31(1):57–62.
71. Penagini F, Dilillo D, Meneghin F, Mameli C, Fabiano V, Zuccotti GV. Gluten-free diet in children: an approach to a nutritionally adequate and balanced diet. Nutrients. 2013;5(11):4553–65.
72. From E, Thomsen K. Dermatitis herpetiformis. A case provoked by iodine. Br J Dermatol. 1974;91(2):221–4.
73. Scialis GF. Letter: dermatitis herpetiformis and iodine. Br J Dermatol. 1976;94(3):343.
74. Douglas WS, Alexander JO. Letter: dermatitis herpetiformis, iodine compounds and thyrotoxicosis. Br J Dermatol. 1975;92(5):596–8.

75. Arduino PG, Farci V, D'Aiuto F, Carcieri P, Carbone M, Tanteri C, et al. Periodontal status in oral mucous membrane pemphigoid: initial results of a case-control study. Oral Dis. 2011;17(1):90–4.
76. Tricamo MB, Rees TD, Hallmon WW, Wright JM, Cueva MA, Plemons JM. Periodontal status in patients with gingival mucous membrane pemphigoid. J Periodontol. 2006;77(3):398–405.
77. Schellinck AE, Rees TD, Plemons JM, Kessler HP, Rivera-Hidalgo F, Solomon ES. A comparison of the periodontal status in patients with mucous membrane pemphigoid: a 5-year follow-up. J Periodontol. 2009;80(11):1765–73.
78. Arduino PG, Lopetuso E, Carcieri P, Giacometti S, Carbone M, Tanteri C, et al. Professional oral hygiene treatment and detailed oral hygiene instructions in patients affected by mucous membrane pemphigoid with specific gingival localization: a pilot study in 12 patients. Int J Dent Hyg. 2012;10(2):138–41.
79. Cram DL, Winkelmann RK. Ultraviolet-induced acantholysis in pemphigus. Arch Dermatol. 1965;92(1):7–13.
80. Igawa K, Matsunaga T, Nishioka K. Involvement of UV-irradiation in pemphigus foliaceus. J Eur Acad Dermatol Venereol JEADV. 2004;18(2):216–7.
81. Reis VM, Toledo RP, Lopez A, Diaz LA, Martins JE. UVB-induced acantholysis in endemic Pemphigus foliaceus (Fogo selvagem) and Pemphigus vulgaris. J Am Acad Dermatol. 2000;42(4):571–6.
82. Rodan KP, Fleischmann H, Nickoloff BJ, Egbert B. Generalized blistering eruption aggravated by heat. Pemphigus foliaceus. Arch Dermatol. 1987;123(3):394, 397–8.
83. Cram DL, Fukuyama K. Immunohistochemistry of ultraviolet-induced pemphigus and pemphigoid lesions. Arch Dermatol. 1972;106(6):819–24.
84. Lee CW, Ro YS. Sun-induced localized bullous pemphigoid. Br J Dermatol. 1992;126(1):91–2.
85. Thomsen K, Schmidt H. PUVA-induced bullous pemphigoid. Br J Dermatol. 1976;95(5):568–9.
86. Jacobs SE. Pemphigus Erythematosus and ultraviolet light. A case report. Arch Dermatol. 1965;91:139–41.
87. Jappe U, Zillikens D, Bonnekoh B, Gollnick H. Epidermolysis bullosa acquisita with ultraviolet radiationsensitivity. Br J Dermatol. 2000;142(3):517–20.
88. Salmhofer W, Soyer HP, Wolf P, Födinger D, Hödl S, Kerl H. UV light-induced linear IgA dermatosis. J Am Acad Dermatol. 2004;50(1):109–15.
89. Rakvit P, Kerr AC, Ibbotson SH. Localized bullous pemphigoid induced by photodynamic therapy. Photodermatol Photoimmunol Photomed. 2011;27(5):251–3.
90. Cafaro A, Broccoletti R, Arduino PG. Low-level laser therapy for oral mucous membrane pemphigoid. Lasers Med Sci. 2012;27(6):1247–50.
91. Yilmaz HG, Kusakci-Seker B, Bayindir H, Tözüm TF. Low-level laser therapy in the treatment of mucous membrane pemphigoid: a promising procedure. J Periodontol. 2010;81(8):1226–30.
92. Oliveira PC, Reis Junior JA, Lacerda JA, Silveira NT, Santos JM, Vitale MC, et al. Laser light may improve the symptoms of oral lesions of cicatricial pemphigoid: a case report. Photomed Laser Surg. 2009;27(5):825–8.
93. Lehman JS, Murrell DF, Camilleri MJ, Kalaaji AN. Infection and infection prevention in patients treated with immunosuppressive medications for autoimmune bullous disorders. Dermatol Clin. 2011;29(4):591–8.
94. Leshem YA, Gdalevich M, Ziv M, David M, Hodak E, Mimouni D. Opportunistic infections in patients with pemphigus. J Am Acad Dermatol. 2014;71(2):284–92.
95. Boughrara Z, Ingen-Housz-Oro S, Legrand P, Duong T-A, Roujeau J-C. Cutaneous infections in bullous pemphigoid patients treated with topical corticosteroids. Ann Dermatol Vénéréol. 2010;137(5):345–51.
96. Carducci M, Nosotti L, Calcaterra R, Bonifati C, Mussi A, Pelagalli L, et al. Early development of disseminated nocardiosis during immunosuppressive treatment for pemphigus vulgaris. Eur J Dermatol EJD. 2007;17(4):346–7.

97. Asilian A, Yoosefi A, Faghihi G. Cutaneous and pulmonary nocardiosis in pemphigus vulgaris: a rare complication of immunosuppressive therapy. Int J Dermatol. 2006;45(10):1204–6.
98. Kakurai M, Hiraga T, Yamada T, Usui K, Kiyosawa T, Nakagawa H. Subcutaneous nocardial abscesses in a patient with bullous pemphigoid during immunosuppressive therapy: report of a case and review of the Japanese literature. J Dermatol. 1999;26(12):829–33.
99. Ahmed AR, Moy R. Death in pemphigus. J Am Acad Dermatol. 1982;7(2):221–8.
100. Barrick BJ, Lohse CM, Lehman JS. Specific causes of death in patients with bullous pemphigoid as measured by death certificate data: a retrospective cohort study. Int J Dermatol. 2015;54(1):56–61.
101. Gerhart JL, Kalaaji AN. Development of Pneumocystis carinii pneumonia in patients with immunobullous and connective tissue disease receiving immunosuppressive medications. J Am Acad Dermatol. 2010;62(6):957–61.
102. Li F, Jin H-Z, Su F, Jia L, Sun Q-N. Pneumocystis pneumonia in patients with immunobullous dermatoses. Int J Dermatol. 2011;50(9):1144–9.
103. Lehman JS, Kalaaji AN. Role of primary prophylaxis for pneumocystis pneumonia in patients treated with systemic corticosteroids or other immunosuppressive agents for immune-mediated dermatologic conditions. J Am Acad Dermatol. 2010;63(5):815–23.
104. Grattan CE, Small D, Kennedy CT, Scully C. Oral herpes simplex infection in bullous pemphigoid. Oral Surg Oral Med Oral Pathol. 1986;61(1):40–3.
105. Kalajian AH, Callen JP. A typical herpes simplex infection masquerading as recalcitrant pemphigus vulgaris. Australas J Dermatol. 2007;48(4):242–7.
106. Negosanti M, Cevenini R, Ghetti P, Fanti PA, Gasponi A, Tosti A. Severe herpetic gingivostomatitis associated with pemphigus vulgaris. Arch Dermatol. 1984;120(4):540–2.
107. Niederecker C, Tappeiner G, Wolff K. Generalized herpes simplex infection complicating bullous pemphigoid. Br J Dermatol. 1995;132(3):484–6.
108. Cliff S, Ostlere LS, Harland CC. Varicella zoster virus infection complicating bullous pemphigoid. Clin Exp Dermatol. 1996;21(2):174–5.
109. Orenstein JM, Castadot MJ, Wilens SL. Fatal herpes hepatitis associated with pemphigus vulgaris and steroids in an adult. Hum Pathol. 1974;5(4):489–93.
110. Keane JT, Malkinson FD, Bryant J, Levin S. Herpesvirus hominis hepatitis and disseminated intravascular coagulation. Occurrence in an adult with pemphigus vulgaris. Arch Intern Med. 1976;136(11):1312–7.
111. Nikkels AF, Delvenne P, Herfs M, Pierard GE. Occult herpes simplex virus colonization of bullous dermatitides. Am J Clin Dermatol. 2008;9(3):163–8.
112. Svecova D, Chmurova N, Pallova A, Babal P. Norwegian scabies in immunosuppressed patient misdiagnosed as an adverse drug reaction. Epidemiol Mikrobiol Imunol Cas Spolecnosti Epidemiol Mikrobiol Ceské Lékarské Spolecnosti JE Purkyne. 2009;58(3):121–3.
113. Roxana Stan T, Piaserico S, Bordignon M, Salmaso R, Zattra E, Alaibac M. Bullous scabies simulating pemphigoid. J Cutan Med Surg. 2011;15(1):55–7.
114. Ansarin H, Jalali MHA, Mazloomi S, Soltani-Arabshahi R, Setarehshenas R. Scabies presenting with bullous pemphigoid-like lesions. Dermatol Online J. 2006;12(1):19.
115. Brar BK, Pall A, Gupta RR. Bullous scabies mimicking bullous pemphigoid. J Dermatol. 2003;30(9):694–6.
116. Balighi K, Robati RM, Hejazi N. A dilemma: bullous-pemphigoid-like eruption in scabies or scabies-induced bullous pemphigoid. Dermatol Online J. 2006;12(4):13.
117. Hylwa SA, Loss L, Grassi M. Crusted scabies and tinea corporis after treatment of presumed bullous pemphigoid. Cutis. 2013;92(4):193–8.
118. Hsiao GH, Chiu HC. Dermatophyte infection associated with a local recurrence of bullous pemphigoid. Br J Dermatol. 1995;132(5):833–5.
119. Sugiura K, Sugiura N, Yagi T, Iguchi M, Ohno H, Miyazaki Y, et al. Cryptococcal cellulitis in a patient with bullous pemphigoid. Acta Derm Venereol. 2013;93(2):187–8.
120. Yen A, Knipe RC, Tyring SK. Primary cutaneous blastomycosis: report of a case acquired by direct inoculation of a bullous pemphigoid lesion. J Am Acad Dermatol. 1994;31(2 Pt 1):277–8.

121. Martín FJ, Pérez-Bernal AM, Camacho F. Pemphigus vulgaris and disseminated nocardiosis. J Eur Acad Dermatol Venereol JEADV. 2000;14(5):416–8.
122. CDC – Vaccines – Adult immunization schedules and tools for providers [Internet]. [cited 2015 Jun 30]. Available from: http://www.cdc.gov/vaccines/schedules/hcp/adult.html.
123. Kar S, Krishnan A, Preetha K, Mohankar A. A review of antihistamines used during pregnancy. J Pharmacol Pharmacother. 2012;3(2):105–8.

Index

N. Sami (ed.), *Autoimmune Bullous Diseases: Approach and Management*,
DOI 10.1007/978-3-319-26728-9

FSC
www.fsc.org
MIX
Papier | Fördert
gute Waldnutzung
FSC® C083411

Kolibri 360 GmbH
Ferdinand-Jühlke-Straße 7
99095 Erfurt, Deutschland
produktsicherheit@kolibri360.de